Written by members of the Academic Unit of the Wellcome Institute for the History of Medicine, London, the world's leading centre for the history of medicine, this book surveys the Western medical tradition in all its aspects from the Greeks until 1800 AD, and in its transformations and transplantations into the world of Islam and the Americas. As well as describing the diseases, medical theories, and medical therapies of the past, it places them in a wide social context, and discusses religious and alternative healing as well as major advances in medicine, surgery, and pharmacology. It includes the accounts of patients as well as of their healers, the pains of childbirth and the preparations for death. Although major figures are covered in detail, this is not a history of great men and great moments in medicine, but an attempt to understand the limitations as well as the triumphs of medicine in pre-modern society. The very latest findings of medical historians are here presented in a lively form accessible to all who are interested in the formation of modern ideas on health and healing. The book provides essential reading as a new synthesis for all students of the history of medicine.

The Western Medical Tradition
800 BC to AD 1800

The Western Medical Tradition

800 BC to AD 1800

LAWRENCE I. CONRAD, MICHAEL NEVE,

VIVIAN NUTTON,

ROY PORTER, ANDREW WEAR

Members of the Academic Unit,
The Wellcome Institute for the History of Medicine, London

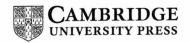

CAMBRIDGE
UNIVERSITY PRESS

CAMBRIDGE UNIVERSITY PRESS
Cambridge, New York, Melbourne, Madrid, Cape Town, Singapore, São Paulo

Cambridge University Press
40 West 20th Street, New York, NY 10011–4211, USA
www.cambridge.org
Information on this title:www.cambridge.org/9780521381352

First published 1995
6th printing 2005

Printed in the United States of America

A catalogue record for this book is available from the British Library.

Library of Congress Cataloguing in Publication Data
The Western medical tradition: 800 B.C.—1800 A.D. / by members of the
Academic Unit, the Wellcome Institute for the History of Medicine.
London: Lawrence I. Conrad... (et al.).
p.   cm.
Includes bibliographical references and index.
ISBN 0-521-38135-5
1. Medicine — History. I. Conrad, Lawrence I., 1949—
II. Wellcome Institute for the History of Medicine.
R131.W47   1995
610'.94—dc20   94-34823   CIP

ISBN-13   978-0-521-38135-2 hardback
ISBN-10   0-521-38135-5 hardback

ISBN-13   978-0-521-47564-8 paperback
ISBN-10   0-521-47564-3 paperback

Contents

Contents

Contents

Illustrations

Acknowledgements

Our first thanks must go to the Wellcome Trust, not only for their un-rivalled support for the development of the history of medicine in general, but also because the Trust and its successive History Panels encouraged the members of the Academic Unit to accept Richard Ziemacki's invitation to write a survey of the whole history of medicine from the Greeks to the present day. But as the project advanced, and grew in size and complexity, it became both practically and intellectually desirable to make a division around the year 1800. By then the coherence of a tradition of medicine that went back to the Hippocratic Corpus had been severely challenged, both as theory and as therapeutics. The social and demographic changes of the nineteenth century, let alone the enormous range of medical developments in the twentieth, mark a new age in medicine, vastly different in scale and in possibilities from what had gone before. Furthermore, to do justice to the achievements of modern medicine and to the historians who have sought to interpret it in many new ways would have extended the size of this volume substantially, and delayed its production still further.

As writers of a textbook we are very aware of the debt we owe to other historians, not all of whom are recorded in the select bibliography at the end of the book. We would like to thank them here for the information and the intellectual stimulus they have given us over the years.

A large number of people have given their time, expertise and encouragement to the writing of the book, and we wish to thank all of the following:

Amal Abou-Aly, Maria Bergmann, Gerrit Bos, Bill Bynum, Elizabeth Craik, Jenni Crisp, Catherine Draycott, Eric Freeman, Faye Getz, Monica Green, Anne Hardy, John Henderson, Frieda Houser, Ralph Jackson, Peter Jones, Helen King, Chris Lawrence, James Longrigg, Michael McVaugh, Christine Nutton, Cornelius O'Boyle, Caroline Overy, Richard Palmer, Dorothy Porter, Andrea Rusnock, Emilie Savage-Smith, Nancy Siraisi, and Richard Smith.

The index, the key to the whole volume, has been prepared by Jean Runciman with her incomparable skill and efficiency.

Finally, we must acknowledge the constant help we have received from the staff of the Wellcome Institute and Library, and from the Reprographics Department of the Wellcome Trust.

Introduction

This volume, written by members of the Wellcome Institute for the History of Medicine, is designed to cover the history of Western medicine from Classical Antiquity to 1800. As one guiding thread, it takes, as its title suggests, a system of medical ideas that, in large part, went back to the Greeks of the fifth century BC, and which, throughout the period covered by this volume, played a major role in the understanding and treatment of health and disease. Indeed even its opponents, whether in Europe or America, at times took their cue from neglected parts of the same tradition, or strove to furnish alternative systems of explanation or therapy that would perform the same function as those they rejected. By the nineteenth century, however, this tradition no longer carried the same force or occupied so central a position within medicine.

The demise of this tradition calls into question the role of modern medicine in the interpretation of the medicine of the past. Whether one is dealing with explanations of disease, the understanding of the body, medical institutions, therapies, or the expectations of patients and doctors, the differences between the medical world of the 1990s and that of the 1690s, to go no further back, are such that one could label the whole of the period covered by this book ancient history, remote in time and, still more, in feel from the present. Even diseases themselves may have changed; contemporaries report occasional 'new' diseases, and both the clinical manifestations and the spread of diseases known from the evidence of written texts or of skeletons (palaeopathology) to have existed long ago may have altered substantially over time. Syphilis, tuberculosis, and smallpox are three examples of diseases with very different histories.

There is thus a temptation to dismiss as remote and irrelevant the medical worlds described in this volume, and to concentrate instead on the few gropings towards the truths of modern medical science at the expense of the mass of apparent ignorance or passivity towards disease and illness that surrounded them. But this is in effect to condemn earlier generations for not being modern, and to single out for praise ideas and discoveries that, in their own day, may not have attracted much attention or approbation. To credit the sixteenth-century physician Paracelsus with the origins of medicinal chemistry is to forget not only his predecessors in distillation, alchemy, and the therapeutic uses of mineral drugs, but also the world of elves and fairies, of astrology and mystical signs, of which his chemical drugs were but one part (pp. 311–17). Yet any attempt to rectify the balance by considering each Age on its own terms and within its own cultural context cannot escape the afterknowledge of modern medicine; we know, for instance, far more about gout or bubonic plague than eighteenth-century or medieval doctors, and our understanding of the anatomy of the body is far more detailed than that of the ancient Greeks. Such knowledge, however, should not be used to denigrate earlier beliefs, but to sharpen an appreciation of the difficulties faced by all those concerned with medicine in the past, and even to emphasise some of the uncertainties in the evidence as revealed in past records. But, inevitably, some of the themes and examples in this book are chosen to illustrate the present, how we have come to our present understanding of the body, in health and disease, and of the consequent responses of both the individual and society in general towards illness.

Yet, paradoxically, modern medicine continues to believe in and to shape the notion of tradition that forms the core of this book. Few writers of medical papers can resist an opening retrospect that sets their discovery in its historical context, few discussions of medical ethics avoid mention of the Hippocratic *Oath* (written *c.* 400 BC), and few physicians are unaware of such famous names as William Harvey (1578–1657) or Andreas Vesalius (1514–64), even if they have never read a page of their writings in their original Latin. The difference between these and similar citations made two hundred years ago lies in the degree of authority conveyed by these names. To a modern physician they are distinguished precursors; to one of 1790 they also imparted sound knowledge and useful practical information. There was then less of the barrier between past and present. An early nineteenth-century physician, writing on fever, could include texts and information taken from the Greeks, the Romans, and his own contemporaries, and argue with a long-dead professor as if he were alive. Such a familiarity with, not to say occasional reverence for, the past is rare today. It has been replaced by a series of historical icons – images that are meant to evoke a great and glorious past that the present will, it is hoped, be led to emulate. The founders of hospitals, the leading professors of medical schools, the discoverers of syndromes or anatomical structures, and the eradicators of disease take on a new status, a status not always deserved or borne out by the historical record.

There is, then, still a tradition to which appeal is made. It is flexible in what it contains, and in what is emphasised. An Englishman may choose Harvey, a German Paracelsus; French historians of medicine focus on the surgical innovations of Ambroise Paré (1510–90), the Italians on Renaissance Padua, the Dutch on Boerhaave (1668–1738) and his Leiden pupils. The perspective from Spain or Eastern Europe is different yet again. But there is equally a sense of the past, and of certain names, as forming the present of medicine, of a tradition that serves as a backbone to medical discovery and, still more, to medical practice. In this volume such a tradition links the eighteenth century with the Renaissance, the Middle Ages, and with Classical Antiquity, and provides both continuity and a means to distinguish between practitioners. The orthodox were those who were familiar with this tradition, which might be called 'formal' or 'regular' medicine, and the unorthodox were those who flouted or disregarded it.

Where and how this tradition began is disputed. Certainly an important role was played in all this by a Romanised Greek, Galen of Pergamum (129–c. 200/216), but even before his time several Greek writers had been singled out for particular reverence and their opinions preserved for posterity, most notably Hippocrates of Cos (traditionally c. 450–370 BC). It was a tradition bounded in time and space, expanding from the Aegean basin to the rest of the Mediterranean region, to Europe, and then to European settlements overseas. It excluded, as this book will do, the medical theories of ancient Egypt and Babylonia, and likewise of India, China, America, and the other civilisations with whom the Europeans later came into contact. The inheritors of the Greek tradition noted the drugs, and occasionally the medical techniques, of non-Europeans, but they largely consigned their theories to the realms of superstition and irrationality. However, the absence from this book of any discussion of these non-European theories signifies merely that they contributed little to the main European tradition of medicine, and is not a judgment on their efficacy, rationality, or historical importance – not least because modern medical anthropologists have demonstrated that many medical procedures, Western and non-

Western, ancient and modern, are determined as much by the preferences and prejudices of a group or society, its general culture, as by
any objective criterion of effectiveness.

Particularly problematic in this regard is the question of medicine in
the Islamic world. Seen from a purely Western perspective, the writers
and translators of medicine who flourished in the Middle East, North
Africa, and Spain between AD 800 and 1200 form one stage in the
transmission of Classical medical ideas to Europe. Their role is that of
conduits and system-makers rather than independent or creative
thinkers, and as such they have a place in the Western tradition of
medicine. But to restrict a consideration of medicine in these regions
and these centuries purely to this transmission process is to miss much,
not least any originality and the variety of ways in which the Classical
tradition interacted with a variety of other traditions and beliefs.
Besides, the medical institutions of the Islamic world, larger and more
sophisticated than anything at the time in Western Europe, are also
worthy of attention, and did not come to an end with the Crusades of
the twelfth or the Mongol invasions of the thirteenth centuries. Hence,
although the Classical tradition of medicine remains the main focus of
Chapter 4, on medicine in the Islamic world, and relatively little space
is given to the other medical theories and practices that existed there,
there is no intention of implying that this is all that is worth knowing
about medicine in the Islamic world, or that the perspective offered is
the only one available.

Nor do the authors of this volume wish to confine the Western medical tradition to a series of 'great names' or, as the title might suggest,
to a tradition of medical ideas alone. That would be to fly in the face of
much recent scholarship, and our own researches. It is now clear that
this tradition, and those who believed exclusively in it, constituted only
the tip of a vast pyramid of healers and healing practices (and, until the
establishment or acceptance of a tradition, any exposition of medical
history in terms of an opposition between one group of healers and
another on the basis of this tradition would be anachronistic). Far from
being a rigid inheritance that passed from one distinguished medical
man to another, European medicine in the pre-modern age demonstrates a remarkable flexibility and variety. The medical market-place
had many stalls and many stall-holders, and patients, as well as their
physicians, could choose what to buy. One of the aims of this book is to
bring this variety to general notice, almost for the first time, and, in a

sense, to subvert the tradition announced in its title by placing it within its social, epidemiological, and historical context. What might appear stable or uniform is greatly qualified by the society in which medicine was practised. Institutions and wider cultural beliefs, as well as medical theories, help determine the relationship between society, disease, and its healers.

Just as the social context of medicine changes over time, so too the vocabulary of healing also shifts, and words take on different connotations. The notion of healing according to nature might constitute a guide to medical intervention, or, in certain periods, be understood as an injunction to avoid it. 'Science', which meant merely 'learned knowledge' in the Middle Ages, only gradually took on its modern resonances. Nonetheless, medical writers, from the Greeks onwards, frequently explained the activities of the body by means of ideas and analogies that encompassed the created world in general and were not confined to medicine, and modern scholars have often thought of them as scientific. The 'scientific revolution' of the seventeenth century thus saw an alteration in these broader explanations for the workings of the universe (pp. 340–59), with attendant consequences for the medicine for which they provided an intellectual context.

This was, on the whole, a literate medicine, one preserved in writing (of whatever level of sophistication, from a farmer's charm to a professor's lectures). We have thus little direct access to the world of the illiterate, which meant most of the population, in both town and countryside. Nor until the fifteenth century, and arguably much later, do we have statistics that enable us to quantify the data on population and disease with the degree of accuracy possible for the nineteenth and twentieth centuries. Estimates of population and similar demographic findings are thus largely qualitative, impressions by contemporary authors or later historians, not exact numbers. The evidence for disease as revealed by archaeology is also patchy in its coverage, and far from easy to interpret. Nonetheless, as modern demographers have shown, these types of evidence, taken together and explicated with care, can supplement the literary record and provide a fuller and richer context for the understanding of health and disease within society.

The vagaries of survival of the written record inevitably mean large gaps in our understanding of the medical history of the past, and render open to criticism almost any interpretation of it. Nonetheless, within the general framework of the Western medical tradition, the authors of this book have endeavoured to reveal the rich variety of the past, and to point out the contrasts, even among writers (and sufferers) who shared many of the same ideas and prejudices. The medical world of pre-modern Europe was no monolithic structure, nor was it the haunt of superstition, ignorance, and bigotry occasionally depicted by those who have not studied it. As this volume aims to show, the struggle against disease and illness has called for resourcefulness, intelligence, and even learning at all periods of history, and one may, on reading this volume, be struck more by the ways in which healers and patients alike coped in an age without modern hi-tech aids than by any obstinate adherence to age-old doctrines. If that is so, then the authors will have succeeded in demonstrating that one of the strengths of the Western medical tradition has been its flexibility both in its response to disease and in its capacity to adapt and to incorporate new discoveries and new ideas.

Note on names, text and illustrations

Names of Greek authors are given in their more familiar Latin or English form or spelling, e.g. Hippocrates, not Hippokrates; Galen, not Galenos. We have not sought to impose consistency on the names of medieval and renaissance authors; generally we have preferred the vernacular or the English to the Latin, e.g. Mondino, not Mundinus, Peter of Spain, not Petrus Hispanus, da Monte, not Montanus. In other instances, e.g. Albertus Magnus, Vesalius, we have retained the more familiar Latin form. Arabic and Syriac authors are usually referred to in Chapter 4 by their vernacular form; in Chapter 5 by their medieval Latin, e.g. Avicenna, not Ibn Sina.

The use of man throughout this text has been used purely in its historical sense.

Every effort has been made to clear permissions for all illustrations reproduced in this book. If there has been a failure to do so, please contact Cambridge University Press. Illustrations from the Wellcome Institute Library, London, are copyright, The Trustee of the Wellcome Trust.

Chronological table for chapters 1–3

The dates of birth and death of most individuals in this period cannot be determined for certain. Unless stated, the date in the left hand column refers to the period at which he was known to be active.

Year	Medical and scientific writers	Year	Contemporary events
(BC)		(BC)	
		753	Foundation of Rome
		c. 700	Homer
585	Thales, first Presocratic philosopher	c. 600	Rise of Athens to prominence
480	Parmenides of Elea	490	Battle of Marathon
		478	Formation of Delian League, later Athenian Empire
470	Alcmaeon of Croton		
460	Empedocles of Acragas		
		431	Peloponnesian War begins
		430–427	Plague of Athens
(428–347)	Plato		
420[1]	Hippocrates		
420	Democritus		
		404	Defeat of Athens
		399	Death of Socrates
385	Philistion of Locri		
		360	Roman expansion in Italy begins
		336	Death of Philip II of Macedon

[1] The historical Hippocrates was a contemporary of Socrates. The Hippocratic Corpus was largely written during the period 420–350 BC; what, if anything, Hippocrates himself wrote of it is hotly disputed.

Year	Medical and scientific writers	Year	Contemporary events
(384–322)	Aristotle of Stagira		
330	Diocles of Carystos	323	Death of Alexander the Great
320	Praxagoras of Cos		
		323–282	Ptolemy I, ruler of Egypt (341–270)
		300	Alexandrian Museum and Library founded
280	Herophilus of Chalcedon		
280	Erasistratus of Ceos		
219	Archagathus in Rome		
(234–149)	Cato	212	Roman capture of Syracuse
		168	Roman conquest of Macedonia
		146	Rome destroys Carthage and Corinth
		133	Kingdom of Pergamum given to Rome
		106–43	Cicero
95	Asclepiades of Bithynia		
80	Heraclides of Tarentum		
80	Apollonius of Citium		
		49–31	Roman civil wars
		31	Battle of Actium
		31 BC to AD 14	Augustus emperor
		30	Death of Cleopatra
(AD)		(AD)	
		4 BC to AD 65	Seneca
(23–79)	Pliny		
40	Celsus		
48	Scribonius Largus		
60	Thessalus of Tralles		
60	Pedanius Dioscorides		
		69–79	Vespasian emperor
		98–117	Trajan emperor
100	Rufus of Ephesus		
100	Soranus of Ephesus		
120	Marinus, anatomist		
(129–200 \216)	Galen		

Year	Medical and scientific writers	Year	Contemporary events
140	Aretaeus of Cappadocia	140	Asclepieion of Pergamum rebuilt
		161–180	Marcus Aurelius emperor
		165–169	Antonine Plague
		193–211	Septimius Severus emperor
		235–284	Roman civil wars
		307–337	Constantine I emperor
		313	legalising of Christianity
		330	foundation of Constantinople as E. capital
(325–400)	Oribasius	350	first hospitals in E.
		360–363	Julian emperor
370	Magnus of Nisibis	364	Roman Empire divided
		330–379	Basil of Caesarea
380	Marcellus of Bordeaux		
400	Caelius Aurelianus		
		476	deposition of Romulus Augustulus, last Western Roman emperor
		493–526	Theoderic ruler of Italy
		527–565	Justinian emperor
530	Aëtius of Amida	541–544	Plague of Justinian
		542	Caesarius bishop of Arles died
570	Alexander of Tralles		
600	Ravenna Commentators		
630	Paul of Aegina		
d. 640	Isidore of Seville	642/646	Arab capture of Alexandria
		672–735	The Venerable Bede
		800	Charlemagne crowned Holy Roman Emperor
900	*Leechbook* of Bald	871–899	Alfred the Great, king of Wessex
		1066	Norman Conquest of England

1 Medicine in the Greek world, 800–50 BC

VIVIAN NUTTON

Introduction

To trace the Western tradition of medicine back to the ancient Greeks is a simple task. Generations of doctors and surgeons have proclaimed their intellectual descent from Hippocrates of Cos and their adherence to a practice of medicine based on ethical, rational, and independent judgment, sound experience, and fine learning. Superstition here has no place; popular fancy and religious dogmatism alike are excluded. Medicine, like philosophy and drama, is part of the Greek miracle.

Such an account, which minimises any influence from the neighbouring cultures of the Near East, might appear unduly Hellenocentric, especially in the light of our present fragmentary state of knowledge of Near-Eastern and Early Greek medicine. The sophisticated medical culture of Egypt, for example, had long been known to the Greeks for its capable practitioners and its drugs, while many therapies and practices in Babylonia – notably prognostication, exorcism, and an emphasis on bodily fluids – have parallels in the Hippocratic Corpus. Nonetheless, many features of Greek medicine cannot be easily found in Near-Eastern medicine, especially its willingness to argue and speculate, and the Greeks themselves, who often acknowledged their debts to other earlier societies, are silent about any such influence on their medicine. If, as some modern writers have asserted, Greek medicine derives from these earlier and medically more advanced civilisations, any borrowing must have occurred so far back in the past that what was transferred was altered beyond easy recognition.

But to define the Greek medical tradition in terms of argument and speculation is also misleading, for it masks the plurality of Greek medicine, in which exorcists, religious healers, root-cutters, folk-healers, and *iatroi* ('healers')[1] co-existed in competition. Beliefs about dirt and pollu-

---

[1] In this chapter the translation 'healer' has been deliberately chosen instead of the more usual 'doctor' or 'physician' in order to avoid some of the modern connotations of these words. It does not imply that only healers offered physical healing or that they differed greatly from their Roman and later successors, who will be called, for convenience's sake, 'doctors'.

11

tion, left and right, or illness as divine punishment were as prominent in the medical world of Hippocrates as was shrewd observation and ingenious theorising, and the results of experience were used as much to confirm presuppositions as to refute them. This plurality of approaches is often forgotten in the face of the unitary (and unifying) concept of a medical tradition, but it was an essential element in the Greeks' struggle against disease.

The social and epidemiological background

The earliest surviving Greek medical writings (parts of the Hippocratic Corpus) date from about 420 BC. By then the Greeks were no longer confined to what is now Greece and the Aegean basin, but had established settlements ('colonies') around the Black Sea to the North and the Mediterranean as far West as Spain. Their characteristic form of political organisation was the *polis* ('city-state'), an independent and ideally self-sufficient community that controlled both an urban centre and its agricultural hinterland. The term 'city-state' is perhaps misleading. Few city-states in mainland Greece had more than 8000 inhabitants, of whom only 1500 may have lived in the urban centre itself. The colonies varied in size. Some were mere trading-posts, but Metapontum (southern Italy) in 300 BC may have had a total population of some 40,000, a quarter of whom lived within the urban centre. City size was limited by the agricultural basis of the area. Larger city-states depended on a large supply of land achieved by conquest or amalgamation or, more rarely, like Corinth and Athens, they relied on commerce and exploitation of the resources of others.

Athens is the great exception. Not only is more known of its social, political, economic, and cultural life than of any other Greek city, but its social and economic structures were vastly different. The total population of Athens and its region, Attica, around 350 BC has been put at 130,000–170,000 at the very least. Such high figures were rarely surpassed in Antiquity. Alexandria in Egypt, the largest city in the ancient world, may have housed 700,000 people around 50 BC; Rome, a century later, half a million; and Antioch (modern south-eastern Turkey), Carthage (Tunisia), Ephesus and Pergamum (west Turkey), over 250,000 at the same date. But these were exceptional. Most urban centres in Antiquity had around 1500–2000 inhabitants, a pattern that

12

continued well into the Middle Ages and beyond. Archaeology can give an overall sense of the size of urban communities, but precise population figures are lacking until the late fourteenth century, and the size of the non-urban population is largely unknown. Fluctuations within populations are hard to track, still more to explain. What matters here, however, is the difference in scale between ancient and modern. Until the mid-nineteenth century, medical practice was generally carried on in what anthropologists term a 'face-to-face', small-town society, not in the anonymity of a metropolis.

The disease profile of pre-modern Europe is equally hard to determine. The extensive palaeopathological investigation of skeletons is a relatively new development and historians of disease still rely mainly on written data. But pre-modern classifications and descriptions of disease do not always correspond to modern ones, and there is no consistency of vocabulary or perception; one author's pimple may be another's pustule. Modern classifications are no longer based solely on temperature, or even periodicity; and the ancient term 'fever' now covers a multitude of conditions. Many modern diagnostic tools were absent; temperature was measured purely by touch; urine was smelled, seen, and even tasted; taking the pulse was unknown before about 320 BC. Investigative results were described qualitatively (e.g. as a soft, quick, or strong pulse), not quantitatively. Hence, what to some ancient observers appeared clear and definite may seem ambiguous to a modern interpreter, and, conversely, modern specific viral or bacillary diseases cannot be easily distinguished among ancient descriptions. The continuing controversy over the identification of the Great Plague of Athens (430–427 BC), which depends on a most detailed description by the contemporary historian, sufferer, and – alas – non-medical man, Thucydides, exemplifies the problem. The spread of any given disease is almost impossible to determine, and an isolated comment, e.g. that the Athenians around 340 BC did not suffer from tapeworms like the inhabitants of the neighbouring region of Boeotia, is hard to interpret. Nonetheless, recent work on ancient nutrition and on palaeopathology, as well as modern understanding of pathogens and vectors, permit a brief recital of diseases likely to have existed in Antiquity.

Famine and pestilence (epidemic disease) were linked by the poet Hesiod as early as 700 BC, and many later medical authors noted amenorrhoeas, oedemas, and digestive disorders in times of hunger, which were distressingly frequent. The prevalence of xerophthalmia in early spring has also been connected with the lack of vitamin A in a

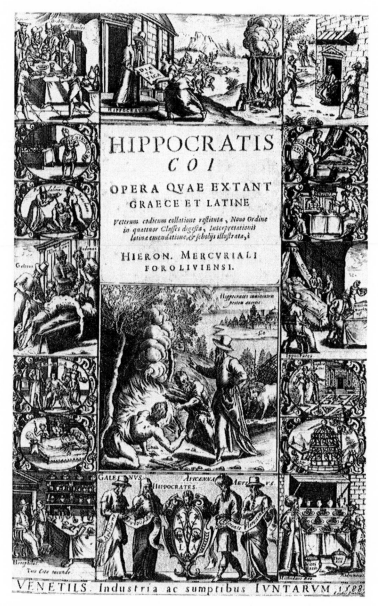

Fig. 1. Hippocrates curing the plague of Athens, a famous, if unlikely story. From the frontispiece to the 1588 Juntine edition of the complete works of Hippocrates (in Greek with Latin translation). (The Wellcome Institute Library, London, W. 3175.)

winter diet (red carrots were not grown, and some medical writers even argued against eating many vegetables in winter). Dysenteries were common, as were a variety of fevers, including typhoid, and malarial fevers formed the model for the understanding of acute diseases. There

14

are early descriptions of tuberculosis, chickenpox, puerperal fever, diph-theria, and mumps; measles and rubella appear to have been absent until the Roman period, and the existence of smallpox is hotly disputed. Leprosy may have arrived during the first millennium BC. Some genetic diseases have also been detected in Classical Greece, including thalas-saemia and sickle-cell anaemia, which may have been a response to endemic malaria. Eye diseases, especially trachoma, seem to have been common, but evidence for sexually transmitted diseases is relatively rare until the Roman period. Even so, these may have taken milder forms, such as genital herpes, or, like gonorrhoea, had a limited spread. Venereal syphilis is not found, but non-venereal syphilis may have existed elsewhere in the Mediterranean world. Other conditions easily identifiable in our sources, e.g. epilepsy, heart failure and rabies, may have attracted attention because of their frightening symptoms and their relative rarity. Breast cancers are mentioned far more often than other cancers, which, like other degenerative diseases, may have been unusual in a population with a life-expectancy of around 40 years.

Whether one should conclude that Classical Greece was an unhealthy place in which to live is debatable. Certainly, life in Athens, as in any other large city, was likely to be far more unhealthy than in a peasant village, simply because of the presence of more diseases and disease vec-tors. But many major killer diseases, e.g. smallpox, measles, and bubonic plague, were absent for long periods, and were certainly not endemic. In Athens, as later in the cities of the Roman Empire, civic organisation was capable of assuring at least a minimum food-supply to avoid contin-ual major outbreaks of famine; prolonged drought in an upland village, however, might have been disastrous. The lack of exposure of the Greeks, largely confined to the Aegean basin, to new diseases may also have helped to maintain a relatively stable disease environment. The later expansion of the Roman Empire into areas with different diseases and, still more, the collapse from AD 350 onwards of many governmen-tal institutions, may have together reduced the life-expectancy of the population. If the chances of a long life in the Athens of Hippocrates were not high, they were even lower in Anglo-Saxon London.

Religion and argument in early Greek medicine

Two features are often taken to mark the Greek approach to under-standing disease – a willingness to indulge in speculation, and a reluc-

15

tance to invoke the gods as the cause of individual disease. This reluctance should not be misunderstood. Throughout Antiquity there existed alongside healers (*iatroi*) others who offered a religious explanation and a religious cure for illness – diviners, exorcists, and various types of priests. Certain diseases, notably epilepsy and pestilence, were often ascribed to the wrath of a god: Homer's *Iliad* begins with a plague sent by Apollo on the Greeks, and some sought relief from the Great Plague of Athens in religious expiation. A comic dramatist *c.* 420 BC displayed a chorus of semi-divine Heroes threatening the unjust with various diseases – coughs, dropsy, catarrh, scab, madness, lichens, swellings, ague, and fever. Belief in divine intervention did not exclude secular healing; those who sought the help of a god for one disease might well consult a healer for another. In turn, few healers rejected the gods. That traditional touchstone of the medical profession, the Hippocratic *Oath*, begins with an invocation to the gods and goddesses, and we know of healers who contributed to the building of a shrine or accepted the orders of the god Asclepius in prescribing for themselves and their patients.

But, at the same time, many healers sought to establish a system of healing that was independent of the divine. The author of the Hippocratic tract *On the sacred disease* (*c.* 410 BC) argued that epilepsy was no more divine than any other disease, or the sun and the winds. Indeed, it was precisely those who championed a religious cure for epilepsy who were impious, for they tried to force the gods to do their will and blamed them for introducing some harmful pollution. Another contemporary remarked that, while prayer was a good thing, it was also necessary for man to lend a hand. This was a bargain for both sides to keep. In the Roman period Galen's anger at the activities of quacks was matched by his amazement at Jews and Christians, whose belief in miracles he thought entailed a capricious deity who could overthrow at will the whole 'scientific' basis of the universe, including medicine.

The relatively amicable coexistence of religion and medicine is one aspect of the pluralism of Greek medicine. Healers, both male and female, competed with root-cutters, exorcists, midwives, bone-setters, lithotomists, gymnasts, and surgeons for patients. There were no examinations to be passed, no lists of forbidden practices, no membership requirements. Doctrinally, too, there was abundant variety. Even within the Hippocratic Corpus (largely written between 420 and 370 BC) there are major theoretical differences among its constituent treatises, and still more can be discerned outside the Corpus. Debates on theory were not confined to practitioners of medicine; important ideas were discussed by the so-called Pre-Socratic philosophers (an unfortunate traditional name for a motley group, few of whom were philosophers in a modern sense, and many contemporaries of Socrates, d. 399 BC).

This openness towards speculation and argument is striking, and it would be foolish to assume that the creative impulse came always from philosophy. Many surviving medical texts are avowedly aimed at asserting (and proving) in debate the truth of their theories against all comers, medical and non-medical alike. They invoke empirical evidence, but rely even more on argument and analogy to carry conviction.

Their theories encompassed both the internal workings of the body and its relationship to the universe at large. The earliest Pre-Socratics in the sixth century BC had attempted to identify the single substance from which all things originated, but after the radical critique of such monocausal theories by Parmenides, the focus of the argument shifted. Parmenides (c. 515–c. 450 BC), who was later honoured at Elea as the native founder of a medico-religious group (*pholeon*), brought to the forefront the problem of change and stability within an ordered universe. It received a variety of solutions. For the Pythagoreans, the basis of the universe was number; for Heraclitus (*fl.* 490 BC) and his followers, it was balanced change itself that was constant, in a world composed of fire, earth, and water; for Leucippus (*fl.* 435 BC) and Democritus (*fl.* 420 BC), the world was made up from atoms and void. Others, like Empedocles (*fl.* 460 BC), imagined it built up from a small number of elements (earth, air, fire, and water), which might form stable combinations – blood, for example, was a proportionate mixture of particles of all four elements. Around 440 BC, Anaxagoras argued that the original mixture of the universe contained an immense diversity of ingredients, coming together as 'seeds', each having within itself parts of everything else, and hence the potentiality for growth and change. In their arguments, as well as in their metaphors, these thinkers drew on evidence from the body and from biological processes. Alcmaeon of Croton (southern Italy, *c.* 470 BC?) is credited with an actual dissection, which revealed the optic nerve behind the eyeball and suggested to him that sensation was transmitted in channels to the brain through the medium of *pneuma*, a form of air or spirit.

It is a small step from thinkers putting forward ideas on how the body was made up and how it worked to healers considering the body

17

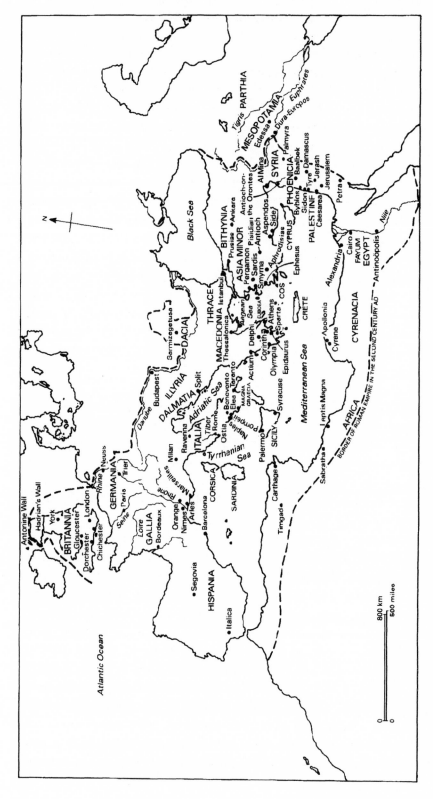

Map. 1. The Greco-Roman world in the second century AD. (Modified from N. and A. Ramage, *Cambridge Illustrated History of Roman Art*. Cambridge University Press. 1991.)

also when it malfunctioned. Indeed, it is hard to distinguish at times who learned from whom, so complex is the interrelationship between the two groups. Some objected to any cross-fertilisation. The Hippocratic author of *On ancient medicine* vigorously denounced philosophical speculation within medicine, but it is debatable whether his own theory of competing 'properties' within the body, e.g. sweetness and sourness, was any less speculative than the philosophers' hot, cold, wet, and dry that he rejected. Like many other writers in the Hippocratic Corpus, he was, in his methodology, covering ground also trodden by others – philosophers, astronomers, and even a historian like Thucydides. All were ready to argue their case in public, and the healer was advised to note the tricks of logic and rhetoric that his opponents might use, and how to counteract them. Greek medicine was not a closed system. In contrast to the medicine of the Near East, it was remarkably open to intellectual influences of all kinds, and, in turn, was accessible to non-healers.

Healers, Hippocrates, and the Hippocratic Corpus

This intellectual openness was hardly surprising, since, in fifth-century Greece, there was little that resembled a medical profession. Only Athens was large enough to have many resident healers whose livelihood depended solely on the fees paid to them by patients. Other healers had either to travel in search of patients around the small towns in Greece, like the author of the Hippocratic *Epidemics*, books 1 and 3, who worked in northern Greece, Thessaly, and the Aegean islands, or to combine medicine with other activities. By 500 BC a few city-states, including Athens, had begun to attract practitioners by paying them a retainer to reside and treat their inhabitants, especially their own citizens. A few places had also gained a reputation for the healers who lived, taught, and studied there, although one need not believe the later theory that all medicine derived from three 'choruses' of healers, Asclepiads (descendants of the healing god Asclepius), at Cos, Cnidos, and, briefly, nearby Rhodes. That such medical clans existed is certain, but by the time of the Hippocratic *Oath*, *c.* 400 BC, the situation had altered considerably. The *Oath* (see p. 29) envisages a quasi-family situation, in which a pupil must regard his teacher and his teacher's relatives as if they were his own, and keep the secrets of medicine within this extended family and those who had sworn the *Oath*. Yet one of the few

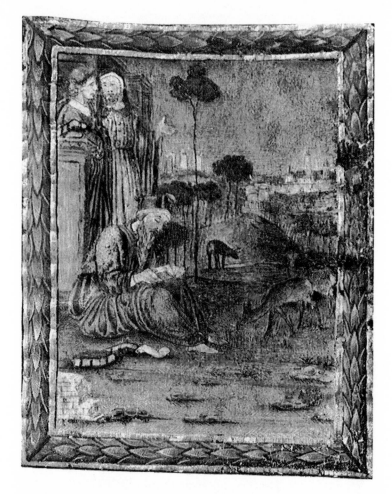

Fig. 2. Hippocrates reading, while two bystanders argue. Opening illustration from a fifteenth-century manuscript of the *Aphorisms* in Latin translation. (The Wellcome Institute Library, London, WMS 353, fol. 3 r.)

certain facts about the historical Hippocrates (*c.* 450–370 BC) is that he taught medicine for a fee to anyone who could pay.

This is reported by Plato (428–347 BC), his contemporary, who also reveals that Hippocrates was an Asclepiad from Cos and that his medical theorising involved a method of logical division. According also to Plato, Hippocrates believed that a disease could not be treated without a knowledge of 'the whole', an ambiguous phrase which may indicate either the body in general or the patient's environment. That Hippocrates enjoyed a great reputation in his lifetime is clear, but beyond this, all is confusion. The Hippocratic *Letters* and *Speeches*, the

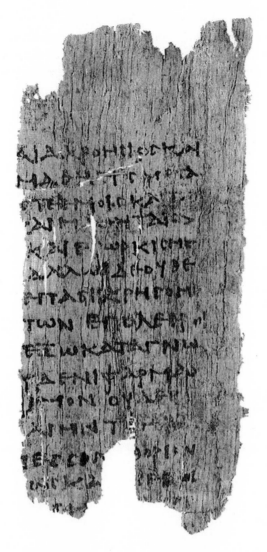

Fig. 3. A papyrus of the Hippocratic Oath, written in Egypt *c.* AD 275. Oxyrhyncus Papyrus 2547. (The Wellcome Institute Library, London, WMS 5754.)

source of much later biography, are now generally believed to have been composed at least a generation after Hippocrates' death, and most are considerably later.

Nor can much information on Hippocrates be gained from the Hippocratic Corpus itself. This is a body of sixty or so Greek medical works attributed to Hippocrates, written mainly between 420 and 350 BC, and largely assembled at Alexandria in Egypt around 280 BC. Even the total number of treatises is not assured, for some were wrongly combined or separated in Antiquity. *On generation* and *On the nature of the child*, for instance, once formed part of the same work, and the seven books of the *Epidemics* were written at three different dates (books 1 and 3 were written in *c.* BC 410; 2, 4, and 6 in *c.* BC 400; 5 and 7 in *c.* BC 350) and, probably, by three different authors.

That some parts of the Corpus go back to Hippocrates himself is likely, but which they are has long been controversial. The explanations of disease given in *On breaths, On ancient medicine,* and *On the nature of man,* each of which has been considered quintessentially Hippocratic, are so different that they are unlikely to have been written by the same man. About AD 170 Galen took *On the nature of man* as the starting point for a complicated classification that related in some degree all the texts in the Corpus to Hippocrates and his family; some were composed by the great man himself, others by his family, others merely retain the spirit of his teaching. Like many, more modern attempts to solve this Hippocratic question, Galen's schema was ultimately circular, although it created an image of the ideal healer that still impresses today. Galen's preferences among the Hippocratic Corpus also defined for generations what Hippocratic medicine was, and how it should be practised, and his methods of identifying the works of Hippocrates were not seriously challenged, or supplemented, until the twentieth century. Many modern scholars are more sceptical in their search for the historical Hippocrates and his writings, preferring to identify earlier strands of material in the Corpus or works commented on by scholars at Alexandria before 250 BC.

This modern scepticism has had the paradoxical effect of opening up the Hippocratic Corpus to scrutiny. Instead of concentrating on a few 'genuine' writings, scholars are now free to consider the Corpus in all its diversity of forms and doctrines. Some texts, like *Dentition*, are little more than a series of easily memorable sentences; others, like *On breaths* or *The art*, are public orations defending a particular medical point of view; some, like *Aphorisms*, were probably used for teaching; others, like *Humours*, appear deliberately obscure. Some, like *On the sacred disease*, propound a definite thesis; others, like *On diseases*, seem concerned merely to list various ailments. Some, like the later *Precepts* and *Decorum*, are written in elegant prose; others, particularly the *Epidemics*, may represent case-notes at various stages of creation. No generalisation can cover all the texts, and no summary can more than hint at the multiplicity of (often conflicting) theories contained therein.

Hippocratic theories

The authors of the Hippocratic Corpus all presume that bodily processes, health, and disease can be explained in the same way as other natural phenomena, and are independent of any arbitrary, supernatural interference. Man is subject to the same physical constraints as the rest of the ordered cosmos, and an understanding of the body, within itself and within its whole environment, provides a way to control it when things go wrong. Even frightening diseases such as apoplexy and mania can be cured by the application of reasoned remedies, in the form of surgery, drugs, or, more usually, diet. This appeal to rationality and argument, however justified in theory and however neglected in actual practice, is a major characteristic of Hippocratic medicine.

By contrast, how the body worked, and what disease was, were questions that divided the Hippocratic healers. While their surface anatomy and osteology was generally accurate, they gained their empirical knowledge of the body's internal arrangement and processes only by an occasional observation of a gaping wound or animal dissection. Water found in the skull of an apparently epileptic goat confirmed an explanation for epilepsy; hen's eggs furnished a model for human foetal development. But nothing suggests that these animal 'experiments' were carried out frequently, or even repeated; the consistency of the analogy was considered convincing enough. Hence the invisible workings of the body could only be deduced from visible processes in the cosmos in general. The eye was compared with a lantern; the stomach with an oven; the kidneys with a cupping glass, drawing fluid to themselves and filtering it off as if through sand. Some authors explained disease as the result of harmful material floating around the body until it alighted in one spot, which thereby became diseased. In a variant on this, the writer of *On the sacred disease* argued that epilepsy was caused by phlegm blocking the movement of air around the body, which then agitated the body as it struggled to find a way round. This often happened when the South wind blew, for it made the brain moister, just like wine in jars.

Another common idea in the Hippocratic Corpus was that of health and illness as some form of balance and imbalance. This type of explanation was given by many of the Pre-Socratics in their attempts to understand the stability and the changeability of the universe. Balance

23

and imbalance were regarded by the Hippocratic writers in two separate ways. The author of *On regimen* thought that the whole body was in a perpetual state of flux, and health consisted in keeping this flux within certain limits. By contrast, the author of *On the nature of man* argued that the body remained in a stable balance until something, external or internal, occurred to overturn it. On both views, once the individual balance was understood, this knowledge could be applied by the healer to its preservation or restoration.

The balance was primarily one of fluids, *chymoi,* a word usually translated as 'humours', although it equally denoted the sap in a plant or the juice of a fruit. Two fluids in particular attracted attention as the causes of illness; bile and phlegm. Not only were they naturally present in the body, but at specific seasons they regularly appeared to flow out during illness. Winter colds were ascribed to phlegm, summer dysenteries and vomiting to bile. By analogy, it was then easy to regard other diseases as dependent on these two fluids. In epilepsy, phlegm generating in the head formed a thick barrier to the passage of air; in mania, bile overheated the brain. National characteristics were ascribed by the author of *Airs, waters, and places* to the effects of these humours; the white, cold, flabby, and phlegmatic inhabitants of the Ukraine were contrasted with the dark, hot, scrawny, and bilious Libyans, and, still more, with the well-balanced Greeks in their well-balanced climate.

Bile and phlegm were visible only when excreted during illness, and hence might be considered permanently dangerous. Other fluids were more ambiguous. Blood, which since Homeric times had been associated with life, was also expelled from the body in nose-bleeds or piles, to say nothing of menstruation. Here was a fluid which Nature (and following her, the healer) removed when in excess. Similarly, water, necessary for life, was in some illnesses excreted as copious urine or, as in dropsy, made the body enormously distended. All these could be associated with specific ailments, foods, and even seasons of the year. The fact that the body itself sometimes rejected them gave further grounds for suspecting them of causing disease, and for taking them into consideration when contemplating any therapy.

The fourth of the celebrated humours, black bile or melancholy, comes relatively late into this picture. Early classifications emphasised bile and phlegm, and although 'sufferers from melancholy' are mentioned, black bile is not considered a specific humour, but rather a depraved form of (yellow) bile. Only with *On the nature of man*, the text

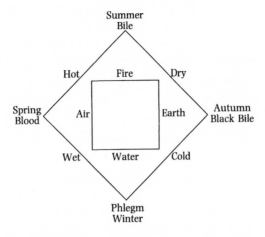

Fig. 4. Plan of the Hippocratic humoral system in *On the nature of Man.*

which Galen and subsequent generations believed was quintessentially Hippocratic, does black bile become an essential humour. By contrast with beneficent blood, black bile was regarded as mainly harmful – it was visible in vomit and excreta, and later authors described how it hissed and bubbled on reaching the ground, burning up whatever it touched. Modern scholars disagree on what black bile actually was (perhaps some form of dried blood), but once proposed as a humour, it fitted neatly into a rational scheme made even more credible by the ease with which it could be extended to cover a whole range of circumstances. The four humours – blood, bile, black bile, and phlegm – could be linked to the four seasons; to the four ages of man – childhood, youth, adulthood, and old age; and to the four primary qualities – hot, dry, cold, and wet, see Fig. 4. By the Roman period, the humours were associated with the four elements – air, fire, earth, and water; four types of fever; four periods of the day; four colours; four tastes; and medieval scholars added the four temperaments, the four Evangelists, and four musical tonalities. This was a schema that had great explanatory power. By understanding, for example, that blood predominated in spring and in young men, one could take wise precautions, by eliminating foods that contained much blood or by letting blood to relieve the expected excess. It was a schema capable of almost infinite variation, unfalsifiable on its own terms, and often corresponding to the facts of observation.

Hippocratic practice

The doctrine of balance, particularly of the humours, provided the healer with a rationale whereby to manage disease – and the patient. The word management is appropriate, because several Hippocratic healers deliberately avoided some therapeutic procedures. The *Oath* forbade cutting, even for bladder-stone, and another author recommended leaving surgical intervention to those experienced in war wounds, perhaps for the very good reason that inexpert intervention might make matters worse rather than from any rejection of surgery itself. The tract *On head wounds* shows a good understanding of cranial trauma, while the author of *On joints* has a sound knowledge of the principles of orthopaedics (and the difference in treatment between reducing a dislocation immediately and doing so when some time has elapsed), even if some of his suggested treatments, e.g. suspending the patient by the neck, or fixing him upside-down on a ladder and then banging it on the ground as a cure for a hunched back, would only have aggravated the condition and might have proved fatal. Hippocratic drug therapy offers a similar prospect, for the potentially dangerous effects of emetics and purgatives were well-known, and one might best preserve one's reputation by referring a patient for treatment to a specialist 'root-cutter'. Against a spectacular treatment and cure one had always to balance the possibility of failure, disgrace, and a law suit.

Most favoured of all types of treatment in the Hippocratic Corpus, however, was diet or regimen. By this was meant far more than the mere prescribing of food and drink; diet indicated a whole life-style, including the way one slept (and dreamed), took exercise, and reacted to one's environment. It is no surprise that some ancient authors linked this medical therapy with the training regimen of athletes or with the austere sect of Pythagorean philosophers, who notoriously disapproved of beans, or that some Hippocratic writers sought to distinguish their dietetics from that of the trainer or the cook. They stressed that diet was more than the treatment of disease; it involved prophylaxis even more than cure. Since disease was a process of change, it was essential to devise a regimen that would alter, reverse, or, even better, forestall that process. The doctrine of the humours offered the possibility of foretelling what conditions were likely to occur at any particular season of the year, and of introducing a contrary (allopathic) regimen that would reduce susceptibility to illness. In both sickness and health, the healer

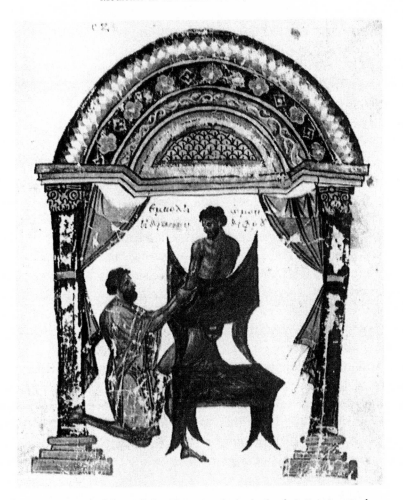

Fig. 5. Resetting a dislocated shoulder, using the back of a chair to gain extra leverage, from the commentary of Apollonius of Citium on the Hippocratic treatise *On
Joints*. (Florence, Biblioteca Medicea Laurenziana, plut. 74.7, fol. 190 r.)

who understood how the body worked would prescribe appropriate
foods or exercise to maintain the body's balance. Balance was what
Nature sought, and, so the author of *The art of medicine* argued, what
might seem to an outsider a spontaneous cure was only Nature's way
of proceeding like an expert healer, albeit more slowly.

This emphasis on diet, which distinguishes Greek medicine from that
of the Near East, also involves the idea of illness as a process, with a
beginning, middle, and end. Just as, after surgery, a patient might be
given liquids, then gruel, and finally solids during recovery, so one

could devise appropriate diets for the various stages of any and every illness. It was the mark of the expert healer to be able to target the precise stage of whatever acute disease required attention. (Chronic illness is mentioned only rarely in the Hippocratic tradition.)

The model for this was malarial fever, whose regular pattern and seasonal onset made it eminently explicable in terms of a regular cycle of humours and seasons. In its mathematical precision it appealed to those who believed in an astrological medicine, or simply in a natural cycle of the stars and planets bringing about climatic changes that affected the individual. The arrival of a quartan or tertian attack could be predicted nicely, and appropriate precautions taken in advance. Its regularity also guaranteed the system used to explain and manage it.

Dietetic medicine demanded careful observation of all that might affect the patient. The more one observed, the more likely one was to pick out crucial signs, and to be able to predict, and, where necessary, change the course of disease. Indeed, the author of *Airs, waters, and places* took it as axiomatic that an advance understanding of the effects of certain environments would enable the healer arriving at a strange town to tell immediately the diseases he was likely to find there. The authors of the *Epidemics* included at length detailed observations of individual cases, some of which they later incorporated into broader discussions of the diseases of their community over a year. In these so-called *Constitutions* they tried to correlate diseases with the seasons and the weather, an impressive achievement in a society with few written records.

Many Hippocratic writers proclaimed the importance of close observation, especially as it formed the basis for the art of prognosis, which, as the author of *Prognostics* put it, encompasses past, present, and future. Modern *diagnosis* is thus subsumed under the heading of *prognosis*, foreknowledge, which indicates the Hippocratic bias. The interest of the healer lies in controlling the future at least as much as in understanding the past or present.

Prognosis had also a social function. By declaring that death was almost certain, a healer could escape blame for apparent failure – or censure for refusing to give any treatment beyond a temporary palliative. As well as a form of insurance, prognosis served also as advertising. To declare correctly at first sight a patient's past history was to create an immediate impression of competence, and to give the confidence that, so Hippocratic writers asserted, lay behind any successful cure. Such a prognosis provided an immediate guide to the abilities of an itinerant healer who arrived at a small town in the course of his travels. Without such guidance, patients, particularly in the back-woods, were at the mercy of those who offered to cure them, and they might prefer to trust in Nature rather than the hands of a stranger. Where there was a choice of medical craftsmen, a correct prognosis, like elegant bandaging, distinguished the good healer from those who were mere wordsmiths, or relied on flashy instruments to attract patients. In such circumstances, medical ethics could be equated with effective practice: a healer's philanthropy, which might include occasional free treatment, not only made the patient feel better, but also imparted a love of medicine.

Most of the ethical writings in the Hippocratic Corpus are concerned to demarcate the good practitioner from the bad by the application of a simple criterion: whatever is best for the case in hand. Appropriate behaviour, dress, and manner all play their part, and the healer is enjoined to do always what is helpful, or at least will not harm. Hence there is no stigma attached to non-intervention or leaving a patient to others (or the gods). Although medicine is called 'holy', the healer is viewed as a public figure, debating and consulting with others in view of the patient and others. The Hippocratic *Oath* by contrast seeks to restrict the practice of medicine to those sworn to secrecy, or, as the author of the *Law* put it, initiated into the holy mysteries. The *Oath*, however, alone of the ethical texts, raises moral problems, not least in its prohibition of abortion, the use of the knife (even for lithotomy), and the provision of a deadly drug on request, and it defines ethics in terms of the obligations involved in belonging to a group. But there is plenty of evidence for healers assisting without qualms in abortions or suicide, and plying the knife, and the generally religious language of the *Oath*, especially its opening invocation of the healing deities, has suggested to many scholars that it was devised for a small, and perhaps unusual, group. Indeed, far from being the touchstone of medical ethics in Antiquity, the *Oath* is rarely mentioned, and may not have been generally sworn until the sixteenth century at the earliest. (For the development of ethical ideas in medicine, see pp. 47, 323, 446.)

As the *Oath* itself reveals, the healer in the Hippocratic Corpus is male, although that neither prevented him from deriving information from midwives and other women who treated female disorders, nor necessarily indicates that such women confined their services to women. The presence of gynaecological treatises in the Corpus (more, indeed, than survive from any other period of Antiquity) demonstrates co-operation, as well as the generally lower level of female literacy. These treatises show the strengths and weaknesses of early Greek medicine; a combination of acute observation, especially of physical symptoms, with explanatory schematism. It was believed that children born at seven months have a more favourable chance of life than those born at eight; the mobile womb is a cause of frequent illness; and the whole female constitution is a weaker version of the male. There are disputes over the function of menstruation and over the female role in generation, neither easily resolved from the anatomical and physiological information to hand, and disputed by philosophers as well as healers. Arguably, the medical view of woman rested far more on what, to modern scholars, seem taboos, prejudices, and inherited folk-wisdom than on any physical external examination or accumulated experience. It is no coincidence that women's diseases, and particularly the impure womb, are treated with excrement, asphalt, sulphur, squill, and laurel, materials found together elsewhere only in Greek religious purificatory rituals.

Part of the explanation for this doctrinal fluidity, and the highly individualistic nature of Hippocratic medicine, is the relative absence of one fixing agent, written documentation. That some doctors took and preserved case notes is clear from case histories contained in the *Epidemics* (a misleading translation of a word meaning 'visitations', of either disease or doctor). But the patient's history always begins with the disease under treatment, not with a summary of earlier medical experiences; the medical past is still only the very recent past. Some authors, most notably in *Epidemics* 1 and 3, combined individual data to give a more general picture of the diseases within a community over a year, but without a complex recording system little more was, or could be, done. Not that epidemic diseases were unknown, or left unexplained by medical writers. Bad air, miasma, was seen as their main cause; and their effects might be prevented by breathing in less air or changing one's environment. Non-medical authors, notably Thucydides, were well aware that those in close contact with the sick were liable themselves to fall ill (and Thucydides also remarked that sufferers from the Athenian plague, once recovered, were rarely reinfected), but no surviving Greek medical text remarks on this or discusses contagion. From a Hippocratic perspective it was not a city that suffered in an epidemic, but an individual, and one's energies should be channelled towards maintaining or restoring the health of that individual.

Plato, Aristotle, and their contemporaries

The Hippocratic writers maintained a largely physicalist view of mental disorders, ascribing physical causes to frenzy and mania, and treating them by physical means. This type of explanation was extended by the philosopher Plato, who used complex and interlocking analogies with bodily processes and civic organisation to define and justify his doctrines of virtue and knowledge. Plato knew of Hippocrates, and may also have derived considerable medical information from Philistion (*fl.* 380 BC), a philosopher and healer from Locris (southern Italy). In the *Republic* and, more influentially, in the *Timaeus*, Plato divided the human soul into three parts, the reasoning, the spirited, and the appetitive, located respectively in the brain, the heart, and the liver. The parts of the human body were purposefully created by the Demiurge (the divine workman) out of the four Empedoclean elements, earth, air, fire, and water, which themselves were transformations of an original matter of geometrical shapes and particles. Disease resulted from excess or deficiency within the elements, but also from the decomposition of a bodily part into its original elements. In addition, breath (*pneuma*), bile, and phlegm were each responsible for a specific range of disorders. The tripartite soul was affected directly by bodily changes; moisture in the bone marrow caused sexual intemperance, and phlegm and bile produced bad temper, cowardice, even stupidity. The philosopher, the healer of the soul, needed also the aid of the physical healer to restore the body by diet, exercise, and, in extreme cases, drugs.

Plato's debt to earlier or contemporary medical writers is a vexed question, for the Hippocratic Corpus contains only a fraction of the medical literature of the time, and only a mere handful of works remains of those written between 380 BC and AD 100. Any reconstruction of the opinions of Philistion, for example, rests on fragments mediated through much later authors, with consequent hazards of bias, misquotation, and lack of context. Galen assumed that the good physician in AD 177 could recite the main theories of the fourth-century BC writers Diocles, Pleistonicus, Phylotimus, Praxagoras, and Dieuches, but there is little evidence that any of their books survived until then, and even Galen may have relied only on medical doxographies (collections of past opinions on disputed problems). Reconstruction of their theories (and importance) is thus more than usually problematic.

But these fragmentary healers are arguably less significant than the two philosophers, Plato (whose *Timaeus* Galen believed was based on Hippocrates' own teaching) and Aristotle (384–322 BC). Aristotle, the son of a doctor, wrote, and through his pupils organised research, on a wide variety of topics relevant to medicine, although except for Meno's collection of the opinions of earlier healers, none relates directly to medical theory or practice. Three main areas are significant here. Firstly, Aristotle's logic provided the scaffolding for subsequent scientific and medical argument in Late Antiquity and the Middle Ages. Secondly, his discussion of psychology, in *On the soul* and *On sensation*, attracted doctors and philosophers alike for many centuries. Thirdly, above all, whereas Plato in his philosophical speculations had played down the evidence of the senses, Aristotle carried out a series of empirical studies of the natural world, on fishes, birds, and animals, including man. His comparative approach involved detailed observation of a wide range of phenomena in an attempt to answer questions about how (and why) living beings functioned. Taking his cue from Plato, Aristotle declared that Nature did nothing in vain, and hence sought an explanation for bodily parts in terms of their purpose (teleology). His investigations involved corporate investigation and, not least, the deliberate and organised use of dissection of plants, fishes, and animals. His associate Diocles is credited with the first book to bear the title *Dissections*, presumably of animals, not of man. The results are not always easy to interpret. Aristotle claimed that the heart had three chambers, not two or four, and, again in contradistinction to Plato, he saw the heart alone as the seat of a unitary soul, leaving the brain to act as a sort of bodily cooling system. His studies of motion and generation, however, as well as his shrewd observations of minor details of zoology, marked an enormous advance over what had gone before. His achievements also redounded to the glory of his patrons, among them the kings of Macedonia, Philip II (reigned 359–336 BC) and his son, Alexander the Great (reigned 336–323 BC), and helped ensure a prominent place for science at the courts of the various dynasts who divided among themselves the empire of Alexander after his death. Chief among them was Ptolemy (reigned 323–282 BC), who established his family's rule over Egypt with its new capital at Alexandria. Ptolemy's main cultural foundations, the Alexandrian Library and the Museum ('shrine of the

Muses'), were designed to preserve and support Greek learning in its new environment.

Hellenistic medicine

Alexander's conquest of the former Persian Empire took Greeks and Greek civilisation as far as northern India, and created city-settlements that looked back, in cultural terms, to Greece, even though their inhabitants were rarely Greeks by race or language (hence the word 'Hellenistic' – 'Greekish' – to describe this wider Greek civilisation and period). The Greek world stretched from southern Italy and Sicily (and even Marseilles, France) to Mesopotamia, and for a while even beyond, and within it Greek became the common language of the ruling elites. There was a remarkable accession of new information, on plants, minerals, and animals, some of it deliberately collected and sent back to Greece by Alexander's own army, and it is likely that, particularly in Egypt, which traded with Africa and India, this also included new drugs.

But the medical men of Hellenistic Alexandria are renowned less for pharmacology than for anatomy and physiology. The step from Aristotelian animal to human dissection is credited to Herophilus of Chalcedon (c. 330–260 BC) and his contemporary Erasistratus of Ceos (c. 330–255 BC), both linked with Alexandria. The most important ancient accounts of their activities, by the Roman medical encyclopaedist Celsus around AD 40 and the Christian polemicist Tertullian around AD 200, state that they practised human vivisection, a claim hard to check since the reported results might have been obtained from a combination of human anatomy and animal vivisection. But the story is not impossible. Certainly royal support was necessary, not least in providing the bodies of condemned criminals for experiment, and some have imagined that the actual dissections took place within the protective walls of the Museum. How much these Greek anatomists owed to Egyptian mummifiers is hotly debated. Linguistic differences would have made communication difficult, even with an interpreter, and the Egyptian method of mummification and removal of the organs differs somewhat from what Herophilus and Erasistratus were doing. But mummification at least showed that the Egyptians had no taboo on mutilating an Egyptian corpse – unlike the Greeks, who retained such prohibitions in force on Ceos even during the lifetime of Erasistratus. In the early days of Alexandria, from whose citizenship native Egyptians

33

were for long legally excluded, Greeks may well have taken advantage of their colonial domination to dissect the bodies of their inferiors, especially when, as convicted murderers and criminals, they were arguably inhuman. Two generations later, when Egyptians were becoming assimilated into Alexandrian society, such considerations may no longer have applied, one possible reason for the apparent absence of human anatomical experimentation after 250 BC. Henceforth, although Alexandria continued to be famous for anatomy, this was carried out by demonstration on a human skeleton, supplemented by human surface anatomy and by animal dissection.

The results of the investigations of Herophilus and Erasistratus were little short of revolutionary. For the first time, the internal structures of the body were revealed, and its parts named – Herophilus had a penchant for neat parallels with everyday objects, e.g. the 'wine-press' (the *torcular Herophili* in the skull). He paid particular attention to the various coats of the eye, described the gross liver, differentiated between various parts of the spermatic duct, and investigated the ovaries and at least part of the Fallopian tubes. He continued an interest of his teacher, Praxagoras of Cos (*fl.* 320 BC), by distinguishing on anatomical grounds between nerves, veins and arteries, although he apparently rejected his opinion that only *pneuma* (spirit), the vehicle of sensation, was carried in the arteries, in favour of a mixture of blood and *pneuma*. His most impressive anatomical work was performed on the brain, where through careful dissection he revealed its various coverings and distinguished between its ventricles. His anatomical knowledge was put to therapeutic use in surgery and, following Praxagoras, he was particularly interested in pulsation as an indication of illness, devising a portable water-clock by which to time the pulse. But some of his therapies may not have been effective. Among drugs, which he called 'the hands of the gods', the near-poisonous emetic hellebore was a favourite, and later healers disapproved of his practice of copious venesection.

By contrast with Herophilus, on whom the verdict of posterity has been universally favourable, Erasistratus was far more controversial. Even now, it is hard to penetrate behind his opponents' rhetoric to his own ideas, and both sides in later debates manipulated his words and discoveries for their own purposes. Galen was ambivalent about him, to say the least. While he quoted with approval Erasistratus' injunctions to practise anatomy constantly, and dwelt at length upon his remarkable investigations of the anatomy of the heart and brain, he was scathing about other aspects of his medicine. The idea that the arteries contained air alone, blood being drawn into them as if by a vacuum only when they were damaged, seemed to Galen ludicrous, and he repeated an experiment of Erasistratus, who had inserted a cannula into a ligated artery to investigate pulsation, precisely in order to show the unreliability of Erasistratus's conclusion.

This Galenic ambivalence also masks the extent to which Erasistratus departed from theories Galen associated with Hippocrates, especially over the humours and the teleological approach to anatomy. Certainly, Erasistratus, unlike Herophilus, did not comment on Hippocratic opinions, and, although he mentioned humours in some explanations for disease, his formulation apparently excludes the qualitative approach of the Hippocratics as well as any belief in the four cardinal humours. For Erasistratus, purpose did not determine form: the biceps muscle became large through work; it was not created large in order to do that work. In his view, the body was like a machine: the stomach ground and crushed ingested food, and if the stomach still continued grinding after the food had been finely milled, then sensations of hunger resulted. The heart functioned like a pump, with ingress and egress controlled by the valves, which Erasistratus may have been the first to describe accurately, while liver, kidneys, and bladder acted as filters. Growth and nutrition were mechanical processes, in which the principle elements formed a threefold rope of vessels – nerves, veins, and arteries. This image reflects contemporary theories in mechanics and artillery-design, just as Erasistratus's opinions on the movement of blood reflect his contemporary Strato's discovery and exploitation of the vacuum. Even if the tradition that Erasistratus had studied with the great scientist and successor of Aristotle, Theophrastus (c. 370–288/5 BC), is unprovable, in the wide range of his activities, the incisiveness of his speculations, and his passion for experiments (e.g. weighing a bird and its excreta to determine loss through per- and transpiration) Erasistratus would have been an apt pupil.

Medical sects and professionalisation

Of other medical developments within Hellenistic Egypt only the briefest of glimpses are possible. The successors of Herophilus were interested in pharmacology, and Alexandrian surgery enjoyed a reputation that lasted for centuries. In Alexandria, from the time of Herophilus onwards, there developed a medical tradition based on the Hippocratic Corpus. First in the compilation of glossaries and later in the writing of commentaries, of which one on *Joints*, by Apollonius of Citium (about 80 BC), survives today, Alexandrian scholars expounded the dark sayings of the Hippocratics, although their interpretations hardly constituted a unified orthodoxy. One can also discern dimly in the Hellenistic world a process whereby literate medicine, like philosophy, began to fracture into 'sects', groups of healers adhering to particular theories and appealing to earlier authorities. There were Herophileans, Erasistrateans, and Hippocratics, to be joined later by the Pneumatists (who regarded *pneuma* almost as a fifth element, responsible above all for maintaining vitality as well as for causing disease). Knowledge of their doctrines circulated in short catechisms or collections of opinions of earlier healers on medical and philosophical problems.

These sects were all later classified as 'rationalist' or 'dogmatic', not because they alone possessed rationality or uttered dogmas but because they opposed the Empiric (or, better, Empiricist) sect. This group of physicians, who claimed intellectual descent from Acron of Acragas, a Sicilian doctor of the fifth century BC, became significant from 200 BC onwards, and in Heraclides of Tarentum (*fl.* 80 BC in southern Italy) they had a leader of ability, although his writings and ideas survive today only through the reports of others. They rejected a medicine based on reasoning from hidden causes of disease in favour of one based solely on experience: what mattered in disease was not its cause but its cure. To this end they preferred to collect case-histories, accounts of successful remedies, which might be re-applied in similar circumstances. Anatomical knowledge was valuable only where it aided therapy, and was gained through medical experience more effectively than through dissection. Besides, so they argued, the dissection of a corpse, logically, revealed information about the dead, not the living; it dealt in structures, not in the processes of life, health, and disease. Speculation about the workings of drugs was equally idle; all one needed to know was that a particular drug had once worked, and hence that it might be re-employed in a similar case. Reasoning was subordinate to the evidence of past experience, a claim that their later opponents, principally Galen, worked hard to refute, while also acknowledging their therapeutic skills.

This increasing intellectual rigidity of medical theory accompanied an increasing professionalisation of medical practice. 'Workshops' with

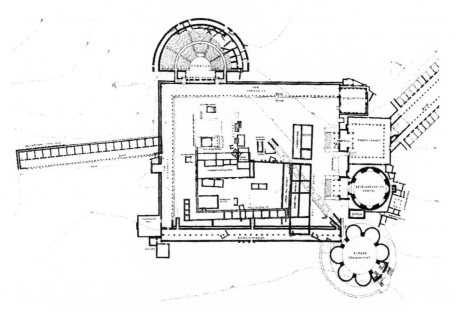

Fig. 6. Plan of the shrine of Asclepius at Pergamum as rebuilt in the time of Galen. The sick, after purification in the spring, and visiting the temple, would retire to the small 'incubation rooms'. The shrine had a library, a theatre, and long porticoes where visitors could walk and talk. It was connected to Pergamum itself by a mile-long colonnaded street. (Based on O. Ziegenhaus, G. De Luca, *Das Asklepieion*, Berlin, 1975.)

20 or more healers, public medical appointments, public medical lectures within a town gymnasium, medical taxes (at least in Hellenistic Egypt), the growth of medical dynasties, and the urbanisation of medicine (exemplified by that most immobile of objects, the Hippocratic orthopaedic bench), all suggest a greater formality, and greater opportunities. An Egyptian apprenticed his son to a 'medical clysterer', confident that he would gain 'an income for life'. In religious healing, the cult of Asclepius, which in the fifth century BC had been a local cult in Thessaly, Epidaurus, Cos, Athens, and a few other centres, had by the third century BC spread all over the Greek world. Patients came to the temples of the god to sleep overnight (incubate) and receive a visitation from Asclepius in a dream. Sometimes immediately, sometimes after the dream had been interpreted by a religious official (who was rarely a medical man), the individual might be cured of paralysis, blindness, suppurations, and the like. The major shrines of Asclepius, in particular Epidaurus and Cos, displayed magnificent temple complexes, and the cures obtained there were celebrated in poetry and recorded on stone

memorials (see further p. 52). Local healing cults, like that of Amphiaraos at Oropus (Greece), also flourished. Yet one may wonder how far this apparent transformation of medicine merely reflects the increasing survival of inscriptions, buildings, and (from Egypt) papyri, and the (equally fortuitous) loss of almost all Greek literature (including medical writings) between the early Alexandrians and the first century of the Christian era.

The problem is neatly exemplified by the 'public physician', a healer appointed by a community. The earliest known is Democedes of Croton (*fl.* 510 BC), who was reportedly hired by both Aegina and Athens before, in what is almost an oriental romance, he endured a hazardous sojourn at the Persian court. A century later, healers were being chosen (for various public purposes) by the assembly of Athens. The inscriptional record of such appointments does not begin till 322/1 BC, and generally refers to special privileges rather than normal activities or obligations. Saving a town from an epidemic, serving for 20 years, or being granted a front seat at a festival and a gold crown was hardly an everyday occurrence. Better evidence for this is provided by the Egyptian papyri, which, from 250 BC onwards, reveal healers as part-time farmers, as well as (in the Roman period) performing such semi-official duties as acting as an expert witness in cases of death or wounding. But it is still an open question how far the activities of public doctors in Egypt (and, mainly, during the Roman Empire) also applied to their predecessors on Hellenistic Cos, let alone in classical Athens.

Yet our inevitable ignorance of details should not hide what is the single greatest development within Greek medicine in the Hellenistic period; its expansion throughout the Mediterranean, and beyond. Even before the conquest of the Greek world by Rome in the second century BC, Greek medicine had been transplanted into Italy to flourish as part of Roman medicine.

2 Roman medicine, 250 BC to AD 200

VIVIAN NUTTON

First contacts with the Greeks

To reconstruct the medical map of Italy around 250 BC is not easy. In the South, along the coast as far north as Naples, were Greek cities whose inhabitants spoke Greek and shared in the intellectual traditions of the Aegean World. At Elea/Velia, Tarentum, and Metapontum, substantial numbers of doctors associated together in institutions that would not have been out of place in Athens or Alexandria. Inland, in the upland regions of central Italy, lived the Marsians, renowned for magic and for medicine, particularly involving the use of snakes. North of Rome, in Etruria, there is evidence for specialist healers, and for medical theories that included both prediction and some emphasis on the liver, but beyond that our ignorance is total.

Later Latin authors, notably Cato (234–149 BC) and Pliny (c. 23–79), believed in a specifically Roman type of healing based on the herbs, chants, prayers, and charms easily available to any head of a household. This practical medicine they contrasted with the worthless theorisings and restrictive specialisms of Greek doctors. Subsequent historians of medicine have repeated this division and these Roman prejudices. But while admittedly the Roman tendency to deify misfortunes such as blight or fever contrasts with a Greek preference for ascribing them to Zeus or Apollo, the split between Roman practicality and Greek intellectualism should not be exaggerated. Indeed, the division is less between Roman and Greek, than between urban and non-urban environments. The medicine of the Greek countryside, when it appears, differs little from that in Cato's *On Agriculture*; and the medico-magical recipes from the villages of Graeco-Roman Egypt are closer to those of Pliny than to the Hippocratic Corpus. For most of the population of the Mediterranean, medicine was necessarily agrarian self-help, based on whatever local remedies were available. Only in the towns, where lived specialist purveyors of healing and drugs, do we find the development of theoretical discussion and intellectualising of the process of cure.

From this perspective, the arrival of Greek medicine in Roman Italy is linked with urbanisation, the mushrooming growth of the city of Rome in the third century BC and the development within northern and central Italy of other urban centres, and with an increasing economic and cultural Hellenisation that, within little more than a century (282–146 BC), drew Rome and its ruling classes into contact with, and domination of, the Greek world. This was a process both public and private. Wealthy Roman senators visited Elea, or brought back from Eastern campaigns Greek intellectuals, including physicians, to the horror of their political enemies like Cato. Both the introduction of the healing god Asclepius to Rome in 291 BC (a cult at Antium (Anzio), south of Rome, existed a generation or so earlier) and the arrival in 219 BC of Archagathus, traditionally the first Greek doctor in Rome, were the result of public decisions. The Roman Senate sent an official embassy to Epidaurus to invite Asclepius to come and cure the epidemic then raging; while in granting Archagathus Roman citizenship and a public surgery at a main crossroad, the government of the city of Rome was acting like the council of any Aegean town to attract a public physician. That Archagathus did not stay – he was subsequently vilified as 'the butcher' – is less significant than the manner of his arrival.

Two other features of Latin accounts of the arrival of Greek medicine call for comment. Firstly, Cato's claim that medicine formed part of the knowledge of every head of a household, and his inclusion of medical material in his book on farming, meant that medicine came in the Latin world to form part of handbooks of the practical arts. From Varro in the first century BC and Celsus and Pliny in the first century AD to Bishop Isidore of Seville in the sixth, non-medical men purvey medical information, theoretical as well as practical, within larger handbooks for the benefit of an interested, educated, and wealthy readership.

Secondly, Cato and Pliny depict Greek medicine as foreign and deeply un-Roman. The social reality was little different. Doctors, *medici*, were generally outsiders, marked off from Roman citizens by their absence of civic rights. Before 212 AD very few doctors in Italy were full citizens by birth. Many were immigrants, some of whom later gained citizenship; even more were slaves or ex-slaves, captured in war or bred and trained as physicians for their owners to hire out. There are no medical dynasties, as on Cos or in some of the towns of Asia Minor, and relatively little involvement of doctors in local civic political or religious activity. In short, the practice of medicine was far from being a high-status occupation.

Asclepiades and the rise of Methodism

After the departure of Archagathus, darkness descends for a century. A few medical jokes in Latin plays and a general Hellenisation of the Roman upper classes provide a poor context for understanding the first notable Roman practitioner, Asclepiades of Prusias-on-Sea in Bithynia (northwest Turkey), who was active in Rome in the early 90s BC. Almost everything about Asclepiades remains controversial – his dates (perhaps dead by 91 BC), his original occupation (allegedly a teacher of rhetoric), and his theories – but this is hardly surprising. He was combative, bombastic, and fond of memorable slogans; a doctor who claims, like him, always to heal 'swiftly, safely, and pleasantly' will not lack enemies. Since none of his actual writings survive, any reconstruction depends on quotations or interpretations by later authors, often in the context of their own polemical arguments. Nevertheless, Asclepiades clearly made an enormous impact on Rome and was credited with an ability to awaken the almost dead. In his therapeutics he rejected drastic measures such as strong drugs in favour of baths, wine, and massage. He approved of gentle exercise (e.g. riding or sitting on a swinging bed), but not everyone agreed with him in starving the patient as a preliminary to other intervention.

His medical theories were equally controversial. He held a mechanistic view of the body that may have been derived from Erasistratus, and although he accepted that health was a sort of balance, he reduced the importance of humours in favour of a corpuscular or atomist theory of the body. Disease usually resulted from changes in the relationship between the corpuscles and the pores of the body, which led either to blockage in the pores or to excessive fluidity. This, he believed, explained both mental conditions, such as *phrenitis* (frenzy), and physical ones, such as *pneumonia* and heart failure. This strongly physicalist linkage of mind and body was not unique to Asclepiades, and even his opponents approved of his attention to the psychological environment of healing.

Although many details of his teaching remain obscure, his success is beyond doubt. He attended many leading senators at Rome and doctors

41

calling themselves Asclepiadeans flourished for at least three centuries. His influence can be traced even further among the so-called Methodist school of medicine, which, established by Thessalus of Tralles (*fl.* AD 60), traced its intellectual origins to his follower Themison of Laodicea (first century BC). Both Themison and Thessalus were Greeks from Asia Minor who practised in Rome among the aristocracy, but their precise contributions to Methodism are hard to define. It may have been Themison who turned the theory of constriction or dilation of the pores or an intermediate state (the so-called 'three common conditions') into a method of explanation for *all* disease. Thessalus went further in his bid to be, as his tombstone put it, 'champion doctor'. He condemned alike the Empiricists' refusal to search for causes and the Hippocratic claim that to establish an aetiology was a complex process, demanding long experience and training. In his view, there were no hidden causes, only the common conditions, easily perceived and understood after a mere six months of instruction in the Method. Dissection he considered of little value, for it revealed nothing about the essential combinations that caused disease (the Empiricists had rejected dissection for providing information only about the dead, not the living), and he favoured instead a simple correlation of visible symptoms with the three causes and their treatment.

Thessalus' method of altering treatment according to changes in the visible phenomena, and his rejection of philosophical reasoning, incurred the wrath of Galen, who poured scorn on the Methodists' preference for fasting on alternate days and on similar over-simplistic therapies. His objections were as much social as intellectual, for in some diseases Methodist treatments differed little from Hippocratic. By 170 AD, the Methodists were Galen's most prominent rivals, in Rome and elsewhere, and emperors employed Methodist doctors alongside a Galen. It suited Galen's own case to ascribe to the founders of Methodism a humble origin, a preference for the uneducated, and a disregard for all that made Hippocratic medical science effective.

Yet even he admitted that some of the later Methodists, notably Soranus of Ephesus (*fl.* 100 AD), had modified Thessalus' tenets for the better, accepting anatomy if only to show off their learning. Methodism had also become intellectually respectable. M. Modius Asiaticus, 'physician, champion of the Method', who lived at Smyrna about 80 AD, was no provincial Dr. Slop, and at least one contemporary of Galen's thought Methodism an appropriate medical theory for a Sceptical

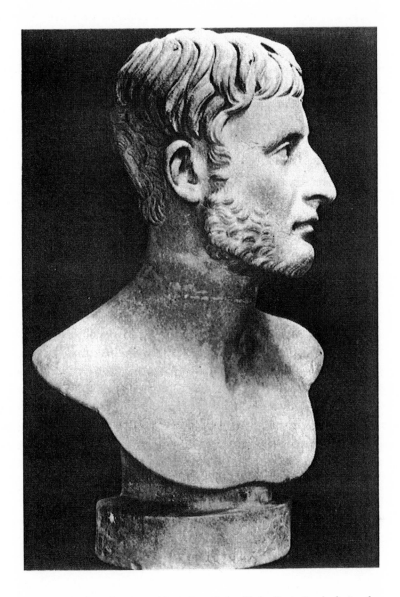

Fig. 7. M. Modius Asiaticus, 'champion of the Method'. A Greek doctor from
Smyrna c. AD 80. (Bibliothèque Nationale, Paris.)

philosopher. Galen's hostile references to disagreements among the
Methodists over the major tenets of their sect indicate development, not
an iron-bound adherence to a fixed body of doctrine.

The Methodists, likewise, could have made the same points about the

43

Hippocratics, whose interpretation of the words of Hippocrates did not always coincide with Galen's. Aretaeus of Cappadocia (*fl.* 140 AD) proclaimed his adherence to Hippocrates by writing his books on acute and chronic diseases in Hippocratic Greek (the Ionic dialect) and by alluding often to the Hippocratic Corpus, but the theories that lie behind his careful descriptions of conditions such as asthma, ileus, diabetes, and stroke would have been rejected by Galen as unfaithful to Hippocrates.

Aretaeus was a 'rationalist' physician, an epithet encompassing a variety of theoreticians and a multitude of theories, with little in common save an opposition to Empiricism (p. 36) and Methodism – whether Asclepiades counted as a rationalist or not seems to have been hotly disputed. Other rationalists included the Pneumatists, members of a sect founded by Athenaeus of Attaleia in the first century AD, who attributed changes in the body principally to changes in its *pneuma* (spirit), a sort of super-element permeating and controlling the whole world, an idea taken over from Stoic and even some Presocratic philosophy. It is not surprising that many Pneumatists, notably Agathinus and Archigenes (both *c.* AD 100), wrote on epilepsy and stroke, afflictions characterised by a sudden loss of control, and were interested in the pulse, which in their view revealed much about the body's *pneuma* in both health and disease. Other 'rationalists' extended the notion of meteorological medicine to include a close fit between the configurations of the heavens and an individual's condition. There were other medical writers more independent or more exotic. One would like to know more about Leonides the Episynthetic ('Super-compiler', *fl.* AD 50) and his contemporary Tiberius Claudius Menecrates, described by his followers as 'doctor to the Emperors, and founder of his own logical perspicuous sect in 156 books, for which he was honoured by notable cities with splendid testimonial decrees'.

The variety of medical practice

This impression of considerable medical diversity in the Roman world is due to two factors. The first is a massive increase in the amount of information available for the first two centuries AD over what had gone before. We not only have the first surviving major Latin surveys of medicine, by Celsus and Pliny, but the Greek medical authors of this period, whether famous like Galen or Soranus or anonymous writers of

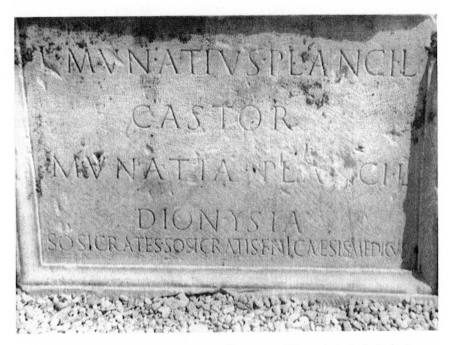

Fig. 8. Tombstone of Dr. Sosicrates, son of Sosicrates of Nicaea (now Iznik, Turkey), who died *c.* AD 20, a Greek immigrant to Rome. His name is squeezed onto the base of the tomb of two freed slaves of the Munatius family. (Photo: V. Nutton.)

catechisms, frequently took issue in detail with their opponents. Ubiquitous records of doctors (male and female) on tombstones, public inscriptions, and Egyptian papyri supplement the evidence provided by writers of history, *belles-lettres*, and other literature to offer a broad view of medical life that is not available again for a thousand years.

This abundant diversity of medicine has also a social or legal explanation; there were no effective means of controlling either the content or the personnel of medicine. Although certain centres, most notably Alexandria, enjoyed a reputation for medicine and attracted students from far afield, there were no medical degrees or officially recognised qualifications. While the authorities, both civic and imperial, were sometimes interested in defining who was or was not a doctor (eye- or ear-specialists were; exorcists were not, however effective), this was in the context of civic obligations and taxation, not medical care. From *c.* 40 BC (and earlier in the Hellenistic world) doctors throughout the Empire were legally excused from having soldiers billeted on them and from paying certain taxes. Subsequent rulers confirmed these and similar privileges. Around AD 150, the emperor Antoninus Pius restricted the

number of doctors eligible for tax-immunity to five, seven, or 10 depending on the size and status of their communities, but other rights continued in Rome and elsewhere. Significantly, the decision over who
qualified for these tax-concessions was made by non-professionals, town
councillors or a governor, and not fellow doctors. While this offered
some form of control, it is doubtful if it guaranteed competence. In Egypt
in AD 142–3, the governor allowed a doctor to claim certain immunities
simply on his own attestation that he was a doctor, even though his
patients apparently distrusted his capabilities. Even where there were
'officially approved' doctors, the administration was less interested in
securing treatment for its citizens than in having access to medical
advice for its own purposes, notably in certifying violent death or injury.

There was thus little official involvement in the control of medical
knowledge or medical personnel – tales abound of cobblers and gladiators becoming doctors overnight – and methods of medical instruction
encouraged a similar fluidity. The quasi-religious *pholeon* continued at
Elea (above, p. 17) with doctors at its head into the Imperial period, and
the Hippocratic *Oath*, with its affirmation of a close-knit family of medical student and teacher, was copied and read. But there are also public
anatomical displays, and lectures on medicine held in a town gymnasium. Some students attached themselves as pupils to individual teachers, sometimes formally with an apprenticeship contract, sometimes
informally accompanying a doctor on his rounds as a friend. What was
available varied from place to place: to a young boy in a small fishing
village in southern Greece, to travel the 50 or so miles to Sparta to learn
medicine seemed wonderful, yet that town hardly features in our historical record of physicians. By contrast, Galen was taught at Pergamum
and Smyrna by teachers who had themselves studied overseas, at
Alexandria, 'the foundation of health for all men' and the one place
where, around AD 100, one could learn skeletal anatomy.

Instruction was inevitably largely oral. Although some teachers
allowed their lectures to be transcribed and put into circulation, and
although Galen implies the existence in his day of a substantial amount
of medical literature, others refused or confined their words to a small
number of favoured students. Even among the audience, there might be
considerable doubt as to what had been said, and, still more, over what
it meant. Galen wrote at least three tracts specifically to resolve arguments over the authenticity and purport of his own writings, and his
examples of others' interpretations of Hippocrates run from forgery and

ignorance, through copyists' errors, to hypersophistication and unintelligibility. Under such circumstances accurate information was not always easy to find, and there were sometimes substantial disagreements on fundamentals even within the same sect.

The availability of medical assistance

This fluidity of doctrine is mirrored in the variety of medical assistance available, and in the statuses enjoyed by healers within the Roman Empire. Some, particularly in Italy, were slaves or ex-slaves, others, especially in Asia Minor, came from dynasties of doctors, related by birth or marriage to provincial magnates. T. Claudius Demostratus Caelianus held a series of civic offices at Ephesus that culminated in AD 153 with the High Priesthood of the province of Asia. The son of Lucius Gellius Maximus, an imperial doctor from Pisidian Antioch (modern Central Turkey), even dared to raise a military revolt in AD 219 against the emperor Elagabalus, a social as well as a political *faux pas* in the eyes of a senator-historian. True, doctors to the wealthy, at court or in a city like Ephesus, were themselves likely to become wealthy; and apparently successful doctors, whoever their patients, would be better regarded than the less successful. But beyond these banalities, it is hard to generalise about the status of doctors, other than to place them alongside teachers and engineers (who often joined the same intellectual clubs) – below lawyers but above cobblers.

Likewise, only the most basic answer can be given to the question of what patients thought of their doctors; that depended entirely on the success of the treatment. Nor can one talk meaningfully about a medical profession. Scribonius Largus, writing in about AD 48, regarded a doctor's 'medical *professio*' as determining his whole ethical approach to healing (e.g. he would not use magic or kill an enemy of the state by his drugs) but his phrase refers to a *declaration* that one was a doctor, not to any external professional association. His discussion drew on philosophical theories about 'duties', some Hippocratic ideas (p. 29), and his own experience of military 'discipline' (in the invasion of Britain in AD 43). There is no evidence that others accepted his conclusions, or thought of healers as constituting a unitary profession, even though *medici* or *iatroi* might come together for banquets, religious festivals, and, occasionally, medical competitions. At Ephesus, the winners' names were inscribed for permanent (and possibly public) record.

But how and from whom was help obtained in the event of illness ? Self-help or assistance from within the extended family was the most common response. Although some medical writers advocated their own specialist terminology, neither the ideas nor the language of learned medicine formed a barrier to wider understanding. In his *On Medicine*, Celsus wrote for a wealthy readership that was equally interested in agriculture and military affairs. Although he had used some of the therapies he described on his family and on his estate slaves, he was no *medicus*, at least in the sense that he did not treat others for gain. His contemporary, the philosopher Seneca (4 BC to AD 65), displayed a sophisticated understanding of medicine, while another contemporary, Athenaeus of Attaleia, recommended to the layman a knowledge of medicine (and medical history) for intellectual stimulation as well as practical benefit. In the next century, it was considered a social blunder for an educated man to mix up his veins and his arteries, while Galen's advice on how to choose a doctor implies that the patient had absorbed as much medical information as the potential therapist.

In large cities, according to Galen, there were many healers (not all of them reputable) and the substantial numbers of potential patients allowed specialism to flourish. In the smaller towns doctors would be fewer, although, he claims, less likely to act dishonestly or incompetently because of the pressures of life in a face-to-face society. Egyptian papyri show doctors farming their own plots of land just like other villagers, a pattern of dual or multiple activity unlikely to have been confined to Egypt. A list of the providers of medical recipes gives a cross-section of society; boxing trainers, grooms, schoolteachers, wise-women, members of the gentry (both male and female), as well as doctors like Lucius the Professor, who taught pharmacology at Tarsus (southeast Turkey), a city where such teaching can be documented for a century, from *c.* 30 BC to AD 70. In the backwoods, one might encounter a doctor on a journey (like St. Luke) or a medical 'crowd-puller' at a fair, like L. Sabinus Primigenius of Gubbio (central Italy), an ex-slave doctor who 'travelled around many markets'. In Gaul, where towns were more scattered, the archaeological survival of 'oculists' stamps' (stone stamps used to impress the names of doctors and diseases onto sticks of ointment for use in eye diseases) may indicate that these practitioners made definite circuits from a base in larger towns. (Some doctors in late Antiquity were also called 'circuit-makers'.)

A similar variety can be found among female healers. Soranus' ideal midwife was a paragon of learning and experience, whose soft hands and long fingers complemented her nimble wit and hard work. Galen approved of the testimony of experienced midwives and nurses, and reported without apparent distinction the remedies of both female and male healers. At the other extreme, the local barmaid might also act as the local midwife, and a 'little African woman' in Rome sold Scribonius Largus a remedy for stomach colic. Women were not necessarily confined to treating women's diseases (male midwives were far rarer), nor did their training, often under a male partner or patron, differ from that of males. Antiochis of Tlos was honoured *c.* AD 50 with a public statue by her fellow citizens for her medical expertise; one of her recipes is preserved for us by Galen. The writings of a certain Metrodora (1st century?) also circulated widely, while much medical information was reported in the celebrated cosmetic treatise ascribed to Cleopatra (ruler of Egypt 51–30 BC), although her authorship is as unlikely as the later tradition that she taught Galen pharmacology.

Two social groups received special medical attention, slaves and the army. By the late first century BC slaves were becoming more expensive; breeding was replacing conquest as the main source of supply, so it was in the interests of owners to provide better care and facilities. In the larger slave-households, especially those of the imperial family, there were slave physicians who cared for their fellow slaves in special units, *valetudinaria* ('hospitals'). The degree of attention available there did not satisfy Celsus, who had a slave-hospital on his own estate, for it did not allow for individualised treatment, but attention was given.

Even better arrangements pertained in the Roman army. During the Roman civil wars of the first century BC, the legions had, like previous armies in Greece, been looked after by volunteers or conscript doctors. The wounded were treated in tents on the battlefield, or left behind in a friendly or a captured town. The campaigns under Augustus (reigned 31 BC to AD 14) brought the Roman armies across the Alps to the Rhine and Danube, into regions where towns were few. Besides, no longer were the legions casual visitors. Deep in unfriendly territory, there was a need for permanent protection, forts or fortresses, which might serve also as refuges for the sick. Archaeologists have uncovered specific buildings set aside for the reception and treatment of the sick (*valetudinaria*), staffed by medici and their assistants. The earliest dates from *c.* AD 9, and by AD 50, a definite plan of considerable sophistication had evolved, with individual small rooms arranged round a long

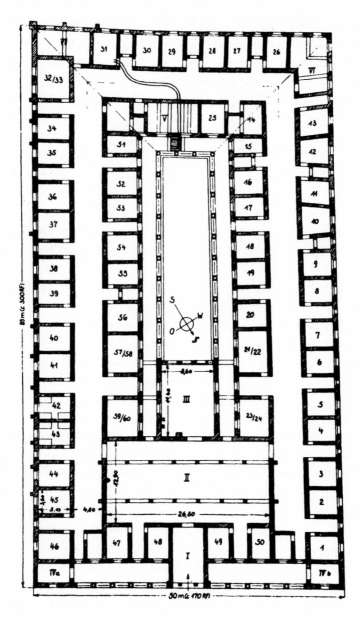

Fig. 9. Plan of the hospital at the legionary fortress of Novaesium (Neuss, Germany). Built in stone *c.* AD 50, it served the 5600 citizen soldiers of the sixteenth legion. The sick were brought into one of the large halls, which may have also been an operating room and dispensary, and slept in small cubicles off a corridor, which reduced draughts and gave added quiet. (The Wellcome Institute Library, London.)

rectangular corridor, and a large hall (for reception or operations) illuminated from above. There was also a good water supply, befitting an army that paid close attention to sewers and latrines. Particularly good examples have been excavated at Xanten and Neuss (Fig. 9) in Germany and at Inchtuthil in Scotland. Smaller forts housing non-citizen troops (e.g. Housesteads in England, and Fendoch in Scotland) had similar hospitals, but on a reduced scale.

Three points need emphasis. Firstly, military hospitals are known mainly from the less urbanised Western half of the Empire and the Danube frontier before the mid third century. When military strategy began to change *c.* AD 250 to a system based on local levies backed by a mobile field army, large hospitals within permanent fortresses were no longer required. Sick and wounded, when not left behind, were treated in field hospitals or accompanied the rest of the army in wagons. Secondly, the capacity of the hospitals varied. When the military situation was still fluid, a camp hospital, like that at Hod Hill in England, occupied from AD 44 to 51, might have beds for 12–20% of the force. When stability seemed assured, as at Inchtuthil, a legionary fortress, the maximum occupancy may have been as low as 2.5%. Thirdly, the legionary hospitals (in Britain at Caerleon, Chester, York, and, more briefly, Gloucester and Inchtuthil) were many miles behind the frontier and even more from any actual fighting. They served only the legionaries, in peace and in war, by providing somewhere for the sick to go for better food and treatment in areas where towns were sparse. Sickness was not a prerogative of fighting. At Vindolanda (a fort near Hadrian's Wall, northern England) a recently discovered roster shows that on 18 May, AD 90 (?), out of 752 men in the unit, 15 were ill, six were injured, and another 10 were suffering from eye problems.

Both the Roman army and navy had a medical service, although precise details are not always available. We hear of doctors serving on a particular ship, in a legion or a cohort, and of 'camp doctors', as well as bandagers and 'pupils'. One might posit a progression from pupil, through bandager, to doctor, a position recognised by lawyers as a valid preparation for civilian life. Some doctors, like the famous writer on pharmacology Pedanius Dioscorides (*c.* AD 60), apparently joined on short-service commissions, for a campaign or to establish good contacts with a wealthy commander. There were also non-medical hospital administrators, army veterinarians, and other assistants concerned with the welfare of the troops and their animals and with the provision of supplies, including such remedies as hoarhound and dock.

Roman hospitals were restricted to slaves and soldiers. Civilians might stay in a doctor's house or his surgery, but provision for the poor was almost non-existent. Their only recourse might be to divine aid, by sacrificing to a healing statue or visiting a healing shrine (see p. 37). Such shrines were common throughout the Empire, dedicated both to local gods (e.g. Sul Minerva at Bath or the Deae Matronae in the Rhineland) and to universal divinities (e.g. Hercules, Sarapis, and, above all, Asclepius). Galen believed that the number and activity of the shrines of Asclepius had increased massively between AD 100 and 150, an impression confirmed by the evidence of coins and archaeology. The big Asclepieion at his home town of Pergamum was rebuilt at this period, and its remains are still impressive today (see Fig. 6). Whether this burgeoning of healing shrines is to be taken as an index of medical failure, religious sentiment, or economic prosperity remains an open question.

The shrines' clientele might range from a poor peasant to a Roman governor, and the god might be asked to relieve a plague, advise an emperor, or confirm that Herminus of Hermopolis was a good eye-doctor. Some suppliants came because they believed their suffering was some form of divine punishment; others, like the orator Aristides (c. AD 117–180), a long-term resident at Pergamum, because they believed they had a special relationship with the god; others because human healers had failed or refused to treat (an attitude widely commended among doctors, and easily compatible with a belief in the power of divine healing). Sometimes the god's advice agreed perfectly with the therapies of a secular healer; at others, it shocked the patient (and any medical acquaintances) by its apparent disregard of medical proprieties. But the records of cures that survive from shrines in Asia Minor, Rome, Crete, and elsewhere, or are validated by Galen, himself a patient of Asclepius, show that many sufferers found health and healing from heaven, and considered divine aid a necessary and welcome supplement to that of human hands.

Diseases and therapies

The diseases of the Roman world are almost identical with those of the Greek (pp. 12–15). Fevers, eye diseases and nutritional disorders predominate in the medical literature, and authors of the second century AD have no qualms about citing descriptions and remedies of the fourth century BC. There were apparently new diseases (e.g. *lichen*, a facial skin disorder), ascribed by some to the consequences of a novel and increasingly luxurious lifestyle. There were also localised diseases – one such epidemic raged in Asia Minor in the AD 170s – but the eastern Mediterranean bias of the surviving literary sources means that we know little of diseases north of the Alps or west of Italy. Likewise, few northern therapies entered the Mediterranean medical handbooks – Alpine yoghurt (*melka*) and the British dock are rare exceptions – in sharp contrast to drugs from the East.

This epidemiological pattern of predominantly local and individual disease was seriously disturbed only once, in the mid-160s, when a plague, almost certainly smallpox, was brought back from modern Iraq by a retreating Roman army, and proceeded to ravage the whole of the Empire. There followed a series of more localised outbreaks. Estimates of mortality vary – some Egyptian villages show a substantial population decline (over 20%) between AD 162 and 180 – but undoubtedly this was the most lethal invasion of disease in Antiquity.

Explanations of disease remained the same. The Hippocratics emphasised individual susceptibility and bad air (*miasma*), and drew attention to diet as both cause and therapy. Galen, an experienced traveller, noted the poor quality of foodstuffs in various regions, and not only in times of plague and famine, when peasants, at the mercy of the army and the big landlords from the city, were reduced to eating shrubs and grasses. In a big city such as Rome, food, although generally kept carefully in surplus by the government, was not always of the best; the scrawny fish from the polluted Tiber contrasted with the plump trout from its upper reaches. In the countryside, although shortage was common, famine was rare, precipitated by a series of bad harvests, wars, or plagues. In the middle-sized towns, the willingness of local magnates (and the occasional emperor) to subsidise special deliveries of corn may have reduced the worst effects of shortage.

Drastic famines and plagues were often ascribed to the gods, and a full panoply of religious rituals might be employed to mitigate divine wrath. During the Antonine plague, local and imperial authorities made public processions, formally consulted various gods and oracles, and sacrificed to city-protecting deities. Doctors reflected on the randomness of epidemic disease (or of sun-stroke) and concluded that possibly some seed of disease had been implanted in particular individuals. Lay authors (and veterinarians) also talked a good deal about contagion (particularly of plague and, metaphorically, religious dissent) and the need to separate affected persons or animals. Galen and other writers in the Hippocratic tradition, on the other hand, say nothing at all about contagion. This omission can hardly have been accidental, and reflects their preference for explanations and treatments that concentrated on individual susceptibility to potentially harmful environmental changes. Besides, slaughtering animals with contagious diseases was not a remedy easily transferable to human plague; it was, as one author put it, against the humanity of medicine.

There is also continuity between Greek and Roman therapies, both in the range of treatments available and in the preference for diet and nursing rather than drugs, and for drugs rather than surgical intervention. The last was highly dangerous to the patient, and to the doctor's reputation if things went badly, although the law punished only criminal intent, not professional incompetence. Dietetics altered little over the centuries, although there were fads and fashions. Antonius Musa's 'cold-water treatment' saved the life of the Emperor Augustus in 23 BC, but fell into disfavour when, the next year, it failed to cure his heir Marcellus. Seventy years later, Charmis of Marseilles had a brilliant success with a similar therapy, and, in Late Antiquity, Jacobus Psychrestus (c. AD 460) gained fame, fortune, and political influence by a similar refreshing technique. Charmis' douche supplanted in Roman favour the astrological medicine of a fellow-townsman, Crinas, which in its turn had ousted briefly the new Methodism of Thessalus (p. 42). Crinas's massive fortune, partly spent on rebuilding the walls of Marseilles, was gained from his ability to regulate the diets of his patients by the motions of the stars as predicted in astronomical almanacs. He was not alone in his liking for astrological medicine. It was associated in particular with Egyptian healers, one of whom had his own horoscope carved on his tombstone, and medical horoscopes feature prominently among the so-called magical papyri. Surviving tracts on astrological medicine are ascribed to Thessalus the astrologer, often identified with the Methodist of that name, and to Galen. But Galen rejected astrological number medicine scathingly, just as he rejected medical divination from the flight of birds or the magical mumbo-jumbo of Pamphilus and Xenocrates of Aphrodisias (both fl. AD 50).

Not everyone shared Galen's scorn. Pliny protested about the magical remedies of Pamphilus and the Persian magus Ostanes, but he still reported them effective. Traces of Xenocrates and Pamphilus can be found within even the Galenic tradition, while the medico-medical *Stone-Book* of another Xenocrates (from Ephesus, *fl.* AD 80) survived long enough to be translated into Arabic. A remedy for epilepsy involving the blood of a dead gladiator, warrior, or street-brawler, although disdained by Scribonius Largus, Celsus, and Galen, nevertheless was singled out as an 'excellent and well proven remedy of Marsinus the Thracian' by Alexander of Tralles, writing around 570.

This citation, appearing long after gladiatorial shows had ended, exemplifies two things: the literary survival of drug recipes, often divorced from their original setting, and the fluidity of the boundary between magic and medicine both over time and among contemporaries. Galen, for example, accepted the phenomena of astrology and bird-divination, but explained them differently: the flight of birds revealed, and the movements of the heavens imposed, changes in the weather that altered individual humoral patterns, and hence caused disease. On another occasion, Galen refused to believe in an Egyptian remedy for a weak stomach, a green jasper stone carved in the likeness of King Nechepso (a fabulous Pharaoh) placed over the pylorus; it worked just as well uncarved. Similarly both he and Celsus rationalised the use of amulets to explain their efficacy, and cast doubt on chants and charms. Archaeological and papyrus finds confirm that not everyone shared their scruples, and later learned writers like Marcellus of Bordeaux (*fl.* AD 380) and Alexander of Tralles willingly included such remedies alongside those of Galen. To take Celsus or Galen as typical of attitudes towards magical healing is unwise.

If dietetics and magical healing changed little throughout the Roman period, important developments can be seen in drug therapy. True, not every *medicus* favoured such treatments, and those who did might contest their use in a particular case, an open invitation, said Scribonius Largus, to ignorant druggists to rush in and gain credit simply for activity. The number and choice of drugs coming to the big cities, especially Alexandria and Rome, increased substantially between 100 BC and AD 100, with a consequent increase in complexity of preparation. Theriac, a confection originally given as an antidote to snakebite and occasionally later as a general tonic, gained ever more ingredients. In the version ascribed to Mithridates VI (King of Pontus 120–63 BC), it

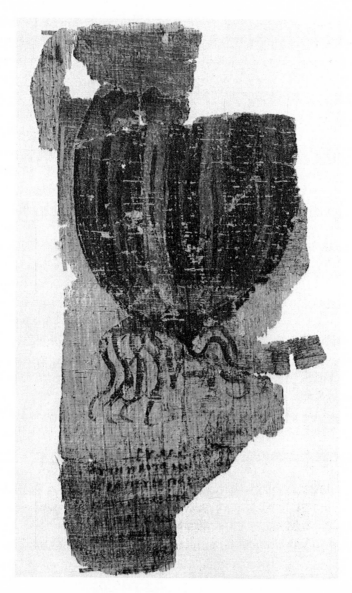

Fig. 10. A page from an illuminated herbal papyrus, written in Egypt *c.* AD 400.
This side shows comfrey, *symphytum officinale;* the reverse *phlommos,* perhaps
mullein. Johnson Papyrus. (The Wellcome Institute Library, London, WMS 5753.)

had 41 ingredients, increased to 48 by Servilius Damocrates (*c.* AD 50),
and to 64 by Andromachus (*c.* AD 68). Galen's own preferred preparation had 77 ingredients, and there were others still more complex.

How theriac and similar preparations were thought to work can be
dimly glimpsed from the remnants of academic writings on pharmacy.

Most authors assumed that drugs produced qualitative changes within the body, e.g. by heating or cooling. Within these broad categories, the choice depended more on accessibility and the patient's preferences (a plutocrat would despise a cheap drug, however effective) than on more theoretical concerns. Pedanius Dioscorides of Anazarbus (southeast Turkey), writing around AD 60, arranged his major study of materia medica according to drug properties, but the later reorganisation of his work into alphabetical order and the survival of several A-to-Z drug books suggest that memorability took precedence over complicated theory. Galen incorporated large sections of the works of Dioscorides and others, organising them according to the disease site and, in another tract, the type of remedy employed. Typically, he ventured his own hypothetical scheme, a classification of drugs into 12 grades or degrees of drug action, but, equally typically, he neither finished his listings (only 161 out of 475 botanical simples were given grades; Arabic pharmacologists added more; see p. 118) nor succeeded in correlating them with an explanation of illness in terms of intensity of disease. Relatively little attention was paid to dosage, a reflection of the many different weights and measures around the Mediterranean, and of a general preference for qualitative over quantitative explanations in a technologically primitive society.

Surgery, by contrast, appears remarkably modern. The basic principles of orthopaedics were well known, and artificial limbs and teeth have been discovered in archaeological excavations. In operations, tourniquets and special hooks would have reduced bloodflow, sutures would have often held, swabbing with wine would have lessened the chances of sepsis, and opiates might have reduced pain a little. Increasingly specialised and well-made surgical instruments ranged from vaginal specula to needles, hooks, and arrow-extractors, some made to order, others by the operator himself. Operations might be complex: Galen successfully sewed back an omentum into the abdominal cavity, and extracted surgically a suppurating breastbone from the slave of a comic playwright. An anonymous contemporary described surgical treatments for breast cancer, piles, varicose veins, and hydrocele that compare favourably with similar operations in the 1970s, while his recommended procedure for bladder stone would have worked swiftly and, if sepsis was avoided, effectively. The cataract operation described in Roman texts and reconstructed from surviving instruments would also have restored some degree of sight. Even the list of eye operations that Galen expected the average practitioner to perform (and which was less than what he himself had done or hoped from the expert) is impressive testimony to the manual dexterity of his contemporaries. But in this hymn to the knife, one should not forget the bunglers – the man who accidentally sliced through an artery, or who produced paralysis because he did not know where a major nerve ran – or the pitiful tombstones of wives, husbands, gladiators, and slaves, killed by those who had attempted to cure them. No wonder that a man might curse a doctor for killing his brother, or turn to the ministrations of a god after 36 human healers had failed. It is important, too, to note that even Galen emphasised that the best surgeon was the man who treated surgically only as a last resort: the expert knew how to correct surgical conditions by drugs and caustics, as well as by fire and the knife.

Galen of Pergamum

INTRODUCTION

The central figure in the development of the Western tradition of medicine is arguably Galen of Pergamum (129 to *c.* 216). His centrality lies not only in the fact that subsequent generations accepted his opinions as correct, gradually squeezing out alternatives and preserving the writings of others, for the most part, only when they passed under his name (like the *Introduction to Medicine*, the source of the examples of surgery on p. 57) or filled in perceived gaps (e.g. Soranus' *Gynaecology*). Equally important is the fact that much of our information on early medicine depends on Galen's interpretation and sifting of the evidence. His view of the historical Hippocrates (p. 22) was scarcely questioned until the twentieth century, even though some ancient followers of Hippocrates held very different opinions of what their teacher had written. Modern scholarship on Erasistratus and Asclepiades has had first to pierce the fog of Galenic prejudice. Yet without his information any reconstruction would be immensely the poorer.

There are other, more subtle ways in which Galen's influence lives on. His willingness to talk about himself, his prolixity, and the relative paucity of other medical sources, mean that it is only too easy to accept his rhetoric and see him as the typical physician of Antiquity. His opponents or his reluctant allies are thus beneath contempt, 'snotty-nosed individuals' as he called them, charlatans, quacks, and medical murder-

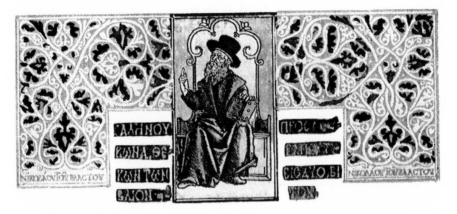

Fig. 11. Galen of Pergamum, 129 to *c.* 200/216, depicted as a learned physician on a heading to his *Method of Healing*, Venice, 1500, the first printing of a genuine work of Galen in its original Greek. (The Wellcome Institute Library, London, W. 2525.)

ers. But Galen was unlike most medical practitioners, not least in his family wealth, his education, and his practice with the court in Rome. Not all agreed with him that the good doctor was (or should be) a philosopher, however much later generations endeavoured to translate this educational ideal into reality (p. 157). In the spectrum of medical activity in Antiquity, Galen stands at one end, not in the middle as he wants his readers to believe.

Galen's friends are treated even worse than his enemies. Much of his pharmacology was taken over, unacknowledged and in large sections almost verbatim, from previous authors such as Statilius Crito (*fl.* AD 100, an imperial doctor who also wrote a memoir on Rome's wars with the Getae (in modern Romania). One may suspect that many of Galen's reports of the opinions of Hellenistic physicians were taken from more recent summaries, not the originals. How much, if anything, he copied from Soranus of Ephesus, the one Methodist of whom he has anything good to say, is unclear, but some of Soranus' views on the therapy of acute and chronic diseases are not incompatible with Galen's.

The author who suffers most from this suffocating friendship is Rufus of Ephesus, a Hippocratic physician of the late first century. The few works of Rufus that survive in Greek include treatises on gonorrhoea, anatomical nomenclature, and kidney disease, as well as an essay on bedside medicine, *Medical Questions*. But much more was translated into Arabic, and scholars have rediscovered from this source his *On Jaundice*, as well as much of his *On Melancholy*, some case histories, and sections from a large book on medicine for the layman. His interpretations of Hippocrates and his sympathetic approach to the problems of such generally despised groups as homosexuals and slaves confirm Galen's praise of him as scholar and physician. But Galen's own increasing authority meant that Rufus' relatively similar ideas and therapies were gradually extruded from the Greek tradition.

GALEN'S LIFE AND WRITINGS

The creeping tyranny of Galen was partly the result of Galen's own prolixity. The latest bibliography lists 434 titles of works, over 350 of which are authentic. They range in length from 30 to 500 pages, on average two or three pages written (or dictated) a day over some 50 working years. The standard edition of his writings contains 133 tracts in Greek (some spurious) in roughly 8000 quarto pages, to which later discoveries have added another hundred pages in Greek. These new finds, although impressive, are dwarfed by the vast amount of material translated into a variety of (mainly Oriental) languages in the Middle Ages and now becoming accessible again. They include, for example, fragments of the genuine text of *On Remedies Easily Prepared* (Syriac), the later books of *Anatomical Procedures* (Arabic), the commentary on Hippocrates' *Airs, Waters, and Places* (Hebrew summary; the complete Arabic version is in preparation); *On Cohesive Causes* (Latin and Arabic); and *On the Eye* (fragments reported in Armenian). In short, more words survive of Galen than of any other writer from Antiquity.

It is not just the sheer amount that impresses. Galen ranged widely, from studies of the vocabulary of comic poets of classical Athens to discussions of the soul, from advice to an epileptic boy to accounts of anatomical dissection, from arguments on the body's elements, faculties, and humours, to compilations of drug lore, and from polemics on bloodletting to a tract on slander (subtitled *On My Own Life*). Galen did not keep his interests in neat compartments. His linguistic studies illuminated his Hippocratic commentaries; his views on logic pervaded his clinical practice; his anatomical findings confirmed the truths of philosophy (and vice-versa); and even his surviving autobiographical and bibliographical treatises can be considered contributions to therapeutics. It is precisely this interlocking of authorial fluency, philosophical and logical argument, technical expertise, practical experience, and, not least, book-learning that made his arguments increasingly difficult to refute, once the social and intellectual conditions for their repetition had passed. Later ages lamented that one could no longer obtain such a mastery of the whole of medical knowledge.

Galen was indeed fortunate. He was born in AD 129, the son of a wealthy architect and farmer, Nicon of Pergamum (now Bergama, Turkey), culturally and economically one of the richest cities in the Greek-speaking half of the Roman Empire, and then at the height of its prosperity. Galen enjoyed a typically upper-class education, studying grammar, rhetoric, and various competing theories of philosophy. He was saved from confusion, he said, only by his discovery of the certainties of (Platonic) geometry. He may well have been intended for a career as a fashionable public speaker and intellectual, but, when he was sixteen, his father was visited in a dream by Asclepius, after which Galen turned to medicine.

From his medical teachers, first at Pergamum and then at Smyrna, he learned of the Alexandrian (and Hippocratic) tradition of medicine. It is thus not surprising that, like other rich young men from his region, he should have decided to study with Alexandrian teachers. Numisianus, whom he had sought in vain at Corinth, had died before Galen reached Alexandria, but his family and pupils preserved some of his teaching. There were other reasons for going. Alexandria was *the* centre for medicine. Even if Galen subsequently derided its teachers as worse than useless, its food and drink as loathsome, and its inhabitants as stupid, he remained there for four or five years. He travelled widely in Egypt, learning about the drugs imported from India, Africa and elsewhere from the shippers who brought them. One is tempted to believe that his father's death in AD 149/150 also kept him away from Pergamum, for their relationship had been unusually intense (Nicon had sat with him on the school bench) and contrasted with the often violently irrational behaviour of Galen's mother.

Not until AD 157 did Galen return home, to be swiftly appointed doctor to the gladiators owned by the High Priest. Although he wrote his first surviving medical treatise, *On Medical Experience*, in Smyrna, c. AD 149, he did not practise extensively until he was 28. His medical education is the longest on record, and was begun at an age (16) when others were already calling themselves doctors. He readily admitted his own passion for book-learning, justifying his wealth by explaining that it enabled him to have books copied and to avoid charging fees (although 'presents' were certainly acceptable). As a member of Pergamum's elite, he would have been known to the High Priest even

61

before he returned with the cachet of an Alexandrian medical and surgical education. He claimed an almost total success in his gladiatorial post - two deaths under five High Priests compared with his predecessor's 60, none the result of wounds received in the arena.

But for a man as ambitious (and obnoxious) as Galen, Pergamum was not big enough. In 162 he left for Rome – there are hints of some civic disturbance at Pergamum in which Galen was on the wrong side. In Rome he quickly found himself among friends and fellow Pergamenes, and with a reputation for philosophy as well as medicine. His medical fame also spread following a series of public anatomical displays, later held in private allegedly because of the animosity they aroused among his competitors. His cure of his old philosophy teacher Eudemus in the winter of AD 162–163 was crucial in establishing him as a fashionable healer. Leading men of Rome, intellectuals, the city prefect, and even imperial relatives demanded his attentions, attended his lectures and anatomical displays, or asked him for treatises. He engaged in public debate with Erasistrateans and Methodists, and expounded the truths of anatomy in ways that were acceptable to Platonists and Aristotelians.

His sudden departure from Rome in AD 166 'like a runaway slave' took friend and foe by surprise. Writing 11 years later, he blamed it on the animosity of his rivals, and the ending of a civil commotion at home. Thirty years later, he offered another explanation: he wished to avoid the onset of 'plague' (perhaps a smallpox epidemic), which may well be true (and discreditable), even allowing for the fact that it was still raging in Asia Minor on his return there. In AD 168 he was summoned to attend the emperors Marcus Aurelius and Lucius Verus in a military camp in northern Italy. The sudden death of Verus brought the postponement of the campaign, and in AD 169 Galen returned with the rest of the army to Rome.

From then on, Galen was in imperial service, first with the emperor's son Commodus on his tours of Italy – Asclepius had fortunately intervened to prevent Marcus Aurelius taking Galen on the campaign against the Danubian invaders – and from AD 178 onwards with successive emperors. He made at least one visit (alas undatable) to Pergamum, but after AD 169 specific incidents can rarely be fixed with precision. He was in Rome during the failed conspiracy of Perennis (185), perhaps the occasion when he was consulted by senators worried that the emperor Commodus was going to murder them (Galen recommended tact and caution). His (lost) *Public Pronouncements During the Reign of Pertinax* suggests he was in Rome during the civil wars of AD 192–193. He certainly attended the emperor Severus (reigned AD 193–211), and was alive at least in AD 198. A Greek dictionary of the tenth century has him dying aged 70, i.e. *c.* 200, but the Oriental tradition, which may well go back to a remark of a contemporary opponent Alexander of Aphrodisias, places his death much later, aged 87, perhaps in AD 216. If the tract *On Theriac, for Piso*, is authentic, and counter-arguments are weak, he was still alive in AD 204, for it mentions the Secular Games of that year.

Galen's accounts of his own career are masterpieces of special pleading. His cases are held up as exemplary, and described with all the skill of a practised orator. Literary allusions, careful organisation, and choice vocabulary all contribute to an artful self-presentation. His fellow-doctors to the imperial family are largely dismissed in silence, or characterised as incompetent fools. In his dealings with patients, Galen is inevitably right. If he is not, then unforeseen circumstances are to blame, or his advice has been deliberately disregarded. Wealthy patients, in particular, did not always treat Galen with the respect he thought he deserved – and paid the penalty. His medical life was shared with competitors, but with few colleagues. Those who attended his dissections were wealthy intellectuals, and, although he dispensed advice, and even instruments and cash, to colleagues, actual pupils are hard to discern, although he claims to have helped many to get on in society and never charged for instruction. One man who alleged that he had learned a dubious remedy for toothache from Galen was promptly arrested and flogged. Save for practical remedies, for which he did not hesitate to consult imperial root-cutters and even peasants, Galen avowedly learned nothing from formal teachers once he had left Smyrna. His self-image is of the independent, self-taught expert.

GALEN'S ACHIEVEMENT

To conclude, as some have done, that Galen's self-praise prevents us from knowing anything of his achievements is over-exaggerated. Galen was a success; he did become an imperial doctor; and his works allow us to see his strengths and his weaknesses. Bombast, prolixity, ambition, deceit, and self-delusion are all there, but they are only part of the story.

Even allowing for exaggeration and silent plagiarism, Galen was a learned man in an age that prided itself on learning. Alexander of

Aphrodisias, avowedly no friend, listed him alongside Plato and Aristotle as an example of 'high reputation', and his productivity was warmly appreciated by another contemporary, Athenaeus of Naucratis. To compare Galen's learning with that of respectable contemporary intellectuals like Aulus Gellius, author of the *Attic Nights*, and Aelian, who surveyed natural history in his *Variegated Enquiry*, is to pass from profundity to trivial pursuit.

Galen was also a philosopher of considerable independence and merit. His arguments for teleology, for example, have been considered superior to those of Aristotle, and his logic and his attempt to create a science of demonstration have been warmly appreciated by modern philosophers. He was aware of the limitations of logical proof – he accepted the existence of a creator god, but could not see how one could decide for certain anything about His essence or eternity, or about the immortality and corporeality of the soul. He was, however, sure that Man had a soul that required both ethical and intellectual training. Hence he acknowledged the morality of Jews and Christians, while denigrating their logic and their willingness to accept miracles in what to him was an ordered, stable universe.

His philosophy was closely tied to his medicine. He used his discoveries about the body to resolve philosophical disputes – so, for example, anatomy proved the truth of Plato's tripartite soul, with its seats in the brain, heart, and liver – and philosophy illuminated medicine. Aristotelian, Stoic, and, to a lesser extent, Platonic physics explained the world in which the body functioned, with its elements, qualities, and the like. Philosophy was no ethereal pursuit, but an integral part of medicine; the best doctor was also a philosopher, whether he knew it or not. The healer who lacked the power to reason was maimed and useless; and a doctor's proper behaviour was simultaneously morally good and medically effective. Even logic and linguistic analysis had their place in medicine. Clarity of terms avoided unnecessary confusion, while Galen's bedside practice has revealed, to at least one modern observer, an impeccable rigor and consistency of applied logic.

Whether in debate or at the bedside, Galen's logic was no feeble tool. Galen, like Rufus and other Hippocratics, believed the co-operation and trust of the patient essential in the battle with illness. They could be gained by adopting an appropriate bedside manner, by careful explanation in language accessible to the patient, and by the art of prognosis. Pointing out to a patient things already known but not yet told to the doctor would produce confidence that here was a proper doctor. Similarly, an accurate assessment of a doctor's abilities might be made by comparing his forecasts with his actual results. Despite Galen's assertions of its simplicity and Hippocratic precedent (p. 28), contemporaries apparently viewed prognosis as something quintessentially Galenic. Certainly its employment demanded a high level of experience, whether practical or codified in book form, logic to perform the essential steps of inference and differential diagnosis, and, above all, immense powers of observation. All these Galen undoubtedly had. It is often tiny and unexpected details that impress – herbs in a pot on a window, the habits of weasels, mineral ores left at an old mineshaft – all of which Galen tried to fit into a pattern. To understand the patient was not easy, but by observation and thought Galen claimed to have reduced the limits of uncertainty.

Galen was far more sympathetic to the virtues of experience than his detractors have allowed. He was no ivory-tower theorist, for patients came in large numbers from all levels of society. He was called in to examine sports injuries by gymnastic trainers at Ostia, the port of Rome, and sufferers from eye-diseases wrote to him from France and Spain (if not further afield). His busy practice involved all types of diseases – ulcers, fevers, pleurisy, styes, and dietary disorders. He was particularly proud of his insight into mental illness. Taking a Platonic line that strongly linked mind and body, he described mental changes brought about by physical illness (melancholia, the result of a surfeit of black bile, is a famous, if somewhat rare, example), and their converse. Stress syndromes were his speciality, whether among potential defendants in a trial, children before a test, teachers whose libraries had been lost, sons with recently deceased parents, administrators fearing that, without them, the world would collapse, or those with guilty secrets, whether gluttony or illicit love. There was, however, in his view no special sign of love; changes in colour or pulse were typical of all emotions, and specificity depended on a range of other factors.

Galen's experience was not confined to the bedside. The manual dexterity gained in childhood from building little toys he employed in later life in dissection. He had been introduced to animal anatomy at Pergamum by Satyrus, who had been trained at Alexandria with its long anatomical tradition. Galen mentions a great revival of anatomy there 'in our grandfathers' day' under Marinus (c. AD 120), whose writings he summarised and commented upon, and implies that this was one of the reasons why he went there to study.

From the earliest medical training onwards, Galen performed dissections, mainly of apes, sheep, pigs, and goats, but, on one famous occasion, of an elephant's heart. He knew human surface and some skeletal anatomy, but little internal human anatomy, although more than many critics have believed. Under these circumstances, it is hardly surprising that he applied many features of animal anatomy to humans, e.g. his female womb has cotyledons like a dog's; his thyroid cartilage is that of a pig; and his belief that the right kidney was situated higher in the body cavity than the left is true of apes, not humans. Two errors were particularly significant for subsequent physiology. His dissections of ungulates had revealed a network of nerves and vessels, the *rete mirabile*, at the base of the brain, which he believed also existed in humans and was where the so-called vital *pneuma* in the arteries began its elaboration into the psychic *pneuma* of the brain. He also misleadingly described the liver, in his view the origin of the veins, as grasping the stomach with its lobes as if by fingers, an image derived from the dissection of an ape or pig and easily interpreted to mean that the human liver had five lobes. By contrast, in his descriptions of bones or muscles his errors are far fewer. Similarly, Galen's explanations of anatomical phenomena in terms of their purpose (teleology) in a divinely organised universe, which earned him the approval of Aristotelians, were both more solidly grounded than theirs and stimulated him to pursue his investigations further. The final book of *On the Use of Parts of the Body* is a hymn, an 'epode', to the wonders of the creator, and a moving testimony to both his science and his religion.

More impressive still is Galen's experimentalism. He stressed the need for dissections to be repeated over and over again, in order to verify results and to improve with practice. If he did not always comply with his own advice to dissect daily (even in the midst of a busy life), he did embark on a sustained programme of anatomical research. He repeated experiments on bloodflow made earlier by Erasistratus (p. 35), and he modelled his dissections of the brain and nerves on those of Herophilus and Erasistratus. In a spectacular series of animal anatomies, he ligated or dissected the spinal cord at each vertebra to see and compare the results (which led him to discover the recurrent laryngeal nerve). Discovery was only one side of these experiments. They were also spectacles, designed to impress. Hence a preference for noisy animals, like pigs, whose silence and subsequent recovery of voice would astonish the audience; equally, in experiments which produced involuntary distasteful facial expressions, monkeys should be avoided, for their human likeness might offend.

Dissections were also essential for medical practice. One needed this knowledge obviously to avoid mistakes in surgery, but that was not all. Without an understanding of the arrangement and working of the body one would be bound to fall into error or, as in the case of Pausanias the sophist, whose partial paralysis Galen traced to a fall from a chariot, be unable to embark on a proper cure.

The visible evidence of gross anatomy offered one path to understanding. Touch, smell, hearing, taste, and sight provided another, hinting at the imperceptible micro-world of the body, an individual balance, mixture, or temperament of qualities, humours, and elements. Although in his clinical writings Galen mentions the four elements rarely, the four humours frequently, and the qualities, e.g. hot and cold, the perceptible manifestations of underlying changes, most often, he was not limited to the perceptible. From combining his own observations with the conclusions about the physical world at large reached by Plato and Aristotle, Galen derived 'plausible hypotheses' about the remotest structures of the body. Each action of the body had its cause, which operated only when its basic elements were correct, and any change in their combination, organisation, or mixture resulted in a loss of function, injury or disease. These (largely unknown) causes and combinations, called by Galen 'faculties' (or 'potentialities'), were determined by the divine Creator and were present throughout the body. Although later derided as mere verbiage (p. 352), Galen's theory of remote 'building blocks' determining bodily activity no longer seems as ridiculous in an age of hormones and DNA as it did a century ago.

THE UNITY OF GALEN

Faced with the sheer size of Galen's output, his multifarious activities, and his relentless desire to be right (and to prove others wrong), it is easy to forget how everything fits together. Hippocrates was indeed Galen's model – some have argued, almost his creation – and much of Galen's activity was aimed at improving on him, at 'perfecting' what he had left unfinished. It was a task that required practical experience, erudition, and thought, and in which the recovery of the sick was proof both of medical skill and of the divine Creator's macrocosmic organisation that allowed one to proceed logically and causally. Galen's patients did not recover through miracles, but through knowledge, understanding, or science.

Galen's pulse-lore exemplifies the unity of his medical and intellectual life. His 16 books on the pulse, written in the early 170s, were divided into four separate treatises, each four books long. The first, *On the Differences between Pulses*, set out the terms of the debate. Typically, Galen blamed the need for precise definition on the demands of his Roman competitors, prone to argue about terms and to mistake differences in names for differences in reality. So in book one Galen provided his own definitions, with a brief look at anatomy, and in book two reviewed the various possible types of pulse. Book three was devoted to an examination (and rejection) of the classification of pulses proposed by Archigenes (*c.* AD 100), while in the final book other theories of the pulse were examined, from Praxagoras in the fourth century BC, through Herophilus and Erasistratus, to Asclepiades and more modern writers. These books display his book-learning, his logic, and, above all, his linguistic studies. His familiarity with the language of classical Athenian drama allows him to select appropriate quotations to lighten the argument, and provides him with ammunition against those who misunderstand Greek or, another typical Galenic hate, invent a novel terminology of their own.

From definitions Galen passed to diagnostics. In the four books *On the Diagnosis of Pulses*, he explained how to take and classify the pulse. He raised a variety of interesting questions. How can one tell whether a pulse is 'full', 'rapid', or 'rhythmical'? Is there a perceptible pause when the artery has reached the limit of its contraction and, again, of its expansion ? Is there also a pause when the artery returns to its normal size? Such questions Galen resolved partly historically, by referring to earlier authorities, and partly from experience. His own enthusiasm for studying the pulse, which had been with him since youth, and his hours of practice had given him, he claimed, a most sensitive touch, an example worth imitation.

The third quartet of books, *On the Causes of Pulsation*, reverted to anatomy. Although Galen was convinced that the arteries contained blood coming from the heart, his understanding of pulsation was different from ours. For him, the heart and the artery contracted simultaneously, and arterial expansion and contraction were two separate and active movements. In contraction, sooty superfluities were forcibly expelled; in expansion, atmospheric air was taken in to cool and, mixing with blood in the heart, to generate vital *pneuma* or spirit. This vital spirit was largely responsible for creating and maintaining the pulsative faculty which existed within the actual coats of the artery. Their condition, of hardness or softness, was thus a crucial factor in any pulse, along with the strength of the pulsative faculty, and the physiological need of the organism. These positions Galen established to his own satisfaction by a combination of rigorous argument and anatomical experiment. If his conclusions do not always agree with those of modern physiologists, one might argue in his defence that determining the chronological relationship between contractions of the heart and arteries without modern aids is not easy, and modern repetitions of Galen's experiments to determine whether pulsation was the result of changes in bloodflow or of something transmitted through the arterial coats have supported Galen's conclusions as much as they have refuted them.

From a clinical standpoint, Galen's misunderstanding of the causes of pulsation is pardonable, for he strongly adhered to the view, first expressed by Praxagoras around 320 BC and then by the Alexandrians, that there was a strong link between pulse, arteries, heart, and illness. What the doctor needed above all was to understand this relationship and the meaning of the various phenomena in the pulse. This Galen provided in *On Prognosis from the Pulse*, adding examples from his own practice to those gained from reading. He adopted a double strategy. His first two books described the disease conditions that a type of pulse might reveal, e.g. the 'double-hammer pulse' was a frequent sign of weakness in the heart; the last two detailed the sort of pulse that should be found in a particular disorder, e.g in hectic fevers the pulse increased in size, frequency, and speed. Yet even in the midst of these clinical phenomena Galen found time for a recondite quotation from the *Hecale* of Callimachus (a poet active around 250 BC) to justify his use of metaphor in sphygmology.

Twenty five years later, around AD 195, Galen returned to the theme. He admitted that the 16 books were prolix, hard to assimilate, and, one might add, expensive to have copied. So, for the benefit of those who might otherwise be tempted to leave this important subject alone, he produced his own summary in a single book (in length, the equivalent of two).

Throughout, Galen was clear that what mattered above all was the usefulness of the pulse in medical practice. That was what people wanted to know, and why they consulted Galen. But equally, a proper understanding could not be gained solely by linking pulse and disease. The true doctor must know the whole process, both physiologically and historically. A correct interpretation of past writers would lead to the avoidance of medical error, almost as much as instruction in actual pulse-taking. Anatomy, logic, linguistics, and experience together contribute to the unity of medicine. Galen's ideal doctor is more than a medical specialist or even, in the modern sense of the word, a philosopher. He is the upholder of an impressive creed, the unity of eye and hand, of reason and experience, of past learning and future performance. To say that Galen endeavoured to fulfil his own ideal, and in large part succeeded, is to pay him the compliment of genius.

3 Medicine in Late Antiquity and the Early Middle Ages

VIVIAN NUTTON

Introduction

Any analysis of the transition from Classical Antiquity to the Middle Ages depends on whether one's standpoint is Gaul, Rome, Constantinople, or the frontier lands of Mesopotamia. East of Italy, in the Byzantine Greek world down to the fall of Constantinople in 1453, continuity is more striking than change. The fearsome plague that ravaged the Mediterranean world in 541–44 was described by contemporaries as if it were the Great Plague of Athens a millennium earlier (p. 13). Medicine as taught in thirteenth-century Constantinople resembles that of second-century Alexandria. Innovations are few: some medicaments and recipes from Persia and India entered the Byzantine pharmacopoeia, and a handful of Arabic medical writings were translated into Greek by 1300. John Zacharias Actuarius, a leading teacher and doctor at Constantinople in 1320, stands recognisably in the same tradition of Aristotelian philosophy and Hippocratic medicine as Galen himself. Byzantine surgeons performed complicated operations with specialist instruments, and may even have dissected, on the Galenic model (p. 66).

There are similar continuities in the legal status of Byzantine doctors in these regions. In the small towns of sixth-century Syria doctors enjoyed the same legal rights and privileges as their Roman predecessors 500 years before (p. 45). Indeed, their social status may have increased, for as the Roman Empire dissolved into a multitude of lesser ethnic groups, their desire to understand earlier Greek medical texts and to communicate with patients enforced a multi-lingualism that enabled them to cross political and ethnic frontiers. In Constantinople by AD 960 there was a medical guild incorporating a variety of practitioners, numerous enough to be mocked by satirists or condemned by biographers of saints. Two centuries later, laymen and doctors elegantly discussed knotty problems in Galen, and, in Constantinople at least, purchased copies of such treatises as Galen's *On the Parts of Medicine* which today no longer survive in the original Greek.

Two qualifications, however, must be made to this picture of continuity. Firstly, the economic, military, and political crisis of the seventh century profoundly altered the infrastructure that had supported the medical life of the Greek East. Cities like Ephesus or Pergamum shrank to mere villages, and the Byzantine Empire contracted over the centuries to little more than Constantinople and its hinterland. Evidence for medical life comes increasingly only from Constantinople, which was hardly typical of the rest of the Empire. Secondly, Byzantine medical institutions had shallower roots than ecclesiastical ones. Official professors of medicine, for instance, required a substantial commitment of government funds that was rarely forthcoming even at the best of times. An illusion of continuity may thus be gained from gazing across at isolated peaks, and forgetting the deep troughs that intervene.

The Greek East had from AD 330 a single capital, Constantinople. By contrast, the Latin half of the Roman Empire was fragile and fissiparous. Rome was its ecclesiastical centre, but at times Trier, Milan, and Ravenna rivalled Rome as the political headquarters of the emperor. Linguistic, cultural, military, and political circumstances combined to break the unity of the Roman Empire. From AD 364 onwards, the two halves of the Empire, ruled by separate (although initially related) emperors, gradually drew apart. By AD 600, the Latin West had fragmented under the barbarian invasions into a series of separate regions. Their economic foundations were weaker than those in the East; towns were fewer, and urban institutions more fragile. Medical practice thus developed in different ways within different societies.

Throughout the Empire, however, the city landscape changed with the advent of Christianity in AD 313 as a religion professed and supported by the Emperors. There was a 'desecularisation' of the ancient world. The claims of Christianity (and later Islam) to universality annexed areas of life formerly independent of religious cult and belief. Galen's religion had been his private affair, and the Methodists' rejection of divine healing had not brought down anathemas upon them. But in Late Antiquity and the Middle Ages religion and medicine interpenetrated in various ways. The Church's insistence on a Christian community that extended from before birth to the grave and beyond left no aspect of life untouched. Determining when a foetus became alive, had both theological and medical implications. To hold a non-religious perspective on healing was to risk being accused of a religious offence, heresy; and a cleric's concern for the eternal salvation of the soul might collide with a healer's concern for the present salvation of the body. This new context, however, was no religious strait-jacket, or necessarily opposed to medicine. Rather, it introduced new relationships and problems, based on belief in a series of sacred texts, the Bible. Hence the need first to look back at the origins of Christianity.

Christianity and medicine

Judaea in the time of Christ was home to a variety of healers. There were intellectuals, acquainted with the philosophical bases of medicine; travelling healers, scarcely distinguishable from magicians; and holy men, convinced that in obedience to the Mosaic Law lay bodily and spiritual health. Jewish healers had an ancestor in King Solomon (reigned 970–931 BC), who was credited with great magical and medical powers, and the injunction of Jesus ben Sirach (c. 180 BC) to 'honour the physician for the good ye may have of him' ostensibly gave them a worthy place in society. Indeed, by AD 400 a community without a healer was, in Jewish law, no proper community. The Jews also had a religious duty to care for their fellow Jews, which extended to the lodging, and occasionally medical treatment, of pilgrims to the Temple at Jerusalem. Temporary medical assistance had been provided in Classical Greece for visitors to the great festivals, but among the Jews this took tangible and permanent form; c. AD 60 Theodotus, son of Vettenus, erected a pilgrim hostel in Jerusalem, an example of the Jewish tradition of hospitality that later Rabbis traced back to Abraham, *Genesis* 21.33.

Some Jews, however, rejected human medical assistance in favour of the divine, aware of the fate of King Asa (c. 914–874 BC), who 'sought not to the Lord, but to his physicians' and whose foot sores grew steadily worse. Skin diseases especially were associated with God's punishment for sin, and were curable by Him alone. Conversely, in a world controlled by the one God, He could heal by a miracle where others had failed.

The Gospel accounts of Christ's healing should be set against this Jewish background. In his activities as prophet and healer, Jesus was not unique, while his careful answers to questions whether sin was the cause of disease reflected contemporary rabbinical debates. The New Testament presentation of secular healing is neutral – or ambiguous. The expensive physicians of Mark 5.26, are balanced by Luke 'the beloved physician'; Paul's advice to take wine for one's stomach by the description, in the Epistle of James, of a Christian medicine of faith, prayer, confession, and the laying-on of hands. Christ's power of physical healing was transmitted to his disciples and those who believed in him. A touch, the hem of a garment, or even a distant command would be effective, if the sufferers, or their representatives, had sufficient faith.

As Christianity developed, the New Testament texts on healing promoted a range of often competing attitudes. Some were entirely compatible with what had gone before: the Hippocratic physician was easily turned to a model of Christian medical charity. Others were vastly different. Stoic resistance to pain was not the same as a belief in the nobility of suffering or disease as some divine trial. Non-Christians would have found ludicrous one preacher's exhortation to welcome plague because it ended overcrowding and provided swift punishment for sinners and a speedy passage to heaven for believers. Few would have agreed with Tatian (c. AD 160) that human medicines were the devil's handiwork, and recovery achieved with their aid, only a snare and a delusion. The scruples of Galen, Scribonius Largus, or the philosopher Plotinus over the use of certain magical remedies in medicine (p. 55) reflect an epistemological, philosophical, and social debate, not a mighty battle in this world between God and Satan.

The Gospel miracles also provided propaganda for the new religion. A few early Christian texts refer to physical healing leading directly to conversion, e.g. the legend, current by AD 300, of the conversion of King Abgar and his kingdom of Edessa (now southeast Turkey) by the apostle and healer Thaddaeus. Most ecclesiastics, however, preferred to interpret Christ as the physician of the soul, a very common metaphor, and rarely mentioned physical healing. Their flock may have been more literal-minded. By AD 400, accounts of healing miracles, particularly those effected with the aid of relics of the saints, become plentiful. Bishop Victricius of Rouen (c. AD 330 to c. 407), joyfully welcoming the arrival of a holy relic, recited a long list of saintly cures. St. Augustine (AD 354–430) was somewhat more reserved. He regarded miracle cures by holy oil, relics, or baptism as marks of special providence, and hence rare, a qualification lost on his congregation, who brought children to baptism to regain physical health, applied the eucharistic host to a child's closed eyelids, and wore the four gospels as amulets to ward off disease.

Whatever learned clerics might think, there was an element of physical healing within Christianity. Hence a distrust of converts who had been formerly pagan exorcists or diviners, and a particular animosity towards the competing cults of Asclepius, many of whose miracles paralleled those of Christian saints, and other healing gods. The Egyptian holy healers, SS. Cyrus and John, established their surgery directly opposite the pagan healing shrine of Menuthis.

Doctors too fell under suspicion, for alongside St. Julian of Emesa, 'a skilled physician of both body and soul', or Dionysius, 'doctor, priest and philanthropist', captured by the Goths in the late fifth century, there were notorious pagans, like the wonder-working doctor Asclepiodotus of Aphrodisias (c. AD 460) and his contemporary, the Alexandrian *iatrosophist* (medical professor) Gesius. Gesius was officially a Christian, but his true sympathies were revealed when he protected a pagan philosopher and doubted the miracles of SS. Cyrus and John. He was afflicted with a disease beyond mortal cure, and recovered only with the saints' assistance after a full and contrite confession of his impiety. Medical chants and charms, apparently amazing cures, and the possession of mathematical, astronomical, and scientific learning in an age of increasing ignorance, may all have contributed to a certain suspicion of doctors, and occasionally even to open hostility.

This does not mean that the Church rejected secular medicine, for the Church as such never pronounced, let alone enforced, any universal opinion on the topic. There were, at best, different strands of opinion, dependent far more on individual beliefs and experiences than on any scriptural text or ecclesiastical decision. The medicine of Galen and the medicine of Christianity were largely complementary. Few sufferers resorted to a healing shrine without first trying a human healer. Human failure was no proof of incompetence, for all parties understood that some diseases were incurable by human means. Even at a healing shrine, the saint could recommend a secular healer, or carry out procedures familiar to a Galenist. According to their biographer, it was one of the strengths of SS. Cosmas and Damian, the patron saints of medicine, that they had 'thoroughly mastered the healing of Hippocrates and Galen'.

Practice also differed from theory over the causes of disease. It was a truth, universally acknowledged, that disease and sin were closely

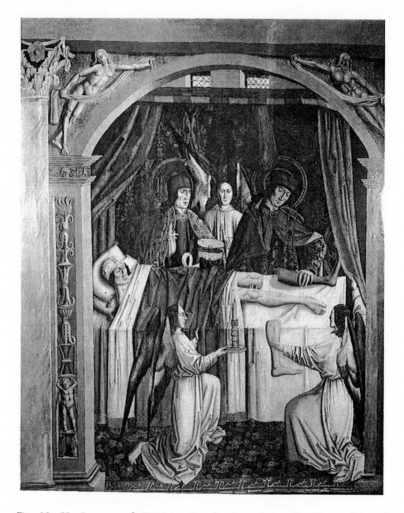

Fig. 12. SS. Cosmas and Damian miraculously replacing the ulcerated leg of a Christian with the undiseased leg of a Moor. The Spanish artist, Alonso de Sedano, *fl.* 1495, shows the medical saints in full academic dress. (The Wellcome Institute, London.)

linked; illness was a consequence of mankind's fallen nature. But writers in Late Antiquity and the Early Middle Ages almost always ascribed their own, or their friends', sufferings to physical causes; those of others, particularly their enemies, to sin.

Early Christian attitudes to the body are equally diverse. The Hippocratic ideal of balance was hard to combine with praise of asceticism and the mortification of the flesh, and with illness as a trial of sanctity. A religious rhythm of fasting and vigil was no harmonious counterpoint to the ordered progression of the humours. The more the body appeared a mere temporary habitation of an immortal soul, the less the need to attend to it. Even if such asceticism was arguably only for the super-Christian, the tension remained, to surface periodically and among minority groups from the second century until our own. Bishop Caesarius of Arles (*c.* AD 470–542, p. 84), St. Bernard of Clairvaux (1090–1153), the monastic reformer, and Mary Baker Eddy (1821–1910), the founder of Christian Science, are but three who set the medicine of faith and prayer above the corrupt worldly material of the body. Some monastic rules forbade drugs and human remedies; others accepted them grudgingly; and even though most Christians agreed with St. Basil (*c.* AD 330–79) that God had put medicines and herbs in this world for human use, many in the fifth century still thought that the truly religious should not need them. True, life in a town or a monastery, wrote St. Diodochus of Photike (*c.* AD 480), might not provide the best environment for an ascetic to have the love and charity towards others essential for Christian healing, but out in a desert a hermit could surely rely on faith and prayer alone.

Charity and the early hospital

The Jewish tradition of hospitality (p. 73) was extended by the Christians. Christ's order to his followers to care for the sick, the poor, the lonely, and the needy was swiftly given institutional form by the creation of 'deacons' charged with the distribution of alms. It was a commitment to all in need, Christians and non-Christians alike. By AD 250 the church in Rome had an elaborate organisation for the distribution of aid. Elsewhere wealthy Christians set aside a room in their house to provide food and shelter as part of a missionary outreach. Their rivals, the heretical Manichees, established similar hostels, and the emperor Julian in 362 unsuccessfully appealed to his fellow-pagans to imitate the Jews and Christians in their charity to outsiders.

With the legalisation of Christianity in the fourth century, charity was given architectural form, at first in the Eastern Empire. Bishop Leontius (AD 344–58) founded a number of hostels (*xenodokeia* or *xenones*) at Antioch and one at Daphne, a fashionable spa nearby. Between AD 357–77, Bishop Eustathius of Sebasteia built a 'poor-house', where those who were 'crippled with disease' could find suc-

cour. At the same time, St. Basil erected outside the walls of Caesarea
'almost a new city', where the sick, the leprous, the poor, and the
stranger could receive care and medical assistance. By AD 400 similar
institutions were common enough to be used for an extended metaphor
in a bishop's sermon. By AD 500, Edessa, a town of 8000–10,000
souls, had three hospitals, all small, which were supplemented in emergencies of plague or famine by beds erected in public colonnades to
house sufferers flocking in from the countryside. Law texts, saints' lives,
and accounts of pilgrims confirm that in the Middle East hospitals, even
if no more than a room off a church courtyard, were now ubiquitous.

They arrived somewhat later in the Latin West – the earliest was
founded by Fabiola in Rome around AD 397 – and do not appear to
have spread widely in Italy, still less beyond the Alps, a reflection of the
economic and social crises of the fifth and sixth centuries. They were
founded under Eastern influence: Fabiola and Pammachius, whose hospital near Rome was erected c. AD 400, had both visited the Holy Land.
In southern France the use of the Greek word *xenodocium* implies, and a
very early description of the hospital at Clermont Ferrand c. AD 550
expressly acknowledges, that the institution came from the East.

Eastern hospitals became ever larger and more complex. Ephesus in
420 had one with over 75 beds; Jerusalem in AD 550 had one with
200 beds; that of St. Sampson in Constantinople was even larger. There
are signs of specialisation. Edessa had a women's hospital by AD 400,
and some big hospitals at Antioch and Constantinople were divided by
AD 600 into male and female wards. By AD 650, surgical operations
were being performed at St. Sampson's, and one section of the hospital
was devoted to ophthalmic patients. The charter of the Pantokrator
hospital at Constantinople, an exceptionally well funded royal foundation of 1136, prescribed a complex hierarchy of physicians, and even
teaching facilities. But there is no evidence that such complexity was
typical or existed much before this date, and the Pantokrator's 50 or so
patients, one to a bed, were only a tiny fraction of the sick of this mega-
lopolis.

Physicians were present as and when necessary. A medical family at
Oxyrhyncus, Egypt, in AD 570 ran their own hospital, but usually the
head was a layman, chosen for probity and efficiency. At Nisibis (now
southeastern Turkey) the king of Persia built a hospital around AD 550
near the Christian theological school to prevent sick students from
being 'plundered and dishonoured' as they went into town for help,

and also to shift the time-consuming burden of care from their fellow-students. Its administrator was a layman, under the director of the school. Statutes of 590 maintain this reserve towards secular medicine. Theology students might be expelled for associating with physicians, 'for the crafts of the world are unworthy to be read with the books of holiness in one light.' But it is never suggested that treatment here was inferior, and some secular institutions also lacked resident physicians: others, no less sacred, gladly employed physicians.

Charting a passage from religious care to medical cure is to adopt a false perspective, even if care and cure could be distinguished. The varied terminology – hospice, hostel, poor-house, sick-house, orphanage, home for the elderly, hospital – indicates a variety of overlapping, even competing, aims. Some institutions specialised in one type of inmate, but only the name proclaims exclusivity. When we penetrate beyond the name, we find a combination of priorities. The Pantokrator's charter established on the same site both a home for the elderly and a medical hospital, and, outside the city, a leper-house unattended by any doctor. The scattered hospitals of Italy, the ubiquitous establishments of Syria, the tiny hospital at Clermont and the giants of Jerusalem and Constantinople, all shared an overall religious framework of care, compassion, and charity.

From Galen to Galenism

The century that followed the death of Galen (c. AD 200/216) is a blank spot in the history of medicine. The Latin medical poem of Quintus Serenus, pseudo-Galenic treatises on medical astrology and *On the Ensoulment of the Foetus*, and a few scraps of veterinary writers in Greek form a poor repast after the feast of the second century. The meagre record of inscriptions and legal texts only confirms that doctors continued to enjoy (albeit with increasing difficulty) their privileges of tax immunity. When light returns, around AD 350, it is almost on a different world. Not only has the Roman Empire gained a second capital, Constantinople, and an official religion, Christianity, but also the type of medical text to survive – summaries, handbooks, and medical encyclopaedias – is new.

Although such works are known earlier, what is found in the works of Oribasius of Pergamum (c. 325–400), Aëtius of Amida (*fl.* AD 530 in Constantinople) and Paul of Aegina (*fl.* in Alexandria c. 630) is different from Celsus, Pliny, and Galen's *Method of Medicine*. The later authors assembled extracts from earlier writers, often verbatim, into a coherent mosaic of opinions, ideas, and remedies. Their compilations can be big or small; Oribasius produced one for his patron, the Emperor Julian, in 70 books, of which over 30 survive, another in nine books for his son Eustathius, one in four books for his friend and biographer Eunapius (AD 340 to *c.* 414), and a single volume (now lost), the fruit of midnight discussions with Emperor Julian while on campaign *c.* AD 358. These medical encyclopaedias show learning, elegant organisation, and practicality, talents not to be despised or necessarily subordinated to novelty. Through them, earlier authors such as Rufus of Ephesus, Athenaeus of Attaleia, or the surgeon Antyllus (*fl.* AD 110), whose advice on aneurysms looks remarkably modern, can still speak in their own words. Paul's Book VI, by far the most informative Greek surgical text, covers everything from hernias and fistulae to sprained ankles and varicose veins, and from battlefield wounds to the surgical reduction of over-large breasts 'when the lady is reproached for their unsightliness'. This text is also a tribute to an Alexandrian surgical tradition, in which complicated operations continued to be performed at least until the seventh century.

But much has been lost. Over time these encyclopaedias became more and more brusque. Alternatives became irrelevant luxuries, and the word of Galen came to dominate. His qualifications were edited out, and the practical and empirical side of his work was replaced by the dogmatic, although a logically structured systematisation of all his many hypotheses was not achieved until Avicenna (p. 114). This transition from Galen to Galenism was assisted by Galen's own rhetoric. His frequent claims to be perfecting medicine were now believed. 'Hippocrates sowed the seed, Galen reaped the harvest', said one author, with the implication that only unprofitable stubble remained. The sheer size of Galen's achievement was also daunting. Few thought that they could now master the whole of medicine as he had done, and preferred either to summarise or to concentrate on only one part of what he had considered a unity.

Galen's influence spread both swiftly and widely. By AD 210 his critical comments on Christian philosophical naïveté had led Theodotus the shoemaker and his followers into heresy, and may have influenced the Egyptian theologian Origen, writing about 230. Papyrus fragments have been recently discovered of Galenic tracts copied in Egypt about

250, just when, in North Africa, the Latin author Gargilius Martialis was quoting Galen's prescriptions extensively in his *Medicines from Fruit and Vegetables*. But the triumph of Galenism should not be exaggerated. There were still Asclepiadeans in the Greek world in the fourth century, and Methodists for some time after that. In the Latin-speaking world Galen, although known, never dominated to the same extent until the twelfth or thirteenth century.

Late Antiquity also saw a progressive split between theory and practice. Such a division of medicine, first recorded *c.* AD 200, became by 400 a standard feature of all medical textbooks. Likewise Galen's insistence on the need for a doctor to understand philosophy was interpreted as a demand for a preparatory training in philosophy, and for a greater theoretical content in medical education. At fifth- and sixth-century Alexandria the same individual might often be found expounding Aristotle as easily as Hippocrates. Stephanus of Athens (*c.* AD 550 to *c.* 630), for example, composed commentaries on three works by Hippocrates and Galen and four by Aristotle, and wrote on theology and astronomy.

The emphasis on theory also aided the move towards a definition of medicine in terms of specific books. Although Galen himself had commented on several Hippocratic texts and singled out the *Aphorisms* as essential, he laid down no canon of set texts. But by AD 500 in Alexandria, there was not only a syllabus of Hippocratic texts (largely those preferred by Galen), but also the appearance of a Galenic canon, the so-called 16 books (in fact 24, some being regarded as parts of larger works). These were taught with formal commentaries (some of which survive), and read in a specific order, beginning with *On Sects* and *Art of Medicine* (see Appendix 3.1, p. 87). Alexandrian scholars also summarised the 16 books for ease of memory, thus imparting a further rigidity to Galenism.

This process can be seen neatly in the career of Magnus of Nisibis, who dominated the medical life of Alexandria at the end of the fourth century. His biographer, Eunapius, the friend of Oribasius, contrasted him with his colleague Ionicus, an expert in bandaging and surgery, but no speaker. Eunapius' preference is obvious, and was shared by the many students who flocked to hear Magnus. No practical physician, he was reputed to defeat death by argument, and to convince the sick they were well purely by the force of his oratory. His book on urines may survive under the name of Magnus of Emesa (a city in the same region). Avowedly based on scattered incidents and ideas in Galen which were selected, organised, and worked up into a guide to diagnosis through the urine, it is an elegant and didactically effective production. It marks a significant shift, for it turns uroscopy, used only occasionally by Galen, into an essential element in medical practice. Henceforth, in both East and West, the urine flask becomes the symbol of the educated physician.

The same period also saw in North Africa an upsurge in learned Latin medicine based in part on Greek sources, principally the Methodists. Whether Caelius Aurelianus (*c.* 420) in his large nosographical handbook *On Acute and Chronic Diseases* was simply translating an earlier Greek Methodist work by Soranus or adding substantial material of his own is disputed, but the result is Latin learned medicine befitting a region in close touch with Alexandria. It is more extensive in its coverage of diseases and more academic in its approach than similar contemporary productions from Italy and Gaul, which emphasised the need for self-help in a society from which the institutions that had sustained learned medicine were rapidly disappearing. Marcellus of Bordeaux, a high official of the emperor Theodosius in AD 394–95, added to the recipes of Scribonius Largus Gallic remedies, chants, charms, and more popular material, to produce a manual of self-help domestic medicine. The differences between this and the similar handbook of Alexander of Tralles (*fl.* AD 570), a cosmopolitan and much-travelled Greek doctor, or the Galenic commentaries associated around AD 600 with Ravenna, the Italian headquarters of the Byzantine Greek administration in the West, mark two very different worlds. The Ravenna commentators imitated (or translated) the lectures of Alexandrian philosopher-physicians; Alexander added his chants and charms to a Galenic synthesis that derived both stability and effectiveness from its roots in a Hippocratic past. There were constraints on what a doctor could now use in a Christian world, but Alexander was still confidently part of a traditional intellectual community within a confident Eastern Roman Empire. One of his brothers was an imperial lawyer, another the architect of the great church of Hagia Sophia at Constantinople. But for Marcellus, despite his links with the court and the leaders of Gaul and northern Spain, many of the old certainties were disappearing in a new landscape. Although he recommended summoning doctors in difficult cases, his readers were expected to rely mainly on themselves; they must, like him, be 'empirics', not as followers of the Greek Empiricist sect, but as experts in what worked. In Marcellus's book, the agricultural tradition of Cato reappears just as the civic structures of Roman Gaul splinter into great medieval estates.

Medicine in western Europe, 500–1000

At first sight, the institutions and practices of medicine in the sixth-century Latin West continue as they had done for centuries. In AD 530 and 531 imperial laws fixed the maximum price of a slave doctor at 60 *solidi* (10 more than a secretary). In AD 534 the Emperor Justinian fixed the salaries of the five *archiatri* (doctors-in-chief) of the province of Africa at 99, 70 and 50 *solidi* a year, roughly equivalent to that of a local judge or a minor bishop. A few years earlier, Cassiodorus had described in flowery prose the duties of the Count of the Roman *archiatri* for his monarch, Theoderic the Ostrogoth (reigned AD 493–526). Like a similar official in Constantinople, the Count exercised an oversight over the doctors in the city, treated the Emperor, judged all medical disputes, and decided who should join the prestigious College of Physicians and gain the title of *archiater*. King Theoderic was attended on his deathbed by a priest-doctor Elpidius (*fl.* AD 510–30), whose varied career had taken him from Lyons and Milan to Constantinople, and given him wealth enough to restore some ruined baths at Spoleto (Italy). His contemporary, Dr. Pegasus of Laribus in Africa, could afford to ransom the governor's son for 50 *solidi*, about 10 years pay for a soldier. In AD 576, Leunast, Archdeacon of Bourges (Central France), sought help for his eye-cataracts from several physicians as well as from the nearby shrine of St. Martin at Tours. Although his pilgrimage brought some relief, he also had himself bled by a Jewish doctor in Bourges. He became totally blind, fit punishment, remarked Bishop Gregory of Tours (AD 539–94), for seeking Jewish help after receiving God's grace through the saint. At Ravenna, in AD 572, a sale document was witnessed by the son of Leontius, 'doctor, at the Greek *schola*', and medical lectures on the Alexandrian model were still being delivered well into the seventh century.

But these apparent continuities mask enormous social and intellectual changes. The legal documents may not correspond to any reality; although their context suggests a specific problem, no slave doctor is otherwise recorded for certain after AD 250, and five *archiatri* could do little in a populous province like Africa. The medical careers reflect what is going on in a few (and, especially in Ravenna, atypical) urban centres. The truth is revealed in a sermon by St Caesarius of Arles (*c.* AD 520). Outside the towns, there are no doctors, only folk-medicine and superstition; inside, medicine is more sophisticated, but extremely expensive and tinged with paganism. In Caesarius' ideal Christian community, blessing and unction replace both types of healing. Scattered records of *medici* survive, however, some in unexpected places, like the Lleyn peninsula in North Wales, but the literary sources show a largely rural population left to their own devices and to the mercy of disease, famine, and war. From Ireland and Wales (where king Maelgwn died in 547 of 'the yellow plague'), through France, Germany, and Spain, to Italy and Africa, authors tell tragic tales of epidemics of fever, boils, dysentery, and the like, which nothing, save the occasional intervention of a saint, could cure. The resources for the maintenance of an active intellectual tradition of medicine were also diminishing. If in the fourth and early fifth centuries pagan and Christian learning were assimilated into a Latin-speaking world, the sixth century saw a retrenchment. Schools were closed; Latin became more and more confined to the church and the monastery. The same Cassiodorus who praised the noble art of medicine before Theoderic advised the monks of his monastery at Vivarium (southern Italy) to aid the sick with medicines and with hope in God. He recommended to the library a few essential medical texts – Gargilius Martialis, *On Gardens*; some Latin versions of Hippocrates and Galen's *Method of Healing, for Glaucon*; an anonymous compendium; an (illustrated?) Dioscorides; Caelius Aurelius, *On Medicine*; Hippocrates, *On Herbs and Cures*; and a few other books, a meagre harvest from Classical Antiquity.

His list is instructive. Firstly, the texts are largely practical; what theory they contain is presented dogmatically, with little room for discursive, Galenic argument. Secondly, the familiar names may hide a variety of unfamiliar or suppositious works. Six tracts from the Greek Hippocratic Corpus were already translated into Latin, including *Aphorisms*, *Prognostic*, and *Airs, Waters and Places*, but *On Herbs and Cures* is not among them, unless it was a compilation of extracts from *On Diet*. Early Medieval Latin manuscripts transmitted, under the heading of Galen's *Method of Healing, for Glaucon*, a partial translation of its two genuine books along with others that were certainly not his. 'Caelius Aurelius' may refer to Caelius Aurelianus or to a popular compendium on fevers ascribed to an Aurelius. The Dioscorides may not be a Latin version of the famous herbal, but the spurious tract *On Feminine Herbs* that survives in seven manuscripts written before 900. This attribution of short practical works to famous names, or to none, is typical of Early Medieval Latin medicine. Thirdly, the combination of guides to diagnosis and therapy with a herbal is common, as in the *Lorsch Book of Medicine*, written about AD 795 in the Benedictine Abbey of Lorsch (southwest Germany), which contains brief introductory texts on anatomy, the humours, and prognostic (as well as an abbreviated Hippocratic *Oath*), and ends with a long series of recipes and practical advice and a letter on diet. Cassiodorus' choice of books may have constituted 'a literature for barbarians', but, equally, they preserved much practical therapy of Antiquity (and no small amount of its basic theory).

Such knowledge was also transmitted through encyclopaedias like the *Etymologies* of Isidore of Seville (d. AD 640). Its sections on medicine (in Book IV on diseases and cures, Book XI on anatomy) summarise learned medicine, and its influence can be traced throughout Early Medieval Europe. Its very title, though, suggests the new context in which its medicine was studied – as words, by grammarians. To understand the meaning of the terms was to penetrate to the very essence of the divinely created world. Its medicine revealed truths about man and God, and the covers of the book protected this knowledge from the unlearned and from decay.

The fact that these manuscripts of medicine were written and read in the libraries of great Benedictine abbeys, like Nonantola (northern Italy) or Reichenau (southern Germany), or, after AD 800, of the revived cathedral schools, such as Chartres (France), indicates the Christian context of early medieval medical learning, as well as the restricted milieu in which any form of book-learning flourished in the early Middle Ages. What was read, copied, and, even more important for the future, preserved must satisfy the needs and the preconceptions of Christians. This does not mean that all early medieval medicine was monastic or that secular medicine was overshadowed by miracle healing – far from it. In his account of St. John of Beverley (d. AD 721), Bede (AD 672/3–735) demonstrates that he and John were well aware of the complementary roles of both types of healing. If doctors broke their own rules for bleeding, it was not surprising that their patient developed nasty complications. The sign of the cross made a dumb man speak, but his instruction in language required only good teaching, and his skin disorder and dandruff were left by John to a doctor. Herebald, who broke his skull in a racing accident, was cured through the prayers and blessing of John and the bone-setting skills of a doctor. Ironically, later retellings of these stories emphasised the miraculous, and left out the doctors.

Although on the fringes of the learned world, Bede and his English monks possessed many of the same medical writings as their contemporaries further South, even if, as Bishop Cyneheard of Worcester put it in 754, the foreign ingredients prescribed therein were unknown or difficult to obtain, even through contacts in Germany or Italy. Anglo-Saxon England, like contemporary Ireland, possessed a written medical literature (from *c.* 900) in a non-Latin language, but this does not mean that the Anglo-Saxon healer, the *laece* or leech, was less competent than the *medicus*. Chants and charms, and explanations of a few diseases as the result of darts hurled by mischievous elves or involving a great worm constitute only a small part of the medicine that survives, and are not unique to the Anglo-Saxons. Similar recipes are found in other regions and in earlier Latin learned texts. Anglo-Saxon knowledge of plant remedies was wide and effective, and authors recognised the problems of identifying Mediterranean with British flora. When the otherwise unknown Bald and Cild wrote their *Leechbook* around 900, perhaps at Winchester, they adapted the best Continental practical medicine to an English environment. Their *Leechbook* has close parallels with both later Salernitan texts and with fifth- and sixth-century medical tracts common elsewhere in Western Europe. They simplified some of their Latin recipes by removing some of the more exotic ingredients, and added remedies obtained from Ireland or Irish scholars. The scientific compendium assembled by Byrhtferth of Ramsey Abbey around 1100 also contained material that reappears in the famous Salernitan *Rule of Health*.

Anglo-Saxon medicine thus exemplifies the practical medicine of Early Medieval Europe. A substrate of classical, mainly Methodist, therapeutics remained, along with a modicum of classical theory, enough to explain diagnosis and treatment. The emphasis, however, was on what worked: recipes, meterological and astrological advice, rules for bleeding and uroscopy. There was, as yet, no room for broad discussions of theory or the wider philosophical context. In medicine, as in literature in general, the scholars of Early Medieval Europe could not afford to dabble in the inessential. Their preference for the practical does not indicate an intellectual torpor, but rather the constraints on medical life in a society where books were expensive and rare, and from which the opportunities enjoyed by a Galen or a Magnus had long vanished.

Appendix 3.1 The Galenic canon, 'the sixteen books', around AD 1000

1. On sects[1]
2. Art of medicine
3. Short book on the pulse
4. Method of healing, for Glaucon
5. Collection I: Anatomy for beginners
   On bones; On muscles; On nerves; On veins and arteries
6. On elements
7. On temperaments
8. On the natural faculties
9. Collection II: The books of causes and symptoms
10. On affected places
11. Collection III: The 16 books on the pulse (p. 68)[2]
12. On the differences between fevers
13. On crises
14. On critical days
15. Method of healing
16. On the preservation of health[3]

[1] Nos. 1 to 4 formed one introductory collection at Alexandria. Nos. 1 and 3 were not translated by Sergius into Syriac.

[2] Not all these books were always studied. The Alexandrians may have studied only four; only six were translated by Sergius into Syriac; and none was included in the medieval Hebrew *Galenic Summaries*.

[3] This work does not appear to have formed part of the canon before the Muslim period.

Chronological table for Chapters 4 and 5

Year	Medical and scientific writers	Year	Contemporary events
541–749	first plague pandemic	565	death of Justinian
		632	death of Muhammad
		630s–640s	Arab conquest of Syria, Egypt and Iraq
		710	Arab invasion of Spain
c.750–1050	Bakhtishu' family of physicians in Persia and Iraq	750	Abbasid revolution
		813–833	reign of Ma'mun
		832	Bayt al-Hikma founded in Baghdad
		847–861	reign of Mutawakkil
873	death of Hunayn ibn Ishaq		
912	death of Qusta ibn Luqa		
925	death of Rhazes		
fl. 940	Albucasis		
c. 999	death of Majusi		
1037	death of Avicenna	1058–1087	Desiderius, Abbot of Monte Cassino
		1066	Norman conquest of England
fl. c. 1080	Constantine the African	1080–1200	School of Salerno
fl. c. 1130	Trota of Salerno	1095–1270	the Crusades
		c. 1180	University of Bologna founded
1187	death of Gerard of Cremona		
1193	death of Burgundio of Pisa		
1197	death of Hildegard of Bingen		
		c. 1200	Universities of Paris and Oxford founded
1204	death of Maimonides	1204	Latin Crusaders sack Constantinople
1214	Ugo Borgognoni public doctor at Bologna		

Year	Medical and scientific writers	Year	Contemporary events
		1215	Fourth Lateran Council
		1222	University of Padua founded
1248	death of Ibn al-Baytar		
c. 1250	first Islamic medical schools in Turkey	1258	Mongol sack of Baghdad, end of Abbasid caliphate
1277	death of Peter of Spain (John XXI)		
1280	death of Albertus Magnus		
1284	Mansuri hospital founded in Cairo		
1288	Sta. Maria Nuova hospital founded in Florence		
1295	death of Taddeo Alderotti		
c. 1313	death of Arnald of Villanova		
c.1315	Anatomical dissection by Mondino dei Liuzzi		
fl. 1317	Pietro d'Abano		
		1321	death of Dante
		1338–1453	Hundred Years War between England and France
fl. 1340	Niccolò da Reggio		
1347–51	Black Death		
1368	death of Guy de Chauliac		
		1374	death of Petrarch
1377	Ragusa institutes quarantine		
fl. 1396	Ibn Ilyas		
1391	first dissection recorded in Spain		
		1400	death of Chaucer
c.1400	Milan institutes permanent health board		
1404	first dissection recorded in Vienna		
1410	death of Francesco Datini		
1424	first recorded regulations for midwives, Brussels		
1452	death of Bartolommeo di Montagnana		
		1453	Ottoman capture of Constantinople, end of Byzantine Empire
1458	death of Jacques Despars		

Year	Medical and scientific writers	Year	Contemporary events
		1464	death of Cosmo dei Medici in Florence
1465	death of Leonardo di Bertipaglia		
1473	death of Puff von Schrick		
1484	*Malleus maleficarum* published		
		1485	Tudor dynasty begins in England
1490	works of Galen first printed in Latin		
		1492	Columbus reaches America
		1492	fall of Granada, last Islamic foothold in Spain
1525	complete works of Galen first printed in Greek		
1525	Hippocratic Corpus first printed in Latin		
1526	Hippocratic Corpus first printed in Greek		

4 The Arab-Islamic medical tradition

LAWRENCE I. CONRAD

In medieval times the Arab-Islamic world developed a medical tradition which ranked among the most advanced of the pre-modern world, not only in its intellectual sophistication, but also in its practical impact in society at large. Over the past century the history of this tradition has come to be recognised as an important topic in its own right, but here our attention will be limited to those aspects of most immediate concern to the history of the Western medical tradition.

The Arab-Islamic medical tradition was founded on Graeco-Roman medicine, the exponents of Arab-Islamic culture translated into Arabic and so saved many classical texts which might otherwise have been lost, and the Islamic world ultimately passed this heritage back to Europe when its medical works were translated into Latin. A primary concern of this chapter will thus be the emergent period of Arab-Islamic medicine and the formation of its medical literature.

But the transmission of literature was only one means by which the West came to know of Arab-Islamic medicine, and possibly also to learn from it. Through most of the medieval period Western travellers came to the Islamic world as traders, diplomats, pilgrims, and sometimes (as during the Crusades) as invaders; in the great cities of the Middle East and North Africa they would have seen the physicians and medical institutions of medieval Islam at work. In some cases they could have seen Middle Eastern physicians in Europe itself, for the latter practised as far afield as France, Italy, and the Byzantine capital of Constantinople. It is thus worth considering this Arab-Islamic medical practice here, not only because some Europeans became familiar with it, but also for comparative purposes – to consider the extent to which various medical customs and practices were simply typical of pre-modern societies, or specific to particular cultures.

The traditional substrate of Arab-Islamic medicine

In earlier chapters we have seen that even in its heyday, Graeco-Roman medicine co-existed with deeply entrenched systems of popular medicine based on folklore and superstition. In seventh-century Middle East a similar situation prevailed. Formal scientific learning, including medicine, continued in the eastern Church, and especially in the Jacobite and Nestorian monasteries of Syria and Mesopotamia; but Christians and Jews, no less than their new Muslim overlords, also had a venerable tradition of deep-seated beliefs in the supernatural and its role in medicine and health. Arab lore is often identical or similar to that of other peoples of the Middle East, and the beliefs and remedies espoused by the Arabs were not specific to them, but part of a substrate of popular medicine which prevailed throughout the region and across religious and ethnic lines. For the sake of description we can label this medicine as 'popular medicine' or 'medical folklore', but such labels should not be presumed to privilege the scientific status of the humoral medicine taken up from the Greeks. The difference was in their means of legitimation: popular medicine gained and kept assent through the power of age-old custom and tradition, the humoral medicine through its associations with circles of formal scholarship and sources of patronage.

People often regarded medical problems from a practical point of view, and if someone lapsed from good health – regarded as the natural human condition – popular lore offered a host of remedies. Materia medica included a broad range of plants and herbs, and it is unlikely that the popular pharmacopoeia of the Middle East in the seventh and eighth centuries was significantly different from that familiar to the area in earlier times. Natural ingredients were used to produce an array of broths, elixirs, liniments, salves, and errhines, and were commonly employed not only to counter medical disorders, but for other purposes as well (e.g. as aphrodisiacs). Inorganic medicaments (such as minerals) were uncommon, but there was considerable use of animal products: meat, gall, milk, and urine. The leaves of the aromatic *arak* bush, for example, were cooked in camel urine to produce a treatment for scrofula. Cupping, cautery, and venesection were widespread medical procedures, as they had been throughout late antiquity, and medical leeches were also used.

The means available to respond to serious physical injury were very limited, however, and such mishaps were often fatal. Broken limbs were massaged, rubbed with salves, and kept immobile to heal; wounds were cleaned with saltwort (high in alkali content), and ashes were used to stop bleeding. Recourse to surgery seems to have been limited almost entirely to simple straightforward cases (e.g. lancing a boil).

Intertwined among these measures was a broad range of beliefs and practices inspired, as in earlier periods, by a deep-seated animism. Deviations from good health, though viewed as ordinary physical problems, were also attributed to forces regarded as animate entities one had to outmanoeuvre, or subject to the power of some greater favourable force. In medicine it was common to see the influence of malicious spirit beings (called the *jinn*) or the evil eye at work, especially where epidemic disease was involved. Avoidance of illness thus involved not only practical therapeutic measures, but also magical precautions and remedies intended to defeat or ward off malevolent unseen forces. Incantations and charms were used for many medical problems, and medical amulets in the form of a necklace, collar, armband, or bracelet could contain defensive devices ranging from rabbit's feet or fox or cat teeth to the sap of the acacia tree, from coloured stones, ornaments, and bells, to menstrual rags or bones of the dead. Phrases used in oral charms could also be written down and worn as talismans, and magic bowls decorated with inscriptions bearing charms or incantations were believed to provide protection from all sorts of misfortune. Though differences on points of detail can often be identified among peoples from different ethnic and religious communities, there are also extraordinary correspondences (e.g. animal teeth as amulets, wolf gall and camel urine in recipes, etc.), and most importantly, the basic framework of juxtaposed and intertwined customs of practical and magical medicine is identical.

Medical practice was equally diverse. In pre-Islamic times the Arabic word-root *t-b-b*, which later came to refer to the administration of medical care within the humoral system, has almost always to do with incantations, charms and amulets – i.e. with esoteric matters rather than with the more empirical and practical alternatives. Someone who was *matbub* had not received medical care, but was afflicted by a spell; *tibb* was not medicine, but the manipulation of incantations and charms; and a *tabib* was not a doctor, but a purveyor of such religious services. One practitioner, al-Harith ibn Kalada, became so famous for his activities that he was known (or so later authorities tell us) as the *tabib* par excellence – 'tabib of the tribal Arabs'. To some extent magical medicine seems to have been practised as a specialisation, and the same may be said of cupping and phlebotomy. The more practical medicine, on the other hand, seems to have been the common stock in trade of society; its remedies were widely known and easily prepared, and self-help and treatment within the extended family continued to predominate, much as they had in ages past.

As some of the popular medical lore was of no use at all in preventing or treating medical ills, it is worth asking how such customs could survive in the face of what must have been repeated proofs of their worthlessness. That people often noticed this themselves is not in doubt, as their popular lore, especially proverbs and poetry, frequently comments on it. That such customs prevailed was thus not due to universal credulity, but more likely had to to with the inclination, in the face of long-prevailing custom, to regard failure in a specific rather than general sense. If an amulet failed to protect a villager in an epidemic, his death would be explained in specific terms – a poorly made amulet or an extremely powerful demon; far less common was the conclusion that amulets and talismans in general were useless.

In the aftermath of the Arab conquests this medical lore continued unchanged; indeed, exponents of the new faith of Islam at first had no reason to oppose it. The Koran says nothing about medicine, apart from a few comments assuring that there is no fault in the lame, the blind, or the sick, advising the faithful how to wash for prayer when they are sick, and claiming curative power for honey. On the other hand, Islamic scripture concedes the existence of spirit beings, especially the *jinn*, and repeatedly refers to their activities in the physical world. Popular medical lore was eventually confined and restrained in important ways in Islamic times – but only gradually, and certainly not in a simple straightforward manner.

Early Islamic medical discussions

The seventh and eighth centuries witnessed the gradual development of Islam from a simple monotheistic creed into a highly articulated religion confronting and resolving a vast array of questions in dogma and theology. As conversion swelled Muslim ranks and Islamic thought became more sophisticated in the seventh century, traditional popular medicine became embroiled in controversy over its animistic tenor; many customs came to be regarded as unacceptable as they came into conflict with emergent religious principles and ideas. People were quick to conclude, for example, that as God's word, the Koran must have magical powers which could be used in charms and incantations, or in 'medicines' consisting of the water used to wash verses off slates upon which they had been written. The early Muslims responsible for these formulations – like the Christian and Jewish exponents of medical folk-lore – would have argued that they were acting entirely within the proper bounds of their religion. But many other Muslims vigorously opposed both the use of the Koran for charms and incantations, and the widespread trend presenting the Prophet as a purveyor of such remedies; early Islam sought to eliminate pagan animism, not to tidy it up in a new monotheistic garb (though this was sometimes the result).

More specifically, numerous aspects of the traditional medicine posed significant dilemmas as the tenets of Islam were gradually elaborated. Here a major problem was the great plague pandemic (i.e. a cyclical series of epidemics) of 541–749. Early views had attributed the repeated epidemics to the *jinn*, set upon the faithful by their enemies. Through the eighth and early ninth centuries, however, this explanation was gradually displaced by arguments intended to orientate the entire problem of epidemic disease within the monotheistic framework of a God who ordained all things (including disease), and yet was just and merciful. Arguments also arose over the extent to which traditional medical beliefs contradicted specific points of emerging Islamic law. Animal bile and intoxicating beverages, for example, figured in both the humoral and popular traditions of pre-Islamic times, but both were anathema in strictly Islamic terms, the first as ritually unclean, the second as disapproved in the Koran. Incantations posed the problem of distinguishing between magic and pious pleas for divine succour, and a concerted effort was made to limit these to prayers to God for strength and relief.

As Islamic awareness and influence in society broadened and became more articulate, the fact that certain practices and beliefs were becoming increasingly questionable in Islamic terms served to weaken their authority as venerable custom. This in turn made it easier to bring other non-religious arguments to bear against them. Certain medical customs were repeatedly collected and commented upon as bedouin superstition and deluded whimsy, and were frequently the basis for proverbs on the theme of futility and ignorance.

Certain points concerning these debates bear special emphasis.

Firstly, they did not represent any official agenda or the interpretation of an educated elite, though by the late eighth century such an elite had formed and was involved in them. The accounts in which these arguments were embedded were in early Islamic times transmitted orally and would have been discussed, like other topics, in mosques, markets, and homes – wherever Muslims tended to congregate. And though their circulation was at first limited to the particular region where they had originated, Muslims by the ninth century were travelling widely on journeys in quest of learning which ensured that the various shades of opinion would eventually reach most parts of the Islamic world. In sum, these debates were not the preserve of the urban literati, but rather expressed the genuine concerns of society at large.

Secondly, the discussions should not be characterised as a systematic attack on magic, and even less on medicine. Indeed, medicine itself was encouraged. 'Should one go to the doctor (*tabib*)?', one saying of the Prophet has a man ask Muhammad; and the response is that he should, for 'God sends down no malady without also sending down with it a cure'. In this account, transmitted in many variant forms and one of the most widespread of medical sayings from the Prophet, a sharp distinction was now drawn between the old-style *tabib*, the master of spells and charms, and a different kind of *tabib* who searches out the cures provided by God, the giver of all things. But the critique was aimed not at 'medicine' *per se*, or even at magic, but rather at specific beliefs and customs which were deemed repugnant to religious sensibilities. 'Contagion', for example, was denied not because it was regarded as a false medical concept, but because the traditional lore viewed it in animistic terms and so exposed it to attack on religious grounds.

Finally, the outcome of these discussions varied. Some targeted practices disappeared, while in other cases the issue remained unresolved; many customs and beliefs formally disapproved by some authorities were not opposed by others, and in any case were still widely practised. Amulets and talismans of all kinds were recommended for protection against disease, most notably the plague (especially in the Black Death of 1347–49), and the belief that the *jinn* cause epidemics has in modern times become less influential only due to the increased control of epidemic disease, not to disbelief in spirit beings. The *jinn* continue to figure prominently in popular medicine, and numerous medical and other publications are devoted to their ways and advice on how to defeat them. Some pre-Islamic medical practices are still to be observed in the modern

Arab world, and Syriac collections of Christian charms and amulets against illness and many other kinds of misfortune were still being copied and used a hundred years ago. The debates served to highlight questions concerning the proper domain of medicine, but they did not – and indeed, could not – fix specific boundaries, much less enforce them.

The background to the revival of humoral medicine

The eastern Mediterranean world into which Islam expanded was a region undergoing profound changes. The reasons behind these patterns of transformation are complex and controversial, but a few salient features are beyond doubt. Prolonged warfare between the Byzantine and Persian empires had drained the resources of both sides and caused enormous destruction and social disruption; in the case of Byzantium, the strain on fiscal and manpower resources was made particularly severe by the efforts of Justinian I (reigned 524–65) to recover the western domains of the Roman Empire, and by his expensive building programmes. The advent of bubonic plague in 541 marked the beginning of a 200-year cycle of repeated outbreaks which devastated cities and wiped out villages throughout the eastern Mediterranean world. Christological controversies and related disputes made religion a focus of division rather than unity, and the centuries before the rise of Islam were characterised by the displacement of patterns of civic autonomy by increasing imperial interference in municipal affairs to satisfy ever-expanding demands for income.

The effects of these developments were profound. The vitality of cities was seriously sapped, and the disruption of agriculture and village life posed grave consequences for all urban centres, which were dependent upon their agrarian hinterlands for both foodstuffs and investment opportunities. Similarly, expanding imperial interference attracted investment away from regional centres to the seat of imperial power in Constantinople. Though much wealth remained concentrated in local hands, widespread urban recession is clear from the archaeological record.

These patterns in turn had an important impact on culture and learning. Local languages – Syriac in Syria, Coptic in Egypt – had long played important roles in Near Eastern society, and their advance was paralleled by a decline in the use of Greek. The provincials upon whom the 'high' culture had flourished ceased to make their way to the great regional centres, and traditional elites and the civic culture they represented were gradually replaced by the Church. In the Byzantine Empire the traditional forms of Greek secular culture had disappeared almost entirely by the end of the seventh century.

The fate of Greek humoral medicine in the sixth and seventh centuries must be viewed against this background, one in which the classical Greek heritage was being reinterpreted within the framework of shifting interests and priorities. Humoral medicine continued to be practised, especially in large centres (such as Alexandria), but its representation decreased as medicine moved into the domain of religion, where disease tested faith and punished sin and the Christian holy man healed all manner of ills by the power of the Lord. An apt and often-evoked image of the times was that of the physician, weak in faith and unable to cure himself, healed by a saint.

Similar changes may be seen in the educational and literary tradition. Teachers such as Asclepius and Palladius were active in the mid- and late sixth century, medical scholarship was in the early seventh century still represented by Paul of Aegina, and formal teaching in Alexandria may have continued after the Arab conquest of Egypt in the 640s. But overall, as interests shifted, the teaching of Graeco-Roman medicine seems to have declined sharply. Certainly, fewer and fewer books of the Greek medical corpus were available for study – only a small sampling of Galen could be pursued in depth, and access to his other works and to those of other scholars often required extensive inquiry, and in many places was probably impossible.

It may of course be doubted whether the Greek humoral medicine had ever displaced popular medicine and folklore at any level below that of the educated elite in the first place. But the increasingly dominant role of more spiritually oriented perspectives, coupled with the recession of traditional classical culture, tended to undermine Greek humoral medicine generally. The interesting juxtaposition of humoral and popular elements evident in the work of Alexander of Tralles (c. 570), which mixed Galenic teachings with charms, incantations, and even Jewish and Christian prayers, was perhaps typical. Though the exponent of secular culture was not an extinct species in the early medieval period, even the Byzantine Greeks of the seventh and eighth centuries looked back at classical times uneasily and used such terms as 'Hellenes' and 'Hellenism' to refer to the bad old pagan ways and those who adhered to them.

It has often been claimed that Arab-Islamic medicine as a formal tradition within a Greek humoral framework harks back to the time of the Prophet Muhammad himself and has connections with a Sasanian hospital and academy at Jundishapur in southern Persia. The Prophet's 'physician' al-Harith ibn Kalada travelled twice to Persia, we are told, was trained at Jundishapur, and engaged in a 'dialogue on medicine' with the Sasanian ruler Chosroes Anushirvan (reigned 531–78). In reality, however, there is no evidence that any academy ever existed at Jundishapur. The hospital there was a foundation of early Islamic times, and all of the medieval material on the ancient glories of the town is late in origin and may best be interpreted as literary invention inspired by the eminence of the Bakhtishu' family of Nestorian physicians (p. 129). Harith figures in the legend because of his reputation as 'tabib of the tribal Arabs'. But as we have seen, in Harith's own day tabib meant a worker of charms and spells. It was not until the late tenth century that material about the medical career of this once-obscure figure began to appear in earnest, and over the next 300 years successive layers of speculation and story-telling promoted him to the formally trained counterpart of the Byzantine and Sasanian court physician.

Aside from the folklore about Jundishapur we have only scanty and dubious information about a limited number of Arab, Greek, Syriac, and Jewish physicians in the sixth and seventh centuries, seldom with any clear indication of what sort of medicine they practised. Clearer indications can be seen in the translation of Greek texts (first into Syriac and later into Arabic) and in patronage of the sciences by a prince of the ruling Umayyad family, Khalid ibn Yazid (d. 704). But these and similar enterprises were individual efforts and limited in their impact. It was not until the early ninth century that the systematic revival of Greek humoral medicine began in earnest.

This revival arose from the confluence of three crucial factors, which explain both why it emerged when and where it did, and why non-Muslims were so prominent in it. The first was social and economic, the growth of an educated elite with broad interests and the financial resources required to fund scholarship, teaching, and the physical production and maintenance of collections of books. This development was especially pronounced in Iraq, where towns such as Basra and Kufa expanded from primitive garrison camps established by Arab armies in the 630s to become, by the mid- to late eighth century, vast thriving cities where cultural influences from places as remote as India and China were felt, and where the resources made available by officials and wealthy merchants and landowners promoted lively and sophisticated scholarship in a broad range of subjects. The founding of Baghdad in 762 led to a further surge of urban growth – within a century the new imperial capital was a focus of incredible wealth and cultural vitality and, with more than a million residents, perhaps the largest city in the world. As had been the case in early Roman Italy (pp. 39–40), patterns of increasing urbanisation were of decisive influence in the development of medicine.

Another key precondition was a specific need which a formal medical tradition could fill (excluding the well-being of the general population, with which the early caliphate was not particularly concerned). In fact, the developments of this period must be viewed within a context of ubiquitous religious disputation – among Christians, for example, over Church law, icons, and Christology, and among Muslims over dogma, theology, and the limits of legitimate political authority. Perhaps most significantly, there was a lively production of polemical and apologetical literature, with both Christian and Muslim seeking to justify their faith against the other. At the beginning, Muslims were at a disadvantage in these exchanges, for while Christians had for centuries used Greek logic and philosophy to elevate confessional quarrelling to an art, the defenders of Islam had no prior experience in disputation at this level. Not surprisingly, then, they began to turn to the same sources of inspiration which their Christian opponents had long used.

At the same time, however, Christians and Muslims had to deal with a common enemy, for equal to the threat each presented to the other was the challenge posed to both by the ancient doctrines of Manichaeism, a gnostic religious system based on a cosmology of opposing forces (matter/spirit, good/evil, etc.) and antithetical to the monotheistic belief in a benevolent, just, and unitary Creator/God. Though the ideas of Mani (late third century AD) were of little appeal to the common man, they did attract considerable attention from intellectuals and in the late eighth century the world view they embodied was espoused by many sophisticated Muslims. As emerges quite clearly in the formulations of Ibn al-Muqaffa' (d. c. 757), their arguments struck at the very heart of monotheistic religion – e.g. a God cannot be just who allows pestilence and famine to ravage the faithful and suffers ruin to spread through His creation. Such propositions brought bitter persecution down on the sect and its members, for not only was Manichaean dualism utterly irreconcilable with the tenets of monotheism in general, its sympathisers were often intellectuals and courtiers who stood (as Ibn al-Muqaffa' did) at the heart of the circles then striving to give direction and form to nascent Islamic culture.

Apart from shared enemies, there was much common ground between Muslims and Christians in this period. The Koran accepts numerous Old Testament prophets, manifests many Biblical parallels, acknowledges the virgin birth and miracles of Jesus, and regards him as a prophet. Numerous concerns over identical medical questions were also being raised: Muslim arguments over whether one should flee from the plague (which had, after all, been sent by God) were paralleled by similar discussions by the Chalcedonian monk Anastasius of Sinai (d. *c.* 700), for example, and Muslim debates about predestination and recourse to a physician were echoed by the Nestorian Hunayn ibn Ishaq (pp. 106–107).

The extent to which medical works could contribute to the religious concerns of the day was considerable. Paradigms for rational inference from empirical data (i.e. for formulating proofs for tenets of faith) were to hand on every side, religiously offensive passages were few and easily deleted or revised with minimal damage to the surrounding context, and Galen in particular offered powerful evidence for the ancient and much-used argument from design – if the parts of the body worked together for the benefit of the whole, for example, and accord to some principle of harmony and order, then this necessarily implied a giver of harmony and order, i.e. God. It did not pass unnoticed that such formulations provided powerful arguments against Manichaean dualism.

Of equal importance was the fact that after the Arab conquests the Arabic language began to spread at the expense of local and confessional languages. A key indicator, the advent of an Arabic translation of the Gospels, can be dated to the late eighth or early ninth century, and in general, by the ninth century a working knowledge of Arabic had become essential for serious work addressed to audiences beyond the confines of the monasteries. Eventually, even Syriac dictionaries and some Church histories were written with facing Arabic and Syriac texts, or in Arabic written in Syriac characters, so that Christians could use them. In summary, in the ninth century both Christians and Muslims stood to benefit from Arabic works which could be used in disputations to defend tenets of their faiths.

The third factor was the existence of a literary corpus to serve as a focus for scholarly work. Here the contribution of the Christian community was crucial, for though books seem to have been scarce in Byzantine lands, they were more accessible in Egypt, Syria, and Iraq. The main ecclesiastical libraries were large and varied, monasteries kept extensive collections of manuscripts (as they do to this day), and many texts were also in private hands. Whole batteries of scribes could be mobilised to produce copies of required works, and books were often loaned and sent long distances to be read and copied. It also seems that Muslim raiding forces sometimes brought back with them books they had found.

The era of the translators

The first phase of the Arab-Islamic medical tradition was thus a major translation movement brought about by these three factors. This is not to say that other considerations – general edification or interests in practical applications – played no role, but the overwhelmingly religious concerns of the day, undoubtedly the key influence on the articulation of Islamic philosophy at this time, were no less crucial in medicine.

The translation movement, already underway in the reign of Harun al-Rashid (reigned 786–809), gained decisive momentum during the caliphate of his son Ma'mun (reigned 813–33). A learned and sophisticated man, Ma'mun was a ruler confronted with the task of uniting and consolidating his authority over a vast empire suffering from the effects of several seriously divisive difficulties – four years of civil war, autonomist tendencies in various provinces of a far-flung empire, controversies over influences on nascent Islamic culture and theology, and socio-political problems focusing on fiscal policy and the legitimate sphere of imperial authority. It was against this background that the caliph took up the cause of the Mu'tazila, an expanding circle of speculative theologians seeking to articulate Islamic doctrine in a systematic fashion on rationalist foundations, and to mount a defence of Islam capable of meeting on equal terms the intellectual challenges posed by other religious systems. The agenda of the Mu'tazila was in no small part aimed to confront Christianity and Manichaeism, but their activities had other attractions as well. Their insistence on laying a rigorous rational foundation for religious discussions undercut the position of more traditional views asserting the literal authority of religious texts (i.e. over the caliph's desire to interpret them according to his own priorities); their receptivity to non-Arab and non-Islamic cultural and intellectual influences opened the way for the foundation of a new culture, Islamic in orientation and articulated in Arabic, but capable of integrating contributions from all the peoples of the empire and from other cultures (especially Byzantium and India) with which they were familiar; and several of their key doctrines, in particular the createdness of the Koran, favoured the aspirations of an absolutist caliph who, advised by an inner circle of select confidants, would himself decide what the nature and content of reform should be.

Such moves provoked a vigorous counter-reaction, and the next 50 years of Islamic history were dominated by controversy over the issues raised by the Mu'tazila. Beginning in the time of Ma'mun, then, those favourable to the Mu'tazila committed extremely high levels of political, social, and financial support to the task of encouraging its exponents and providing them with the materials necessary to support and justify their doctrinal positions.

A landmark in these efforts was the establishment in Baghdad in 832 of the Bayt al-Hikma, where scholars supervised by members of the Munajjim family (renowned as scholars, literati, and personalities at the Abbasid court) worked to collect important texts and to translate into Arabic a broad range of non-Arabic and non-Islamic works which could contribute to the tasks set by the regime. The name Bayt al-Hikma is usually translated 'House of Wisdom', and the institution itself is often regarded as an indubitable imitation of the 'academy' at Jundishapur. But in consideration of the spirit of the times, the title should rather be taken in its more juridical and dogmatic sense, as suggesting not a pursuit of truth wherever it might lie, but a choice among competing, exclusive, and unequivocal formulations on a given issue, one of which is to be upheld as absolutely true while the others are repudiated as absolutely false. In this context *hikma* thus means 'the authoritative alternative' or 'solution', and in social terms it can be traced to ancient Arab tribal custom. The foundation of an institution called 'Bayt al-Hikma' must also be seen as building upon an ongoing library tradition, though having nothing whatever to do with Jundishapur. Hence, while in important ways this development marked a major new turn in agenda, the factors of continuity were also significant.

The translation work associated with the Bayt al-Hikma was dominated by Christians, by virtue of their knowledge of Greek and Syriac and their prior experience in translation and intellectual debates. The most important of these figures was Hunayn ibn Ishaq (d. 873, later known in Europe as Johannitius), a Nestorian Christian from Hira (southern Iraq), long a Christian centre and a focus for Manichaean sympathies in the region. Hunayn was himself a Christian theologian and translator of the Old Testament into Arabic, and the fact that it was possible for him and his circle to play such a major role in the programme pursued by the Abbasids indicates, once again, the common ground between Christians and Muslims and the extent to which non-Muslims could participate in Islamic culture.

Much of what we know about Hunayn's activities comes from Hunayn himself, in particular his *Letter to 'Ali ibn Yahya*, one of the Munajjims, in which he describes his translation technique, comments on past translation work, and discusses 129 Galenic texts made available in Arabic or Syriac by himself and his circle. From this crucial work and his comments elsewhere we learn of difficult and long-ranging searches for desired books, the extreme care taken to render texts accurately, and the enormous materials – impressive in their range as much as in their bulk – which Hunayn and his colleagues produced.

At the same time, however, there is a great deal of fancy and embroidery to be taken into account, both in Hunayn's own descriptions of his work and in later accounts of it. For example, he often speaks of previous translations and their authors in extremely disparaging terms; but earlier translators, working with the paradigm of Bible translation in mind, had simply been anxious to produce a literal word-for-word rendering. Hunayn and his circle recognised, however, that translations so produced were sometimes intelligible only if one already knew the text (as, in the case of the Bible, people often did), and that scientific translations needed to convey the sense of the original, if not in precisely the same words or phrasing. Hunayn also gives a prominent place to Syriac in the translation programme. The part played by Syriac was indeed important in many instances, but for others it is not mentioned at all, and translation directly from Greek to Arabic was often possible – the famous Muslim littérateur Mas'udi (d. 956) refers to Hunayn's Arabic translation of the Old Testament as made directly from the Greek Septuagint and a work 'regarded by many people as the best translation' of it. It cannot be true that Hunayn (as he reports to 'Ali ibn Yahya) made a habit of carefully collating numerous Greek exemplars to produce a correct text before translating, while at the same time (as he repeatedly states in the *Letter*) manuscripts of Greek medical works were extremely rare and attainable only after much searching and enquiry. Such a critical method – the idea probably came to him from discussions by Galen – may have been feasible in certain specific instances, but in many, and perhaps most other cases, it would have been out of the question because of the scarcity of Greek manuscripts of the text – one cannot make a habit of collating numerous manuscript copies of a book when multiple copies of books are not routinely to hand. The surviving examples of Hunayn's translation work clearly establish him as a master, but he had, after all, an obvious vested interest in ensuring that others should appreciate the difficulty of his work and the level of his achievements.

Finally, later accounts of Ma'mun, Hunayn, and the translation movement in general sometimes prove to be the stuff of folklore and legend – Ma'mun, for example, is said to have obtained texts in the ancient sciences by asking the Byzantine emperor's permission to remove representative copies from libraries in Byzantine lands, but the source for this is a tale of a dream the caliph had of Aristotle. We are likewise told that Hunayn journeyed to Byzantine lands in search of manuscripts, travels about which Hunayn himself says nothing. Books were more likely obtained by travels to private collections in Syria, Mesopotamia, Persia, and Egypt (often mentioned by Hunayn), through the venerable custom of loans from monasteries (p. 104), and occasionally by seizure as booty during Arab campaigns in Asia Minor.

The output of the translation movement was vast in both range and content. Hundreds of Greek texts were rendered into Arabic, primarily works by Galen, but also including such authors as Rufus of Ephesus (pp. 59–60), for whom nearly 60 titles are recorded in Arabic. Greek was by far the preferred tradition, but works in Syriac, Pahlavi, and Sanskrit were also translated, reflecting, once again, the rich cultural tradition thriving in ninth-century Iraq.

The era of the translators continued into the early eleventh century, but a major change seems to have occurred by about 900. Through the time of Hunayn, the quest for and translation of ancient texts proceeded at a frenetic pace, encouraged by official sanction, generous patronage, and the immediacy of the debate at hand. But the definitive repudiation of Mu'tazilism by the caliph Mutawakkil (reigned 847–61) meant a sharp drop in the theological temperature; and the gradual demise of the Bayt al-Hikma and the drying up of patronage and financial support probably reflect the fact that as the amount of already translated material increased, the perceived need for further translation decreased. Though individuals continued to pursue translation work on their own, they were just that – individuals. It is revealing that Razi (pp. 112–13), for example, writing in the mid-tenth century, seems to regard the Arabic translations as a closed corpus; he knows of those who can read Greek and Syriac, but he sees them as informants who can check non-Arabic works in response to specific queries, rather than as translators themselves.

The impact of the translation movement was enormous, most obviously for the hundreds of ancient texts which it saved for posterity in Arabic. But beyond the factor of quantity was that of selection – as the favoured author was Galen, it was his work which set the standard for Arabic medicine in centuries to come. It was his system which prevailed throughout the Islamic lands, and even the works of the Hippocratic corpus were known primarily through the prism of Galen's commentaries. Further, the translation movement rose to prominence precisely when Arab-Islamic literary culture was generating masses of texts in many other subjects. Although we are told nothing about any connection, it is difficult to imagine how the high standards set by the translation movement for assessing, copying, and using manuscript texts could have failed to influence the ways in which Islamic culture in general came to set equally high standards for handling codices in all fields of learning.

The movement also provided the decisive impetus for the revival of Greek humoral medicine in an Arab-Islamic context in several ways. Firstly, it made Arabic a language in which original scientific scholarship could henceforth proceed. Prior to the translation movement, Arabic had no formal vocabulary for expressing philosophical or scientific concepts, and no exact terminology for names of diseases or their symptoms (as Hunayn himself observed). The efforts of the translators bequeathed to future generations a mode of scientific discourse in which even the most obscure and complex formulations – not just in medicine but in philosophy and science in general – could be articulated with precision and clarity. This endeavour, which Manfred Ullmann rightly characterises as the 'creation of a language', was one in which the translators received little support from professional philologists, who were more concerned to collect and study ancient poetry and elucidate philological difficulties in the Koran.

Secondly, the movement thrust into the arena of emergent Islamic culture a vast array of scholarship of manifest practical utility, and for the re-emergence of humoral medicine we need look no farther than the ranks of the translators themselves. Hunayn himself is perhaps the best example. The chronology of his works is largely unknown, but it seems that it was his theological interests which in the first instance led him to an interest in medicine as a specialisation; he was the son of a dealer in materia medica, but says nothing about any formal medical training and appears to have learned what he knew from his work as a translator. Eventually he took to composing his own works, often based on Graeco-Roman models (p. 122), and to practising medicine himself, eventually becoming court physician to the caliph Mutawakkil. Both of his sons followed the same path to medical practice, and the transition from medical translator to medical author and physician appears to have been common.

Finally, it must be noted that the translation movement was closely related to the discussions of popular medicine described above, in that both were part of the general debate among Muslims in the eighth and ninth centuries over what the content and direction of Islamic culture was to be. Just as discussions of the former decided, through arguments largely pursued through traditions attributed to the Prophet Muhammad, how and to what extent the old medical folklore would be accommodated within Islam, the translation movement determined, through its selection of specific works and by its adjustments to offensive or troublesome passages (e.g. references to the pagan gods in the Hippocratic *Oath*) the ways in which ancient literary culture was to contribute to that of Islam. The Bayt al-Hikma clearly played a central role in the movement, but patronage of translators extended beyond the Abbasid regime to include many private individuals. The movement thus injected into emergent Islamic thought a profoundly rationalist current which was to dominate Islamic humoral medicine (and science more generally) throughout the medieval period, and even to set the standard for what formal medicine was. Physicians knowledgeable in the Greek tradition looked down on those who were not, and this perception came to be widely shared in high society at large. At the same time, the translation movement, insofar as it made concessions to new religious sensibilities, laid the foundations for a medical tradition which was more generally monotheist than specifically Islamic in tone, indicative, again, of the broad concerns motivating the movement in the first place. The tradition thus, on the one hand, always allowed for large-scale participation by non-Muslim practitioners and thinkers, and on the other, manifested a certain ambivalence which often rendered its Islamic credentials suspect.

The growth of the literary tradition

Though there was no distinct break between the era of the translators and that of the later masters, medicine in about 900 was very different from what it had been in the heyday of Hunayn 50 years earlier. While the earlier period was dominated by efforts to render what was already known into Arabic, later times were increasingly devoted to new scholarship. The result was an entirely new genre of Arab-Islamic literature which was vigorously pursued for nearly a millennium. It generated thousands of works produced by authors ranging from some of the greatest scholars of the age to utterly unknown local figures, and in some parts of the world its classics are still esteemed today as relevant to modern medical needs.

The early translators who wrote original medical works produced mainly specialised treatises. Hunayn, for example, wrote a series of essays on ophthalmology now known as his *Kitab al-'ashr maqalat fi l-'ayn* ('Book of the Ten Treatises on the Eye'). These were pioneering studies in ophthalmology and laid the foundations for future research which established Arab-Islamic science as the leader in this field. A further shift toward original scholarship can be seen in the career of Qusta ibn Luqa (d. 912), a younger Christian contemporary of Hunayn in Baghdad. Qusta collected and translated Greek texts, but primarily pursued his own research in physics, mathematics, astronomy, and especially medicine. Many of the more than 60 titles attributed to him are lost, but those that survive reflect the thought of a broadly learned scholar.

By the late ninth century, researchers in medicine had access to a rapidly expanding corpus of original scholarship. This trend continued for several hundred years and produced many specialised monographs of fundamental importance. One of the most outstanding was the *Fi l-hasba wa-l-judari* ('On Smallpox and Measles') by Razi (pp. 112–13). Here questions of pathology, diagnosis, therapeutics, and materia medica were all brought together in a brilliant contribution (if not the first) to the treatment of smallpox (measles is only a secondary concern).

As the sheer quantity of this material increased, the need arose for

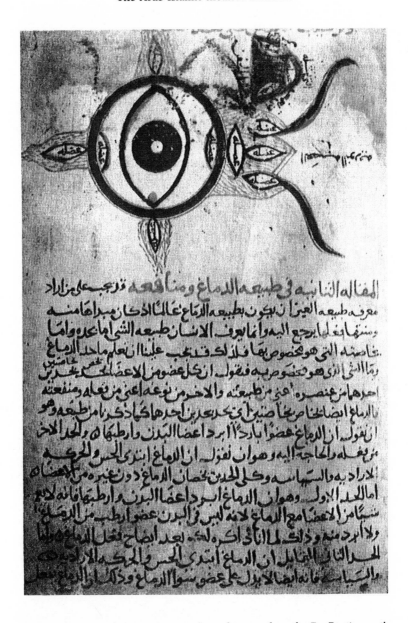

Fig. 13. The eye, with connecting muscles and nerves, from the *Ten Treatises on the Eye* by Hunayn ibn Ishaq, Treatise II. Following Greek thinking, Hunayn believed that perceived images were the result of light reflected from objects meeting in the air with luminous rays emanating from the luminous spirit which streamed forth from the brain and out through the eye. (Cairo, Dar al-Kutub al-Misriya, Ms. Taymur Tibb 100.)

111

more synthetic writing providing ready access to the essential information across the whole range of an expanding discipline. The efforts to fill this need gave rise to the most prominent literary achievement of Arab-Islamic medicine, the medical compendium. This must be viewed within the context of research in other areas in the ninth and tenth centuries, when similar works were appearing in such fields as history, lexicography, *belles lettres*, and Koranic exegesis. In all these disciplines, authors wrote ambitious compendia not just to collect what was already known, but also to pursue its implications to their appropriate conclusions, fill in gaps, and so to produce broadly authoritative works.

In medicine, the first great compendium was the *Firdaws al-hikma* ('Paradise of Wisdom') by Rabban al-Tabari (*c.* 850), in which the author, a Jewish convert to Islam, prepared a 350-chapter summary of the medical knowledge of his day for the caliph Mutawakkil. His sources were Arabic and Persian translations of ancient texts, including not only Greek authorities, but also Indian and Persian writers.

The early date of Tabari's work is evident in his innocent interweaving of rational and magical lore, and even more in his interest in non-Greek medical traditions. The presence of a considerable body of Indian medical lore in his compendium indicates that he considered it possible to make use of various medical traditions within an Islamic framework, and hence also that in his day the Greek tradition had not yet gained the authority it was to achieve later. As Tabari lived and worked in northern Persia, where eastern influences were strong, the possibility of such a synthesis may have seemed very real indeed. These prospects receded, however, as Graeco-Roman medicine became increasingly dominant.

The following generation produced one of the greatest Muslim physicians and philosophers, Razi (known in the Latin West as Rhazes, d. 925). A student of the natural sciences, alchemy, and music in his youth, Razi travelled from his native Rayy (in northern Persia) to Baghdad at about the age of 30 and studied medicine. His career included directorships of hospitals in both Rayy and Baghdad, and he composed about 200 books on medicine, logic, philosophy, theology, the natural sciences, alchemy, astronomy, and mathematics. In addition to his study of smallpox (p. 110), two medical works are of particular importance. His *Al-Kitab al-mansuri fi l-tibb* ('The Mansurian Book of Medicine') was composed for and dedicated to the governor of Rayy, Mansur ibn Ishaq (d. 914–15), and covered the various fields of medicine in 10 books generally adhering to a theoretical/practical mode of organisation which, as we have seen (p. 81), had already become prominent in the medical literature of late antiquity. Books I–VI treated topics Razi regarded as theoretical: diet, hygiene, anatomy, physiology, general pathology, and materia medica, while the last four books dealt with practical matters: diagnosis, therapy, special pathology, and surgery. The work as a whole was extensively used by later authors, and the special pathology of Book IX was especially esteemed for its discussion of diseases and other medical problems from head to foot. In about 1175 the *Mansuri* was translated into Latin in Toledo by Gerard of Cremona (d. 1187) and entitled *Liber medicinalis ad almansorem* or simply *Liber almansoris*; Book IX was extracted and circulated under its straightforward book number in Latin form, *Liber nonus*. The later Latin commentaries on the work, especially on the *Liber nonus*, were extensive and were still being published as late as the seventeenth century. Translations were also made into Greek and Hebrew.

Like many medieval scholars, Razi kept detailed notes and copied potentially useful passages from books he read. These notes on pathology and therapy seem to represent his 'files', each consisting of a quire of pages devoted to a particular subject and gradually filled as Razi added quotations and his own observations. When one quire was filled, another would be added, producing a kind of *aide-mémoire*, well organised at the level of primary subjects but difficult to use at any more detailed level. It is tempting to see in such a system a response to the need for organized access to medical information in an era when comprehensive medical compendia were not yet widely available. Such notes would not have been compiled with broader circulation in mind, but Razi's jottings and reflections were gathered together after his death and published. The resulting compendium, called *Al-Hawi fi l-tibb* ('The All-Inclusive Work on Medicine'), was a vast book of which complete copies soon became rare, but despite its size, problematic organisation, and scarcity it proved influential. In Europe it became available in a Latin translation, entitled the *Continens*, by Faraj ibn Salim.

The development of the Arabic medical compendium culminates in works by two authors of the tenth and eleventh centuries. On one, Majusi (Haly Abbas, d. late tenth century), little is known about his personal life apart from the fact that he was from Ahwaz (southern Persia). He was attached to 'Adud al-Dawla (reigned 949–83), the powerful Buyid ruler of Iraq and parts of Persia, and it was to this prince that he dedicated his only medical work, the *Kamil al-sina'a al-tibbiya* ('The Complete Medical Art'). Following the example of Razi (of whom he was nevertheless a critic), he divided this work into two sections on theoretical and practical medicine, each of which included 10 different treatises on specialised topics; in his introduction he gave an especially valuable assessment of the development of medicine up to his own day. The *Kamil* paid greater attention to certain subjects than Razi had (especially anatomy and surgery), and was both more compact than the vast *Hawi* (and hence easier for the scribe to copy and the scholar to afford) and more comprehensive than the *Mansuri*. An eminently practical work, it was so well organized and accessible that it secured Majusi's medical reputation and eventually occupied a place second only to that of the *Qanun* of Ibn Sina. In Europe the *Kamil* was translated into Latin twice: by Constantine the African (*fl.* 1080) under the title *Liber pantegni*, and then in 1127 by Stephen of Antioch as the *Liber regius*.

The multi-faceted talents of the second author, Ibn Sina (Avicenna, d. 1037), were already evident in his youth, though it may be unwise to trust his claim that he was practising medicine at the age of 16. He served as a jurist and held several government positions in Persia, but his primary interests were philosophy and medicine, and these concerns dominate his bibliography of over 250 titles. In medicine his great work was his *Al-Qanun fi l-tibb* ('Canon of Medicine'), which abandoned the theoretical/practical division of Razi and Majusi in favour of a more rigorous approach. For Ibn Sina, medicine was a subordinate science within the domain of the Aristotelian natural sciences in general, and as such could only be understood and practised in terms of the laws and principles governing those disciplines. In the *Qanun*, this resulted in the organisation of Galen's medical writings into a definitive system governed by Aristotelian philosophy, the most prominent aspect of this being the fusion of Galen's humoral system with Aristotle's doctrine of three life forces – psychic, natural, and human. Arguments and conclusions on particular subjects which had originally been scattered through the vast Galenic corpus were now drawn together into definitive discussions related to one another through a strictly logical hierarchy of five books subdivided into treatises and chapters. Book I covers what Ibn Sina calls 'universals' (*kulliyat*): medical theory, aetiology, hygiene, therapy, and surgery – i.e. a systematic framework for medical practice; Book II presents the simple drugs of Arabic materia medica in detail; Book III discusses diseases from head to foot; Book IV considers general pathology (i.e. medical problems which did not belong in Book III), fevers, pustules and abcesses, wounds, poisons, surgery, fractures, and obesity and emaciation; and Book V covers compound drugs.

The *Qanun*'s primary importance lay in its systematisation of medicine, and it was the precision and thoroughness with which this goal was pursued that gave the work authoritative sway over the discipline for hundreds of years and won its place among the masterpieces of Arab-Islamic science. But Ibn Sina was not creating system for its own sake; he sought to place in the hands of physicians a single exhaustive work which set medical practice on solid theoretical foundations and connected its various subfields in a comprehensive logical fashion. (Galen's works lent themselves very well to this sort of treatment, since the essential link between theory and practice had been a prominent imperative in his thought.) In the *Qanun*, discussions of the four elements and generation and corruption, for example, justify discourses elsewhere on such topics as the preparation of compound drugs for specific diseases, surgery and the dressing of wounds, and obstetrics and gynaecology. It is also worth noting that the work's reception was not limited to assent, but included centuries of discussion and criticism in the form of a broad-ranging commentary literature (p. 123).

The impact of the work was equally great in Europe. About 100 years after Ibn Sina's death, Gerard of Cremona in Toledo translated his masterpiece into Latin as the *Canon*. This rendering was later reworked and improved by Andrea Alpago (d. 1520), a physician and scholar who had worked for many years in Damascus, the seat of the Venetian consulate, and who had access to older Arabic manuscripts. The improved version was published in Venice in 1527, and was reprinted more than 30 times in the fifteenth and sixteenth centuries. A Hebrew translation was also published, and later European commentaries in Latin, Hebrew, and the various vernaculars are practically beyond counting. As the medical historian Max Meyerhof has observed, probably no medical work ever written has been so much studied.

These compendia all originated in Persia, but important work was also produced elsewhere. One from Spain merits special attention. Little is known about the physician Zahrawi (Albucasis, *fl. c.* 940), apart from his authorship of a medical compendium organised in 30 treatises and entitled *Al-Tasrif li-man 'ajaza 'an al-ta'lif* ('The Recourse of Him

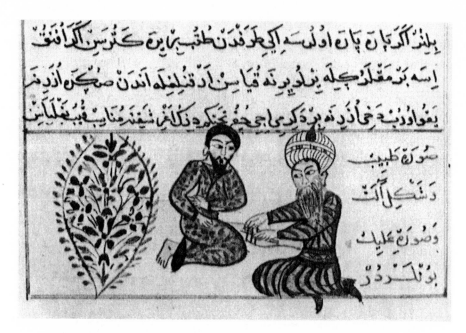

Fig. 14. A physician treating a patient with a broken leg, from the Turkish translation of Zahrawi's *Tasrif*. Note the splints and padding, to which Zahrawi had
attached great importance. (Paris, Bibliothèque Nationale, Ms. suppl. turc 693.)

Who Cannot Compose [a Medical Work of His Own]'). Though similar
in some ways to other compendia, it also considers topics not well covered elsewhere – midwifery, the raising and education of children,
cooking, weights and measures, psychology, and the flora and fauna of
Spain. Its section on surgery is particularly important for its detailed
coverage and nearly 200 illustrations of surgical instruments. The book
was partially translated into Latin by Gerard of Cremona, and its book
on surgery was of enormous influence in Europe.

While it would be anachronistic to judge, in terms of originality,
works from a tradition which took for granted the authority of the
ancient masters, it is worth observing that Arab-Islamic medicine made
important new contributions in numerous areas. In ophthalmology, for
example, scholars from Hunayn to Ibn al-Haytham (Alhazen, d. 1038,
also from southern Iraq), added much to medical knowledge of the eye,
vision, ailments involving the eye, and more generally, to the science of
optics. Also important was the contribution to pharmacology. The
lands conquered by Arab armies were full of plants, animals, and minerals not found elsewhere, and the various cultures in these lands had

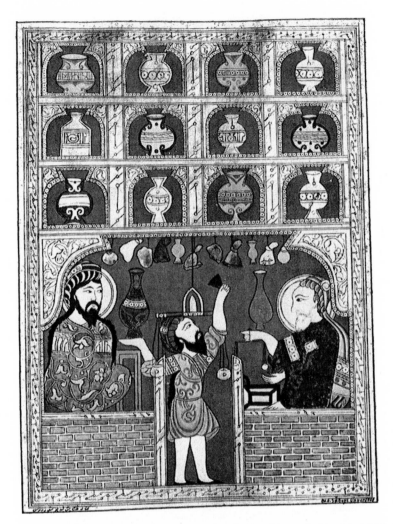

Fig. 15. A Baghdad pharmacist's shop in 1224, illustrated in an Arabic manuscript of the *De materia medica* of Dioscorides. This illustration is probably correct in its (unintended) implication that of the vast range of simples known to the medieval Islamic materia medica collections, pharmacists actually dispensed only a small selection of the most commonly used items. (Istanbul, Aya Sofia Müzesi, Ms. 3703.)

their own systems in which the medical uses and perils of all these were set forth. The rise of Arabic pharmacology, beginning in the ninth century, thus involved the tasks of collating names and descriptions coming into Arabic from many other languages, harmonising diverse descriptions of their nature and use into one system, generating standards for expressing and comparing weights and measures, and unify-

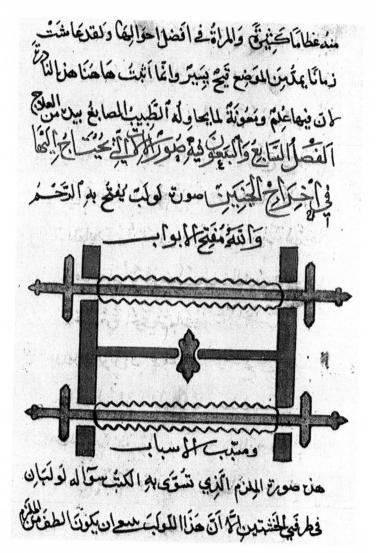

منه عظاما كثيرة والمراثي في أفضل احوالها ولقد عاشت

زمانا يمكن من المضجع تنجح بيسير وانما اثبت هاهنا هذا النا

لان فيها علم ومعونة لما يحاوله الطبيب الصانع بين من العلج

الفصل السابع والبعوذية صور الالي التي يحتاج اليها

في اخراج الجنين اصورة لولب يفتح به الرحم

والله مفتح الابواب

ومسبب الاسباب

هذه صورة الملزم الذي تسوى به الكتب سماه لوليان

فطبق في الخشبتين اعلم ان هذا اللولب سمى ان يكون الطفل

Fig. 16. Illustration of a kind of vaginal speculum from the *Tasrif* of Zahrawi. As this example clearly shows (cf. Fig. 17), the illustrations in manuscripts of the *Tasrif* often represent the results of repeated copying by scribes unfamiliar with the items they were drawing, and thus provide only general impressions of what were certainly precision instruments of a high professional standard. (Berlin, Deutsche Staatsbibliothek, Ms. Or. 91.)

ing the results of scholarship in botany, zoology, chemistry, toxicology, and materia medica. The scale of this enterprise may be gauged from the fact that while the materia medica of Dioscorides (p. 57) had included only about 850 plants, animals, and minerals, that of the widely travelled Andalusian Ibn al-Baytar (d. 1248) listed over 3000,

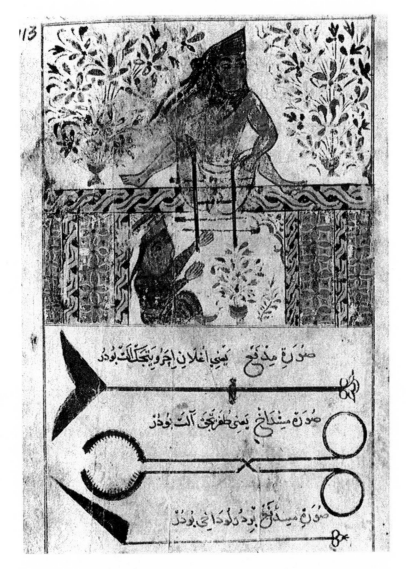

Fig. 17. Use of the instrument shown in Fig. 16 in the delivery of a child. This is one of 140 illustrations of surgical procedures in Sharaf al-Din Sabuncuoglu's Turkish translation of Zahrawi's *Tasrif*, presented to the Sultan Mehmet II, the conqueror of Constantinople, in 1465. (Istanbul, Millet Kütüphanesi, Ms. Tibb 79.)

based on over 250 sources ranging from Dioscorides and Galen to Razi, Ibn Sina, and other Muslim researchers.

In surgery the advances were especially prominent. New medical procedures were developed, including extremely delicate operations for ophthalmological complaints, repair of major abdominal injuries which

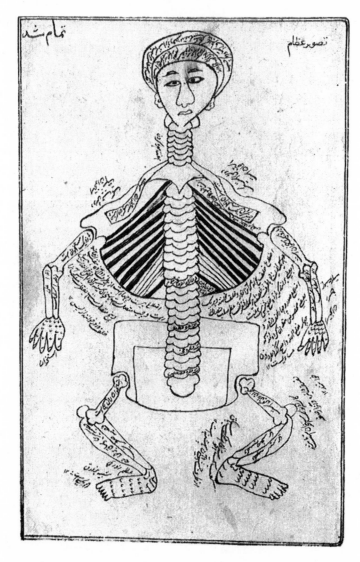

Fig. 18. The human skeletal system, from the 'Five-Figure Set' which appeared in Islamic medical texts beginning with the *Tashrih-i Mansuri* of Ibn Ilyas. This is an example from about the eighteenth century. (London, Wellcome Institute Iconographic Collections.)

previously would have been written off as lethal, and the use, for the first time, of animal gut as a suturing material. Increasingly sophisticated procedures were accompanied by advances in medical instrumentation. The extremely patchy evidence makes it difficult to discern which cases represented new creations, but it is at least clear that there were significant improvements in the design of such instruments as scissors, trocars, syringes, lithotrites, various probes and exploratory devices, and in the field of gynaecology, obstetric forceps.

Particularly intriguing, where surgery is concerned, is the Persian *Tashrih-i Mansuri* ('Mansurian Anatomy'), written by Ibn Ilyas in 1396. This work of descriptive anatomy devoted separate chapters to the skeletal, nervous, muscular, venous, and arterial systems, and was built around a set of five full-body illustrations showing the layout of each system (cf. p. 120), with some manuscripts bearing additional illustrations of a pregnant woman carrying a foetus in a transverse or breech position. (There is also a second female figure marked to show cautery points, but this belongs to a totally different tradition.) Inaccuracies and ambiguities abound in these diagrams, which represent a tradition long pre-dating Ibn Ilyas (a nine-figure set belonging to the same tradition was already known in Europe before his time); but they became very popular and were often tipped into appropriate places in copies of older texts (e.g. the *Qanun* of Ibn Sina). The emergence of anatomical illustration on such a scale is in itself a development of great importance – one of the greatest problems in medieval surgery was the rather rudimentary knowledge of the internal systems of the human body (p. 131), and Ibn Ilyas' diagrams reflect both the state of this knowledge and an ongoing effort to improve it.

One area where the formative role of the Arab-Islamic tradition is as yet little appreciated is that of contagion. That disease could pass directly from one victim to another was known in antiquity, but as a formal medical doctrine contagion was almost entirely ignored in the Galenic tradition. In early Islamic times the notion became a focus of religious controversy (p. 98), and this dispute may well have been the catalyst that drew physicians to its defence. A detailed and sophisticated account by Qusta ibn Luqa in the ninth century seems to mark an advanced stage in the discussion, and by that time contagion, if not always distinguished from simple infection, was a widespread medical doctrine which figured prominently in both literature and practice.

All of these contributions were of great importance, and not least of all to Western medicine, since many of these works were eventually translated into Latin. But the greatest contribution of Arab-Islamic medicine was that it systematised and unified the field of medicine as never before. The greatness of the works of such authors as Majusi and Ibn Sina lies not in their originality, but in the devastating thoroughness with which they drew together what was known in many discrete fields and harmonised it in such a way that it both made sense intellectually and gave the physician ready access to the information he needed for his practical work, all this within the confines of a single (albeit very large) book.

The dissemination of medical learning

The dissemination of this medical learning proceeded in several important ways. Firstly, while leading works in other fields could quickly become rare, medical texts were copied and recopied on a scale which, considering the time, skill, and expense required, can only be described as vast. For example, over 5000 medical manuscripts in Arabic, Turkish, and Persian survive in both public and private libraries in modern Turkey, and cover about 1000 works by more than 400 authors. There are more than 50 complete or partial copies of Ibn Sina's *Qanun*, and manuscripts of the many later commentaries on it are even more numerous.

Secondly, the exponents of medical scholarship as a whole sought to circulate it as widely as possible. Hunayn, for example, wrote a book entitled *Al-Masa'il fi l-tibb* ('Questions on Medicine'), a teaching text written – following a classical model – in a question-and-answer format and composed so as to lead the student from simple to more complex medical problems and issues. This work is also known, quite appropriately, as his *Al-Madkhal ila l-tibb* ('Introduction to Medicine'), and in fact many authors wrote introductory manuals (often with exactly this title) aimed at the aspiring novice. In Europe such texts were often translated into Latin, Hunayn's by Constantine the African (pp. 140–41).

Humoral medical writers also sought to make the results of their work accessible to the literate layman, a trend already evident in Razi's *Man la yahduruhu l-tabib* ('He Who Has No Physician to Attend Him'). The Iraqi physician Ibn Butlan (d. 1063) devotes his *Taqwim al-sihha* ('The Proper Pursuit of Health') to the presentation in terse tabular form of everything he could collect pertaining to the six Galenic non-naturals, and leaves the reader in no doubt as to why he proceeded in this fashion:

> People are dissatisfied at the length to which the learned pursue
> their discussions and the prolixity encountered when these are set
> down in writing in books; what [laymen] need from the sciences is
> that which will benefit them, not the proofs for these things or their
> definitions.

This agenda was widely pursued in the tenth to thirteenth centuries, and a Christian physician like Qusta ibn Luqa found no impediment to writing a book of advice on how the Muslim pilgrim could stay healthy and avoid mishaps on his way to Mecca. These works too were prime candidates for Latin translation.

Thirdly, while the era of the great Arabic medical compendia may be said to have ended with the *Qanun* of Ibn Sina, these works long continued to attract scholarly attention. No fewer than 15 later authors wrote commentaries on the *Qanun* of Ibn Sina, for example, and these commentaries in turn were the bases for supercommentaries and glosses. It has long been customary to deprecate such commentaries, but they are undervalued today because the commentary mode of discourse not only makes them appear to be unoriginal to modern scholars, but also has the deleterious effect of fragmenting the main trends of thought into disconnected comments on discrete points of detail. This meant that many independent remarks, like those on the pulmonary circulation by the Damascene commentator Ibn al-Nafis (d. 1288), were less likely to provoke further discussion, and, in the case of Ibn al-Nafis, in fact did not do so. Still, such works were very useful. To the physician unable to find or afford copies of such massive classics as the *Qanun* they offered ready access to the main arguments and most important points advanced by the masters, while to the student and layman they conveyed the gist of the tradition in a more accessible form.

The medical literature of medieval Islamic culture was thus an enormous corpus sufficiently varied to be accessible to much of literate society, and it was also well distributed. Work proceeded in centres scattered from Spain to India, and once in circulation, books passed from one urban centre to another, carried along the main routes by merchants, pilgrims, and travelling scholars, and with their circulation stimulated by a brisk book trade. Copies of medical texts were widely available in the libraries of mosques and schools (the *madrasas*), and in private collections, even those of individuals who were not physicians. It was this diffusion of scholarship which allowed Qayrawan in modern-day Tunisia, and such flourishing Spanish cities as Cordova, Granada, Seville, and Toledo, to benefit from scientific works published thousands of miles away in the East; Europe's debt to it is just as great, since it was in part through Qayrawan and the Spanish centres that Arabic medical works passed to Italy and France.

Humoral medical scholarship was paralleled by a trend to incorporate medical learning into Islamic culture at a more general level. In his cultural encyclopaedia *Al-Nuqaya fi l-'ulum* ('The Select Work on the Sciences'), Suyuti (d. 1505), for example, included medicine and anatomy among the 14 topics – including Koranic exegesis, jurisprudence, grammar, calligraphy, and rhetorical skills – with which the educated Muslim should be familiar. Especially prominent was the tendency for popular tales and literary narratives to present ancient medical personalities as Islamically unobjectionable sages, and in one branch of Arabic literature the category of 'physician' became the focus of a series of works, culminating in the *'Uyun al-anba' fi tabaqat al-atibba'* ('Pristine Sources of Information on the Classes of Physicians'), a collection of notices on almost 400 medical personalities compiled by the Syrian Ibn Abi Usaybi'a (d. 1270). These works appear to be biographical dictionaries of physicians, and do contain valuable historical information. But their literary tenor is manifest in the entertaining tales and poetry which figure so prominently in them, as also in the fact that genuinely biographical material (e.g. birth and death dates, education or professional interests) is often incidental, highly speculative, or absent altogether. The anecdotal element has wrought much mischief in modern research, but indicates a major way in which medical learning was assimilated into Islamic culture.

Of even greater importance in this regard is the so-called *Tibb al-nabi*, or 'Medicine of the Prophet'. As we have seen (p. 98), traditions ascribed to the Prophet Muhammad were used early on in debates over important issues, including medicine. It was noticed, for example, that humoral medicine sometimes prescribed a medicament that would violate Islamic law (e.g. the drinking of alcohol or the ingestion of potions made with ritually unclean or forbidden substances), so the question was put: Does the prohibition apply in the case of someone whom the substance might cure? Cases calling for amputation raised the problem of whether, on the Judgment Day, God would regard this as an attempt to escape His will. Such issues were addressed not by posing direct questions, but by recalling an identical or analogous situation with which the Prophet or one of his companions had allegedly dealt.

By the mid-ninth century, collections of these sayings and stories, the *hadith*, were including chapters devoted to traditions on medicine. Ibn Abi Shayba (d. 849) has the largest collection of this early material, and his student Bukhari (d. 856) includes in his *Sahih* a selection more conservative in both scope and numbers. The *hadith* collections were extremely influential, and new traditions, addressing new medical questions, continued to appear. These medical materials were ultimately compiled in separate works, the fullest being that of the Syrian jurist Ibn Qayyim al-Jawziya (d. 1350). If Qusta ibn Luqa is representative, humoral physicians in early Islamic times despised this lore, but by the thirteenth century their objections had largely been overcome. 'Abd al-Latif al-Baghdadi (d. 1231), for example, not only wrote important works on medicine and the natural sciences, but also compiled a *Medicine of the Prophet*.

Europe seems to have been unaware of this literature, but it is relevant here since it is often claimed that these works were written to oppose Greek-inspired medicine by providing an Islamic alternative. But the 'Medicine of the Prophet' simply reflects an ongoing interest in medical issues among a religiously educated public familiar with the medical chapters and traditions in the early *hadith* collections. Hippocrates, Dioscorides, Galen, Aristotle, and Plato are quoted as eminent authorities, and the Greek humoral system eventually comes to exercise a very powerful influence. It is also sometimes claimed that the 'Medicine of the Prophet' is bedouin superstition in pious Islamic dress, but this too is wrong. As argued above (pp. 98–9), these traditions – including many favourable to talismans, amulets, and various magical procedures – reflect beliefs and customs common at the popular level among all peoples of the early medieval Near East; further, they represent a process of argument which was not opposed to any category of medical lore *per se*, but rather sought to reduce elements considered inimical in Islamic terms. The 'Medicine of the Prophet' combines humoral medical axioms, aphorisms, and basic precepts with popular folklore, common-sense traditions, and religious dictums, and they offer advice on the use and efficacy of many items of materia medica. As in the literary works about physicians, Islamic society is here appropriating medicine on its own terms, albeit here at a more popular level.

Medicine in Arab-Islamic society

It is often proposed that the formation of a formal medical profession in medieval Europe and the rise of elaborate medical institutions, especially hospitals, was to some extent inspired or even directly influenced by models in the Islamic world (pp. 93, 150–53). Though this is difficult to prove, it is certainly true that there were ample opportunities for Arab-Islamic models to be observed in detail. The opportunity usually cited, the Crusades, may have been of some influence, but was certainly not the only, or even the most important one. The political and religious antipathy between Europe and Islam was often of little impact in other spheres, and there was, for example, usually a brisk trade back and forth across the Mediterranean, especially between the ports of Italy and those of Egypt and North Africa. Merchants, pilgrims, and official embassies all made their way to Islamic lands; and in the other direction, Middle Eastern physicians took advantage of opportunities to render their services in Christian domains. Egyptian doctors practised in the Byzantine Empire, for example, and the great Latin translator, Constantine the African, seems to have been of Tunisian origin. An assessment of medicine in Arab-Islamic society thus serves not only to indicate how the textual tradition manifested itself in medical practice in the lands of its origin, but also to suggest patterns against which developments in Europe might fruitfully be compared.

Medical and public health conditions in the Middle East were as bad as in other parts of the world before the advent of modern medicine and the implementation of public health schemes broad enough to affect the lives of the common man. The vast majority of people were peasants in the agrarian hinterlands, and most of the rest were labourers in urban centres. Poverty, hunger, and malnutrition rendered these people especially and constantly susceptible to illness and physical mishap. Fractures and other injuries which today threaten little more than prolonged inconvenience and discomfort, in medieval times were often fatal. Endemic diseases such as dysentery, leprosy, malaria, scurvy, tuberculosis, and typhus were widespread, and parasitic infections and eye diseases like trachoma and conjunctivitis were common.

It is often claimed that Middle Eastern towns were cleaner than their European counterparts, but the evidence against this is overwhelming. Although there were elaborate sewage disposal systems in some towns (Fustat in Egypt is the most famous example), the effective disposal of refuse and waste always depends on the availability of huge amounts of water and the efficient functioning of elaborate (and therefore expensive) networks dedicated to their removal. In no medieval town were either water supplies or disposal systems ever up to the formidable task confronting them, and we often read of how filthy these places were. Garbage was cast into the streets or nearby bodies of water, dead animals were abandoned without proper disposal, and water supplies were often polluted. Domestic animals in both cities and rural villages were often kept in the home with the family, and vermin infestation of homes, clothing, and hair was almost impossible to prevent or combat.

These problems were of course most difficult in urban centres, where epidemic diseases wrought great havoc. Medieval sources usually refer to outbreaks of 'pestilence', and without details of symptoms it is impossible to identify the disease in question. Smallpox is sometimes specifically named, but the greatest scourge was undoubtedly the plague, which devastated the Middle East in a series of outbreaks between 541 and 749. It then largely faded away, only to return with the Black Death in 1347–49 (about which more will be said in Chapter 5) and to recur on numerous occasions until the advent of modern medicine in the region in the nineteenth century. Plague mortality in the medieval Middle East is as uncertain as anywhere else, but it is clear that epidemics often wiped out entire families and even villages. In large cities one outbreak of the disease could certainly kill tens of thousands of people, and in some cases the mortality was even higher; in the Black Death in 1348, the plague killed about 200,000 people in Cairo alone.

The medical practitioner

To confront the dangers posed by these problems a wide range of medical practitioners and services emerged. Even if one excludes the purveyors of popular folklore, the humoral physicians who remain were themselves a very disparate lot. In the ninth century the profession was dominated by Christians, with a lesser number of Jews and pagans. The Christians were particularly prominent not because of their central position in the translation movement, but rather because of the long tradition of medical learning within the ecclesiastical hierarchy. Many leading churchmen in the towns were physicians, and in both urban and rural monasteries many monks also had some medical expertise. Later trends toward conversion largely eliminated the pagan element and significantly diminished the ranks of the Christian practitioners, while increasing numbers of Muslims entered medical practice and the Jewish element remained (insofar as we can judge such matters) about the same. But as has been stressed above, the rise of Arab-Islamic medicine created a central discipline within Islamic science and culture which allowed for the participation of many non-Muslims. Christians still dominated the medical profession in Palestine in the tenth century, and in Egypt and North Africa Jewish doctors were very prominent throughout medieval times. The well-known North African Muslim physician Ibn al-Jazzar (d. *c.* 1004), for example, studied with the great Jewish doctor and writer on fevers Ishaq al-Isra'ili (Isaac Judaeus, d. 955).

In intellectual terms physicians again display a great deal of variation. Islamic humoral medicine was primarily Galenic in inspiration, but tenth- and eleventh-century sources from Iraq occasionally refer to what appear to be circles of medical thinking which focused on other sources of influence (e.g. the *baqarita*, 'Hippocratics', or the *rawafisa*, 'followers of Rufus [of Ephesus]') or were sufficiently distinctive to gain separate recognition (e.g. the *jundishaburiyun*, the '[doctors] of Jundishapur'). Physicians also engaged in vigorous debates over what rendered them qualified practitioners. Some felt that formal study with a teacher was essential, while others considered that knowledge of the classics of the medical literary tradition was what mattered; certain authorities stressed the importance of experience and empirical observation (as in Majusi's advocacy of bedside training), while others saw the key to medical truth in logical skills and formal reasoning.

The same diversity is evident in professional terms. Many physicians had other occupations, and interests in trade and property appear to have been common; as such trends suggest, many physicians were prosperous and highly esteemed members of society, and certainly far more prominent than their predecessors in late antiquity had been. The most eminent doctors had often benefited from a very broad education, and in some cases are better known today for their literary careers, though in their own time their prominence had been in the field of medicine. The most prominent example of this is Ibn Tufayl (d. *c.* 1185), the influential court physician of the Almohads in what is now modern Morocco, but known today almost exclusively for his tale *Hayy ibn Yaqzan*. Such noted Iraqi scholars as Ibn Durayd (d. 933) and Miskawayh (d. 1030) were both trained as physicians, but this aspect of their careers has in modern times been obscured by other achievements, the former in poetry and philology, the latter in history and philosophy. The links between philosophy and medicine were particularly strong; Razi and Ibn Sina excelled in both, and others, like Maimonides (d. 1204) and his fellow Andalusian contemporary Ibn Rushd (Averroes, d. 1198), were physicians who published their most important work and gained their primary reputation as philosophers.

These trends highlight the fact that, as had been the case in late antiquity, the medical profession in medieval Islamic times was very fluid – there were no specific requirements to fulfil before practice, no fixed curriculum of study or places to which medical education was restricted, and no clear boundaries defining the profession. And as we have seen, medical learning was available to the educated in a broad range of forms. In the final analysis, one could practise medicine provided that and so long as sufficient means of support – patronage or clientele – existed to make it feasible.

The vast majority of practitioners were clearly men, and where women appear at all they tend to be midwives and exponents of various forms of magic and medical folklore. But more evidence is appearing to indicate (if in a very patchy fashion) that women also played a role in the humoral tradition. Cases are known of female physicians establishing thriving practices and taking patients under their direct care, and we are also told of women specialists in ophthalmology and surgery. But while further study will undoubtedly clarify and expand our understanding of the place of women in medieval Islamic practice, it is unlikely to challenge the prevailing consensus that medicine was overwhelmingly dominated by men, even in such fields as gynaecology and obstetrics.

There were various avenues to a medical career. In some instances a great doctor seems to have been self-taught; such were the claims of Ibn Sina and Ibn Ridwan, for example, although their special pleading should be viewed with some reserve. In other cases a physician's son followed him into the profession; this practice assured education without charge and guaranteed access to books, instruments, and clientele. Family lines of medical men were common in all religious communities, but especially among Christians. The families of Hunayn ibn Ishaq and Thabit ibn Qurra (d. 901) were prominent examples, and the most dramatic case is that of Jibra'il ibn Bakhtishu' (d. 769) and his descendents. For three centuries this family from Jundishapur produced eminent physicians, pharmacists, and medical translators, and members of the line served as the personal physicians to numerous caliphs and other rulers of Iraq and Persia. Their renown was such that they became the subject of entertaining and didactic anecdotes which figured prominently in the legends about medical practice in their city.

Other aspiring physicians studied with a formal teacher. In early Islamic times teachers instructed students in their homes, and Muslims sometimes taught in the mosques, which were centres for education in general. Once hospitals were widespread these were logical venues for medical education: patients for examination were immediately to hand, and many hospitals had libraries of medical books. In the thirteenth century medical schools began to be founded (the first in Turkey), complete with hospital facilities, libraries, and student living quarters. The institution of the *madrasa*, or college in a more general sense, may have played a key role on these developments. One can see in the rise of medical schools a more specialised manifestation of the pattern exhibited in the evolution of the *madrasa*, in which the institution of the mosque came to have maintenance and pedagogical dimensions attached to it. And in any case, the number of advanced medical texts to be found in *madrasa* libraries suggests that the *madrasa* itself was a venue where medical teaching took place. None of these venues, however, displaced the custom of study in the master's home.

Students were often young, reflecting the widespread view that adulthood began at the age of 15 or sexual maturity, whichever occurred first. Hunayn ibn Ishaq made his way to Baghdad at 17, Ibn Sina began his studies at 16, and Maimonides was only 13 when he embarked on his.

Teaching methods varied considerably. The mastery of medical and other related texts was very important, but while instruction often focused on the 16 Galenic works in the *Alexandrian Summaries*, what was taught was left entirely to the discretion of the teacher. Mathematics and logic were also studied, and as described above, the novice had at his disposal a vast array of general and specialised manuals, *aide-mémoires*, and other introductory materials, supplemented in the later medieval period by the burgeoning commentary literature focused on the *Qanun* of Ibn Sina. These texts were usually memorised, read aloud, or both, and class work consisted of long sessions with a master, who would correct misreadings, clarify obscure passages, and pose and answer questions.

Clinical experience was available in hospitals, but exactly how such opportunities were pursued in pedagogical terms is unclear. It seems that physicians used patients to illustrate various maladies and problems to students accompanying them on their rounds, and it is sometimes implied that students would assume certain basic duties. At one practitioner's office in tenth-century Cairo, advanced students undertook preliminary examinations of patients waiting outside and performed procedures such as venesection.

It is clear, however, that medical education in the classical tradition concentrated on written texts, and many students must have entered medical practice without ever having treated a patient. We must also conclude that practical knowledge of human anatomy was gradually acquired as a doctor's career proceeded, for knowledge of the internal workings and arrangement of the human body could only be gained in very limited *ad hoc* ways, as and when treatment of individual medical complaints provided access to internal tissues and organs – such a pattern would help to explain some of the anomalies in the illustrations in the *Tashrih-i mansuri* of Ibn Ilyas. Dissection of animals (especially apes) appears to have been fairly common. Yohanna ibn Masawayh (d. 857), the teacher of Hunayn ibn Ishaq, dissected monkeys (perhaps following Galen's lead) in order to gain information for an anatomical work, one which eventually won great praise; and similar cases of animal research are known. But work on human cadavers was abhorrent to both Muslim and Christian sensibilities and, if not explicitly forbidden, was almost always out of the question. The belief was widespread that the dead can continue to feel pain, and that disturbance of a corpse was tantamount to desecration of the dead. These views were related to the doctrine in both faiths that at the Last Judgment the dead would be summoned before God in their physical bodies, at which time any desecration (including amputations or dissection) would be clear to all and would have to be accounted for before God.

While it was widely felt that the competence of physicians should be verified, there was no regular system of examinations or other qualifying procedures which one had to complete successfully before beginning to work. There are numerous instances (especially in the manuals of market inspection, or *hisba*, and in manuals on the examination of physicians) in which an authority enumerates all that a physician should know, but such material is prescriptive rather than descriptive. Closer to the mark is an incident recorded by Thabit ibn Sinan concerning his father, the famous physician Sinan ibn Thabit ibn Qurra (d. 942). In 931, when the caliph in Baghdad learned that one of the common folk had died at the hands of an incompetent doctor, he ordered that only physicians who had been examined by Sinan should practise medicine in the capital. This entailed a comprehensive examination of physicians in Baghdad, exempting only physicians in the imperial service and others too eminent to justify review. About 860 candidates applied during the first year. Among them was an elderly well-dressed gentleman who confessed that he had no formal training and indeed, could hardly read and write, but pleaded with Sinan not to deprive his family of their livelihood by denying him permission to practise medicine. Sinan agreed, provided that he confined himself strictly to simple maladies and ordinary medications. The next day the man's son appeared before Sinan, and was also authorised to practise on similar conditions. As this story illustrates, the examination was aimed not at establishing a uniform standard for admission to medical practice, but at ensuring that practitioners were not engaging in deliberate fraud. The tale also implies that such supervision of the medical profession occurred only sporadically and as *ad hoc* initiatives by concerned authorities.

Overall, Islamic society was prepared to tolerate a very broad range of practioners and remedies, in the first instance because the more popular lore, if not legitimated in formal intellectual terms, was nevertheless upheld by equally (or even more) compelling structures of authority – the approval of the Prophet, for example, or the compelling sanction of long-established custom. Further, humoral remedies were often unavailable in the countryside, where most people lived; in the cities, humoral medicine was often beyond the financial means of the common man. And it could not have passed unobserved that if many folk remedies seemed to be ineffective or even dangerous, the same could be said of many of the humoral procedures and drugs. What society sought to root out was deliberate fraud – the chemist who adulterated drugs with inert ingredients to make a higher profit, for example, or the surgeon who pretended to extract a stone, olive pit, or lizard from a boil he had just incised. But both society and governing authorities tolerated doctors of many sorts so long as suspicions were not raised (e.g. by the unexpected death of a patient) that they were practising beyond their expertise.

Access to a physician could be had in a number of ways. Doctors received patients in their homes or in a 'surgery', an open shop like most other business establishments in the medieval Islamic city. Wealthy or favoured patients would receive special attention, but most people with medical complaints could expect to wait at the door until the master was available, and in the meantime be seen by an attendant or student, who might perform a preliminary examination or simple procedures, such as venesection. On many occasions a messenger would be sent to the doctor with a description of the patient's problem, and on the basis of this (often ambiguous and minimally helpful) account a written prescription would be issued. At other times a physician could be summoned to a patient's home, even in the middle of the night, though it was expected that transportation and a fee in advance would be provided. If a patient required constant attention or was in a critical condition, the doctor might take the sufferer into his own home (a custom already observed for Roman times) until the crisis had passed or the situation was truly hopeless. The documents from the Cairo Geniza (a cache of discarded medieval Jewish documents on a vast range of topics) suggest that doctors must have been very busy and in a high demand, for their advice and assistance were sought even for minor complaints.

Medical examinations involved careful questioning of the patient (and sometimes also of family members and servants), examination and palpation of affected body parts, and in particular scrutiny of pulse and urine. Doctors were routinely advised to exercise prudent judgment in discussing the case with others, who might thereafter reveal confusing or frightening details to the sufferer, and visitors were also a source of concern as potential busybodies who might gainsay the physician's diagnosis and interfere with treatment. Second and third opinions were sometimes sought, however, and if a patient was not fully satisfied with a doctor's decisions and conclusions, he or she would readily leave him for another.

Arab-Islamic medicine always gave highest priority to the preservation of good health, but once this had been lost many means were used to restore it. The vast materia medica of the medieval period included thousands of herbs and drugs, but of these a much smaller number were the staple of the trade. Medications were often prepared by the physician himself, and some prescriptions provided that if the medication was supplied from elsewhere it should be taken only in the doctor's presence. If surgery was required, the doctor would have access to a wide range of specialised surgical instruments, the scope and complexity of which are evident from the drawings in the *Tasrif* of Zahrawi. For the relief of pain both numbing drugs and actual anaesthetic agents were available, although the exact nature of these is unclear.

Payment of the physician seems to have been due upon conclusion of treatment, and fees varied widely according to the means of the patient and the renown of the physician. If the patient died, his family could institute proceedings against the doctor if they felt that his diagnosis

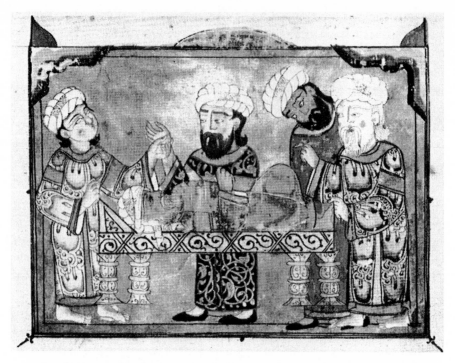

Fig. 19. Examination of a patient by the physician (centre, at the bedside) and his assistants. The illustration is a miniature in a manuscript of a literary work, the *Maqamat* of Hariri (d. 1122). (Vienna, Österreichische Nationalbibliothek, Ms. A.F. 9.)

had been wrong or his treatment inappropriate. Witnesses and the written prescriptions could be produced in evidence, and if found guilty of malpractice the unfortunate doctor could be heavily fined, barred from practice, or both. For Christian and Jewish doctors this system of redress must have posed a serious dilemma, since in Islamic court proceedings the testimony of non-Muslims against Muslims was not accepted.

Undistinguished and even poor people could at times benefit from the best medical attention the tradition could offer. Razi, for example, was not only a prolific author and director of hospitals, but also a medical practitioner in a thriving commercial district of Baghdad. His patients were his neighbours, and from his clinical notes it is clear that he ran what amounted to a family practice for all sorts of people: merchants, government officials, and the nobility came to him, but so also did common labourers and craftsmen. In Cairo several centuries later, Maimonides described his hectic daily routine in a letter to a friend in

France: from the early morning to the afternoon he was busy with the sultan, and then returned to find his house swarming with patients, both Jews and Gentiles, notables and common folk, who occupied his time until after nightfall. The works of most medieval Middle Eastern medical writers betray a background of ongoing medical practice, and there are numerous indications that access to such eminent physicians was not limited to powerful and wealthy patients.

There were also other efforts to extend care to less fortunate parts of society. In the cities, doctors were sometimes appointed to visit prisons and lunatic asylums to tend to persons suffering the effects of the appalling health conditions there. Efforts were also made to extend medical care to rural areas, where most people lived. In Egypt and Syria in the eleventh and twelfth centuries, for example, small towns and large villages usually seem to have had at least one humoral physician, and in Iraq a century earlier specific arrangements were made for medical teams to tour the agrarian hinterland to tend to the needs of the peasantry. References to impassable roads, the need for guides, and raging outbreaks of epidemic disease suggest that these journeys were both dangerous and difficult.

Physicians also had other duties to fulfil, some of them quite bureaucratic. Prescriptions were, as noted above, formal legal documents, and recording and filing them was a major exercise. Doctors were also frequently called upon to make official statements of their findings, as for example, in the case of a leper seeking confirmation of his condition so as to gain access to communal support funds. Jewish physicians were often leaders of their local communities, and Muslims often found themselves in bureaucracy-bound positions such as medical inspector, chief physician of the army, or medical superintendent at a hospital.

The Islamic hospital

The hospital was perhaps the crowning achievement of Islamic medical practice. This institution appears to have been generally inspired by the precedent of poor and sick relief services offered at Christian monasteries and other church-run establishments, although the Islamic hospital was a far more elaborate medical institution. The first Muslim hospital foundation is often attributed to the caliph Walid I (reigned 705–15) and placed in Damascus, the Umayyad capital in Syria, but the oldest accounts of the episode refer simply to the restriction and feeding of lepers, not to a hospital, and this in the Arabian town of Medina, not Damascus. The extant evidence suggests that the first Islamic hospital was that founded in Baghdad by Jibra'il ibn Bakhtishu' on the orders of Harun al–Rashid, *c.* 805. This was followed by similar constructions elsewhere, and by the twelfth century a hospital was an essential feature of any large Islamic town.

Hospitals were established and funded as acts of personal charity and not as matters of state policy, though the founders were most often rulers or highly placed administrators. The founding of a hospital involved formally setting aside the revenues from specified properties as a religious trust (*waqf*) which would defray the costs of providing the services stipulated by the endower. Such endowments were to survive in perpetuity, and as every aspect of the arrangement was spelled out in the deed, a great deal is known about several hospitals (especially the Mansuri, founded in Cairo in 1284) for which these deeds survive.

Hospitals were complex institutions, with separate facilities for men and for women, in-patients and out-patients, and wards for different afflictions and different medical procedures (e.g. ophthalmological complaints, or bone-setting). Some hospitals seem to have specialised to some extent, or at least had more than usually prominent facilities for the insane, the poor, or army officers. The hospital precinct usually included a kitchen and pharmacy, a mosque, and audience or lecture rooms; very often there was a bath, and a library of medical books (measured in terms of shelves, not rooms). The better-endowed hospitals were spectacular places built to the highest architectural standard, with pools, streams of running water, and small groves of trees where patients and staff could relax.

The self-contained medical community so created attracted both students and practising physicians, and association with a leading hospital seems to have been regarded by the public as a sign of particular eminence. Doctors regularly made rounds at the hospitals and used both patients and library facilities to teach their students. As the hospital was established as a pious act of charity, admission to it was free; in some cases provisions were made not only for poor inmates to receive their treatment, lodging, and board without charge, but also to be given a stipend upon discharge, to support them until they could work again.

Impressive as these individual institutions were, Islamic hospitals should not be regarded as having played the leading role in health care

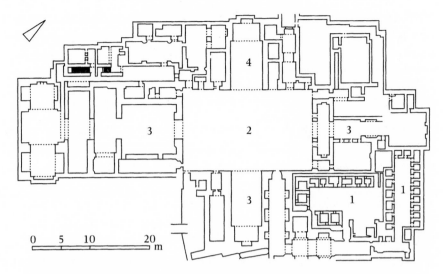

Fig. 20. Plan of the Mansuri Hospital, Cairo 1284. The institution could accommodate more than 100 patients, and had wards for different ailments arranged around
a large central courtyard. Key: 1. Psychiatric ward; 2. Courtyard; 3. Sick-rooms; 4.
Waiting-room for patients in opthalmology. (Michael W. Dols, *Majnun: the Madman
in Medieval Islamic Society*, Oxford, Clarendon Press, 1992.)

in medieval Islam. They were in all cases extremely limited compared
to the vast size of the populations they served (in much the same way
that one shelter in a modern Western city does not meet the problem of
homelessness), and their effective function must always have been
rather to demonstrate and promote ideals of compassion and charity
and to serve as foci for the activities and expansion of the medical profession. Insofar as it was possible to offer meaningful medical care at
all, this remained the effective domain of the individual practitioner.

It is, in fact, as a melange of individual practitioners that medieval
Arab-Islamic medicine may best be viewed. The problems confronting
the physician were enormous, and many of these difficulties must be
put down to the scientific, technological, and logistical limitations of
the era. In many cases physicians were powerless in the face of personal illness, and even the most sophisticated medical measures could
not have alleviated the innumerable hazards of day-to-day life. They
could do little, for example, to change the facts that life expectancy was
not much above 35 years, and that the majority of children died before
reaching adulthood. But in the face of these harsh realities physicians
offered what was arguably the most cosmopolitan profession in the
medieval Islamic world, a concern for their field which was both intel-

lectually rigorous and profoundly humane, and a determination to relieve suffering and promote good health, despite the endless frustrations that such efforts must have suffered in the pre-modern age.

Postscript

As later chapters will show, early modern Europe gradually came to replace Arab-Islamic medicine with its own alternatives, and no longer found inspiration in Middle Eastern medical institutions. And with the onset of aggressive European intrusions, most notably Napoleon's invasion of Egypt in 1798, Middle Eastern regimes would themselves embrace Western bio-medicine as part of their determined efforts to modernise for defence. But in important ways the older traditions continued to survive, and even flourish. The medical folklore described above continues to shape the way many conceive of their medical world; and with the upsurge in Islamic religious sentiment over the past two decades, the 'Medicine of the Prophet' has seen a dramatic revival. A modern Beirut edition of Ibn Qayyim al-Jawziya's compendium on the subject (p. 125) is a bestseller in Arab lands, and even in Britain many Muslims are familiar with these traditions and follow their medical advice.

The humoral medicine represented by the compendia of Majusi and Ibn Sina witnessed a more serious reversal. Deprived of patronage and increasingly marginalised in urban centres, the foci of its intellectual and pedagogical traditions, it had drastically receded as a therapeutic alternative in many parts of the Islamic world by the end of the nineteenth century. In the Indian subcontinent, however, it retained its support and thrived as *Unani tibb*, 'Greek medicine'. There its practitioners are still widely consulted and its doctrines taught, and its remedies are mass-produced and purchased on a large scale.

Even in areas where it was abandoned, however, the literary legacy of Graeco-Arabic humoral medicine remained influential. Majusi's and Ibn Sina's compendia were printed in Cairo in the 1870s as a contribution to modern medicine, not history. And as far away as London, the Sydenham Society in 1848 published an English translation of Razi's *On Smallpox and Measles* with precisely the same goal in mind.

5 Medicine in Medieval Western Europe, 1000–1500

VIVIAN NUTTON

Salerno and the impact of translation

An observer of medicine in 1050 would have found little changed from 550. The intellectual renaissance of the ninth century had had little impact on medicine, save for a general increase in literacy and the availability of manuscripts. But medicine had not gained a place among the new 'liberal arts', and cathedral schools like Chartres (France) with a reputation for medical teaching were exceptional. Indeed, at Chartres medicine formed only part of a wider programme of studies that encompassed the whole world of natural knowledge – it was not intended specifically to produce professional healers, but to lead to a better understanding of God and His creation. Such instruction, both in its clerical context and in its content (largely Methodist in its therapeutics (pp. 82–5), with a minimum of basic theory), differed from that associated with Salerno from the late eleventh century onwards. Salernitan doctors were already famous in France by the late tenth century, when an erudite Frenchman and a practical Salernitan disputed before the French King, and when a French bishop journeyed to Salerno in search of a cure. But it is not until the next century that one can properly understand what was happening in this small southern Italian town.

The tradition that the school of Salerno was founded by four masters – a Latin, a Jew, an Arab, and a Greek who brought with him the writings of Hippocrates – contains a kernel of symbolic truth. Salerno stood at the intersection of several cultural, economic, and political routes. In the eleventh century, it was ruled by Norman Dukes, who constantly played off the Pope, to the North, against the Byzantine Emperor, who still controlled much of southern and eastern Italy. Jewish physicians might be found anywhere, like Shabbetai Donnolo (913 to c. 982), a southern Italian Jew, whose *Book of Wisdom* united Greek anatomy and pharmacology with Jewish mysticism and astrology in a complex of universal interrelations. Arab settlers had by 950 established themselves in Sicily and along the southern Italian coast, and trading relations, particularly through nearby Amalfi, were maintained with both Byzantium and northern Africa. A hundred miles to the north lay the greatest abbey in Europe, Monte Cassino, then at the height of its influence as an intellectual centre under Abbot Desiderius (1058–87), and housing in its library a collection of medical texts exceptional for both quality and quantity.

In 1063, Alphanus, a monk of Monte Cassino, who in his youth had studied medicine at Salerno, and was now its archbishop, travelled on an embassy to Constantinople, where he became acquainted with Greek medical texts. His translation of *On the Nature of Man* by Bishop Nemesius of Emesa (*fl.* 390) introduced into Latin a Christianised Galenic anthropology, while his own writings on pulses and the four humours reflected contemporary Byzantine medicine. Greek influence is also visible in a collection of Latin *Questions* associated with Salerno at this time. Together they offered a new view of medicine, more speculative and more open to (largely Greek) natural philosophy, *physica*, than what had gone before.

The earliest Salernitan teaching texts of medicine continued this exploration of basically Greek ideas in Latin. Some form of anatomical dissection based on animals was introduced around 1120, by which date the custom of medical teaching by means of commentary on another author was well established. The earliest commentators expounded their base text closely and methodically. By about 1180, however, Bartholomaeus in his lectures on the *Articella* (p. 142) was using his base text as a starting-point for a wider exploration of different arguments, incorporating Aristotelian and Arabic philosophical learning. He did not repeat unthinkingly the letter of the text, but tried to augment his hearer's knowledge of the natural world with medicine at its centre.

Salerno is also credited with the introduction of Arabic medicine into Western Europe. Here the moving spirit was Constantine the African, a Tunisian who became a monk of Monte Cassino, and who between *c.* 1070 and his death by 1097 transmitted to the Latin world hitherto unknown texts of Arabic and Greek medicine. His *On Intercourse* (*De coitu*) and the *Traveller's Guide* (*Viaticum*), both from Ibn al-Jazzar, and his rendering of the compendium of Majusi (pp. 113–14), which he dedicated to Abbot Desiderius and became known as the *Pantegni* (*Universal art*) of Haly Abbas, conveyed the sense of the Arabic originals rather than their exact words. His translations, via the Arabic, of Galen's *Art of Healing* (*Tegni*), and his commentaries on the Hippocratic *Aphorisms* and *Prognostic*, and of an adaptation of Hunayn's *Medical Questions* (p. 122), the *Liber ysagogarum* (*Introduction*) of Johannicius, provided an enlarged theoretical basis for medical knowledge. By 1150 manuscripts of these texts had spread widely in Italy and beyond, and separate sections of the *Pantegni* had taken on an independent life of their own.

The importance of Constantine's translations cannot be overestimated. They put the Latin-speaking world in touch with the tradition of Hippocratic learning promoted by Galen and extended by the Arabs. They introduced new therapies (Constantine's drug book, the *Antidotarium* was widely copied) and a new technical vocabulary, as well as a whole range of new concepts, particularly in anatomy and physiology. The *Liber ysagogarum* also provided a structure for medical discourse, for it laid down how to diagnose a patient and organise therapy. Its emphasis on the 'six non-naturals' (food and drink; sleep and waking; air; evacuation and repletion; motion and rest; and the passions or emotions) as the crucial determinants of health and illness played an important role in medical thinking long after the identity of Johannicius and their Galenic origin had been forgotten. Without proper attention to these non-naturals, the body's natural state would turn to the contra-natural state of illness as a result of changes in its humoral balance. Similarly, by regulating the non-naturals one could protect the body in advance of predictable changes; one needed to eat less, or different, food in summer than in spring or autumn. Medieval and Renaissance authors composed their books on diet (or, better, lifestyle; see pp. 26–8) to take account of the non-naturals, and they prescribed for patients in accordance with the rules set out by Johannicius. Their medical counsels (*consilia*), thousands of which survive, mainly from the period after 1300 and ranging in length from a few lines to many pages, dealt in turn with each of the six non-naturals, describing what foods, rest, ambience, evacuations (including one's sex-life), exercise, and emotional state would best preserve or restore an individual's health. Onto the holistic framework set out by Johannicius, doctors and their patients could fit a highly individualised scheme of therapy.

Translation was only one part of the medical activity of southern Italy in the late eleventh century. It was in Salerno, or possibly even at Monte Cassino, that a new canon of medical authority, known in the sixteenth century as the *Articella* or *Little Art of Medicine*, was created. To the *Liber ysagogarum*, the object of learned commentary at Salerno before 1150, were added Hippocrates' *Aphorisms* and *Prognostic*, and two Byzantine treatises, Theophilus, *On Urines*, and Philaretus, *On Pulses*. Before 1200, this collection had been supplemented by Galen's *Tegni*, soon followed (though not necessarily in Salerno) by Hippocrates' *On Regimen in Acute Diseases* as translated by Gerard of Cremona. The *Articella* swiftly became the basis for advanced teaching in medicine throughout Western Europe. It differed from the typical pre-Salernitan medical collection in several important ways. Firstly, it contained few remedies, and was largely concerned to convey the theoretical knowledge essential for practice. Secondly, it was a mixture of translations from Greek and Arabic (a nice indication of the cultural mixture of southern Italy). Thirdly, its discussions linking medicine with a wider world of natural philosophy demanded both a philosophical and a medical understanding. Its largely Aristotelian orientation increased its attractiveness for those who had already studied Aristotelian logic and natural science – i.e. the university teachers from 1250 onwards. Finally, for all its pedagogic merits, the *Articella* paradoxically narrowed the medical focus. Pre-Salernitan compendia included texts drawn from the Methodist and the Hippocratic tradition; Galen featured in them, but he was not dominant. By contrast, the *Articella* was confined to the Galenic tradition – the Hippocratic works in it were often accompanied by the Galenic commentary, and at least one, *Prognostic*, was constructed out of Hippocratic quotations embedded in Galen's exposition. Constantine's translations of Arabic authors added therapeutic information from within the same tradition, confirming the value of the theories put forward in the introductory texts. In short, while the Salernitan commentators of the twelfth and thirteenth century were far more learned than their medical predecessors of the tenth, and viewed medicine against a broader background of natural philosophical enquiry, their Galenism reduced the range of acceptable medical ideas. The appearance of the *Articella* also gave learned medicine its equivalent of a sacred text – a proper doctor could henceforth be defined in terms of knowledge of a series of books.

This process was accelerated by two important developments, the rise of universities and renewed access to earlier medical learning through the medium of translation. The two are interrelated, for ideas newly available in Latin influenced what was taught, and the existence of a learned (and wealthy) clientele encouraged the search for new and better translations.

Five separate stages in the translation of earlier material into Latin can be usefully distinguished. The first, associated with Constantine and southern Italy, involved both Greek and Arabic texts, and was predominantly concerned with medicine. It established a new vocabulary of medicine, e.g. *siphac* (peritoneum), as well as the beginnings of a standard way of medical thinking.

Of equal significance, however, was the great outpouring, from the 1140s onwards, of Latin translations made in Spain from the Arabic, often with the assistance of Hebrew intermediaries. This included, as well as medical texts, many works of science and philosophy, especially Aristotle. Although Gerard of Cremona (*fl.* 1150–87 at Toledo) translated some of Galen's writings, e.g. the *Method of Healing*, he and his colleagues concentrated on major Arabic practical texts, like the *Canon* of Avicenna (p. 114) and the *Liber ad Almansorem* of Rhazes (p. 112). The consequences of these Spanish translations were two-fold. They provided a far wider and heavily Arabised vocabulary for learned medicine in Latin, and they imparted an ever greater Arabic and Aristotelian slant to Galenic medicine. In Avicenna's *Canon*, medicine was systematised within a strongly philosophical and logical framework, with each part carefully related to every other. What in the Galenic original was diffuse or tentative was now reduced to succinct certainty. The new Arabic material was also far more advanced, conceptually and practically, than what was available through the Greek; Kindi's *De gradibus* (*On the Grades of Drug Action*), said Roger Bacon (*c.* 1214–94), demanded a knowledge of mathematics well beyond his own contemporaries in philosophy, let alone in medicine. Arabic pharmacology, surgery, and practical medicine in Latin dress thus formed the foundation for further medieval investigations, and apparently new questions of wider, philosophical interest now occupied teachers of medicine. Whereas for the Salernitan commentators, medicine had remained at the centre of the universe of physic, their successors in Spain and northern Italy discussed medicine as only one part of an Aristotelian philosophical universe, and a subordinate one at that.

Contemporary with Gerard, but operating from Constantinople, was a Pisan merchant, Burgundio (1110–93). A friend of the Salernitan master Bartholomaeus, he had his own collection of specially copied Greek manuscripts, in which one can still read his annotations and follow the development of his technique as translator. His renderings of Galen from the Greek are more accurate than those of Gerard, and covered a wider range of (generally theoretical) writings, including *On Crises* and *On the Natural Faculties*.

A century later came another burst of translation, mainly in Spain and Italy, that brought into Latin other major works of Arabic science (e.g. the *Continens* (*All-Embracing Book*) of Rhazes, in Sicily in 1282; or the *Colliget* (*The Book of Universals*) of Averroes (Ibn Rushd), in Padua in 1283), and yet more Galen. In Spain, Arnald of Villanova (d. 1311) translated Galen's *On Rigour* (1282), as well as Avicenna's *On the Properties of the Heart* (*c.* 1280?); while in Italy, versions of Galen, including portions of *On the Use of Parts of the Body*, were made by another professor, Pietro d'Abano (1257 to *c.* 1315), directly from Greek manuscripts he had brought back from Constantinople. Still more significant was the utilisation of the new Galenic material to review the doctrines found in the Arabo-Latin compendia. Arnald's commentary on Galen's *On Bad Temperament* criticised earlier views of fever, while Pietro's *Conciliator* (*The Reconciler of Differences Between Philosophers and Doctors*) was a celebrated exposition of the basic principles of Galenic/Aristotelian medical science. The Spanish translations clearly influenced the type of medicine taught by Arnald and his colleagues at the University of Montpellier (southern France), and the 'new' Galen seems also to have stimulated Taddeo Alderotti (active at Bologna 1260–95) to original thoughts on disease and internal medicine. His example was followed by several of his pupils, who tended to take Galen's side in university debates with Aristotelian philosophers.

The final translator of importance was Niccolò da Reggio (*fl.* 1315–48), a bilingual doctor and diplomat in the Kingdom of Naples. In all he translated over 50 writings by Galen, many for the first time, including the complete *On the Use of Parts of the Body*. He was remarkably accurate, living up to his claim 'neither to add nor remove anything' from his Greek original, and modern philologists have united in his praise. Some Galenic texts, e.g. *On Procatarctic Causes*, were for centuries accessible only in his versions, but his medieval influence was generally small, perhaps because most of the Galenic treatises he translated are minor, e.g. *On Prognosis*, or highly philosophical, like the two tracts *On Causes*, and appeared at a time when university curricula, and their preferred texts, had already become established. The few who cited them, e.g. the French surgeon Guy de Chauliac (*c.* 1300–68), were already learned men, able to appreciate their subtleties, and, more important, wealthy enough to have such relatively recondite books copied for them. Whether all owners read them is another matter. By 1503, a manuscript in Nuremberg (southern Germany) containing several of Niccolò's versions was located only through the stench of its rotting leaves and binding, a reminder, in more than one way, of the fragility of medieval medical learning.

The literature so far mentioned circulated in Latin, the language of learned Europe. A similar, if far more restricted, transmission of the learning of others can be found among the Jews of Catalonia and southern France around 1300, including some Galen as well as works by such local medical worthies as Bernard of Gordon (*fl.* 1283–1308). Not until the late fourteenth or early fifteenth century can one detect elsewhere the growth of a learned but non–latinate class with interests in medicine. This is not to say that medicine was not written earlier in the vernacular languages – several thirteenth-century manuscripts contain drug recipes written in both Latin, English, and Norman French – but, with the exception of surgery, both the types of text involved and their message rarely rise above the level of basic self-help. By contrast, vernacular writings from 1350 onwards included (a little) Galen and Hippocrates, as well as theoretical discussions. Fifteenth-century German medical texts, in particular, often ally practicality with a sophistication of thought and exposition superior to that of university treatises. Indeed, many of their authors had themselves studied at an Italian university, and could easily have written in Latin, had they so wished. The explanation for their choice lies rather in their intended audience – more local and less dependent on the universities.

Nor do Latin and vernacular texts represent learned and folk traditions respectively. The *Surgery* of John of Arderne (*c.* 1307–70) exists in both Latin and English, and Bartholomew the Englishman's *On the Property of Things* enjoyed a wide circulation in both Latin and English. Although many of the texts translated were severely practical, dealing with surgery, drugs, veterinary medicine, and 'medical forecasting', parts of the *Articella*, for instance, were available in French, English, and Gaelic. Their sponsors were frequently surgeons, especially those resident in major cities, keen to have for themselves in an accessible tongue treatises that were highly praised by other practitioners. Other writers, like Henry Daniel in his English *Book of urines* (1379), were intent on bringing the best of medicine to a wide audience, with charitable or religious aims in mind. Books like these, and, in particular, the many writings by German physicians and surgeons in the fourteenth and fifteenth centuries, show how an audience for learned medical discourse was being created outside the universities.

These translations into Latin, and later into the vernacular, had important consequences for medieval medicine. They reinforced the power of tradition, while at the same time enabling a more sophisticated understanding of medicine to develop within the new linguistic community. New words, new concepts, and new errors alike were introduced. The texts themselves carried a Galenic medicine, frequently within an Arabised and Aristotelian framework. Such medical knowledge was validated by its place within the divinely created order of things; apparent contradictions did not necessarily indicate error, but rather positions to be reconciled by logic, by words, and by better understanding. The heavy Arabism of many Latin translations tended to create a specifically medical vocabulary, which in turn encouraged the separation of medicine as an elite science in the thirteenth century, a development only partially retarded by the rise of learned medical writing in the vernacular, especially on surgery, in the fifteenth.

Religion and medicine in the Later Middle Ages

From the eleventh until the fourteenth century at least, the economic, political, and social power of the Papacy and its dependent religious institutions grew enormously. Older claims to oversee the whole of the life of the Christian community were vigorously repeated, even if local conditions, not least the opposition of kings and local magnates, nullified the effects of many decrees of Popes and Councils. It is significant that the most effective religious action against any type of medicine did not take place until the sixteenth century, when Emperor and Inquisition, acting together in Spain to stamp out heresy, secured the destruction of a medical tradition based on a first-hand acquaintance with Arabic (and occasionally Jewish) sources. In the Middle Ages, neither Church nor State possessed such an efficient mechanism of control, whatever legislators thought to the contrary.

Besides, the Church's priority was the eternal salvation of the soul.

Hence it was concerned to see that Christian midwives, not Jews or heretics, attended births, where they might, *in extremis*, baptise the new-born and thereby help them to Heaven. Hence, too, many Italian regulations for civic doctors specified the number of visits a doctor might make before summoning a priest to administer confession and absolution of the patient's sins. This concern for the soul also involved a certain suspicion of Jewish doctors – the Lateran Council of 1215, the high-water mark of Papal pretensions to authority, forbade practitioners not approved of by the Church from attending to the sick. But this was in theory only, for Jewish doctors were found everywhere, not least in attendance upon Popes and Bishops, and their very marginality made them occasionally a cheaper option than a Christian physician. Their lack of a university degree did not stop them from being licensed by civil authorities.

Most ecclesiastical regulations on medicine, however, are best explained as an attempt to control the religious life and to preserve the dignity of the Church. Several Church Councils banned monks from learning medicine, practising outside their own monasteries, or spending too much time away on this secular (and lucrative) science, a rule frequently repeated and frequently broken. The possible riches from medical practice made it an attractive option – and ecclesiastical lawyers in no way prevented those clerics who were not monks from taking it. Likewise the notorious decree of the Lateran Council of 1215 that forbade clerics in higher orders from shedding blood was not an attack on surgery – for those in lower clerical orders and laymen could still do it – but an attempt to maintain the dignity of the higher ranks of the clergy by dissociating them from the manual (and bloody) craft of surgery. Nonetheless, it did not stop Teodorico Borgognoni, later Bishop of Cervia in northern Italy (1205–98), from becoming the most famous writer on surgery of his day.

Nor did the church authorities intervene to ban human dissection when this was introduced into university teaching in the fourteenth century, although many believed they were not wholeheartedly in favour. As Pope Sixtus IV wrote to the University of Tübingen (Germany) in 1482, provided that the body was that of an executed criminal, and, after dissection, was given proper Christian burial, there was no objection. Regulations against the boiling up of bodies to obtain bones or organs for separate burial similarly were directed against improper religious practices, not against medical investigation as such.

Ecclesiastical authorities were interested in the minutiae of medical practice, because many monks and clerics were also healers. The village pastor, stumblingly literate, might seem to his flock a veritable Hippocrates if he knew a few recipes and snippets of theory; satirists and medical reformers, however, considered him the best ally of Death. At the other extreme, Peter of Spain (*c.* 1205–77), whose *Treasury of the Poor* was a medical best-seller and who had been a medical professor, became Pope in 1276 as John XXI. In the northern European universities from 1300 onwards, many medical graduates were in holy orders, for the income from a religious office, the duties of which could be devolved to an impecunious deputy or vicar, or joining a religious order was one way to finance a long period of academic training. A religious qualification also fitted a doctor for his role as personal adviser to a wealthy patron, and helped to guarantee his honesty and fairness as a practitioner.

Medieval monasteries also served as repositories of medical learning, and until the rise of the universities their involvement with medicine was greater than that of any other institution. Monte Cassino may have played a crucial role in the creation of the *Articella* (p. 142). In England, St. Albans Abbey was the home of two Cambridge brothers, Matthew and Warin, both of whom had studied medicine at Salerno. Warin was succeeded as Abbot in 1195 by 'a Galen in medicine', the Paris-trained John of Cella. John was treated on his death-bed in 1214 by yet another medical monk, William of Bedford, later Prior of Tynemouth and then of Worcester. A century earlier, Abbot Faritius of Abingdon, an Italian medical man and a royal physician, had failed to be elected Archbishop of Canterbury in 1114, despite the backing of Henry I, because it was thought unbecoming that such an important office should be held by 'a man who spent his time examining the urine of women'.

Most monasteries, especially those of the Benedictine Order, had their own infirmaries, where sick monks might be treated, sometimes by a fellow monk, sometimes, as at Westminster, by an outside doctor under contract. Surviving account books show that therapy was almost entirely by diet (in some places with an annual blood-letting in spring). Outlay on doctors and drugs was, in general, a mere fraction of that on the upkeep of the premises; roofs cost more than hernias. The monastic infirmary was for the monks themselves, with perhaps the occasional servant or visitor. The general public was served through the provision of a separate hospital, as at Bury St. Edmund's (England), where between 1150 and 1260 six hospitals were founded to cater for lepers, pilgrims, the sick, and the old.

Bury demonstrates nicely the co-existence of secular and religious healing. The monks of the Abbey, when sick, might pray for healing to St. Edmund, or take advantage of doctors among their own number, one of whom, Walter, was rich enough to rebuild the Abbey's Almonry in 1197 solely from the fees he received from outsiders. Bury was one of the great pilgrimage centres of England, and its chroniclers recorded the healing miracles performed at the shrine – and the construction of the local hospitals. Typically, there is no gulf between religious and secular healing. True, many accounts of healing miracles, like John the Monk's *Book of Miracles*, a popular Latin collection of miracle stories that derives from Egypt by way of Salerno, described the failure of secular help, sometimes with biting words, but their ultimate focus is on the power of almighty God and the saints, not the weakness of physicians.

Healing shrines in the Later Middle Ages almost constituted an industry in themselves. Some saints, e.g. St. Luke or St. Michael, were invoked for a variety of illnesses, while others were more specialised. St. Roch was considered a particularly effective intercessor against plague, St. Blaise against goitre, St. Radegund against ulcers. French sufferers from fever could pray to 108 saints; sufferers from dropsy a mere 11; while those with gangrene or 'an internal decomposition of the humours' were restricted to one, St. Fiacre and St. Amable respectively. These shrines were marketed, with their own souvenirs and protective images of the saint. Sometimes, as at Bury, the cult flourished and pilgrims came in large numbers. Elsewhere, as with the cult of Godric of Finchale (Durham, northern England), response was small and local, or fluctuated in numbers and area. The bones of St. Thomas Cantilupe of Hereford (d. 1282) were at first interred in a modest tomb; in 1287, they were moved to a new and larger tomb in a more accessible part of the cathedral. The first pilgrims were almost entirely local, living within 10 miles, but by 1289, many had travelled 50 miles, a four- or five-day journey. By 1300 most cures are reported to have occurred in the patient's home or away from the shrine, and by 1349, the whole healing cult had faded away. This does not mean that its healings were in some way fraudulent, but rather that the shrine failed to compete: it did not attract the wealthy male sufferer, whose patronage enabled other shrines to flourish.

In their pattern of suppliants and diseases, the shrines of Godric and St. Thomas are typical. Women come usually from the lower, men from all classes. Madness, sterility, 'the flux', and physical impairment are characteristic of women, accidents and woundings of men (which reflects the different lifestyles of the sexes rather than the preferences of the saints). Childhood accidents, fevers, and dysenteries show the hazards of life for the young, while reports of ulcerations lasting for years remind us that medieval Galenic medicine was targeted at acute rather than chronic disorders.

The chronic sick, and those suffering simply from the ravages of old age, might find shelter and sustenance within a hospital. Although in the same tradition as those described above (pp. 77–9) the hospitals of later medieval Europe differ from them and from monastic infirmaries in size, scope, and foundation. Whereas the Western hospitals of the sixth century were small, mainly for pilgrims, and often attached to a bishop's palace, some of their fifteenth-century successors were huge in size and independent foundations. Several in London were founded by merchants or trade guilds and, staffed and run by monks and nuns, fell outside the local parish organisation. But, first and foremost, they continued to be religious refuges for the poor, and strictly medical functions were the last to develop.

To characterise the late medieval hospital is not easy. At the one extreme were hospitals like St. Leonard's, York (England), with 225 sick and poor on its books in 1287, or the even larger civic hospitals of Milan, Siena, or Paris. For these, a model has been suggested in the hospitals of Constantinople or the Islamic world, for they were founded at the time of the Crusades, when knightly orders of Hospitallers, devoted to the care (and protection) of pilgrims to the Holy Land, also came into being. But many hospitals housed very few inmates: at Bury the Domus Dei (God's House) cared for up to seven destitute men, St. Saviour's for 12 poor men and 12 poor women. Their subsequent development shows an equally bewildering variety. Some hospitals, like St. Bartholomew's in London, and many of the great hospitals on the Continent, survive to this day as medical hospitals or almshouses. Others became schools or colleges (like St. John's hospital, Cambridge), or simply disappeared. Few English or continental hospitals escaped episodes of near disaster as a result of financial mismanagement, bad luck, or corruption.

In such circumstances, the provision of permanent assistance from a physician was unlikely. But this does not mean that some of the reli-

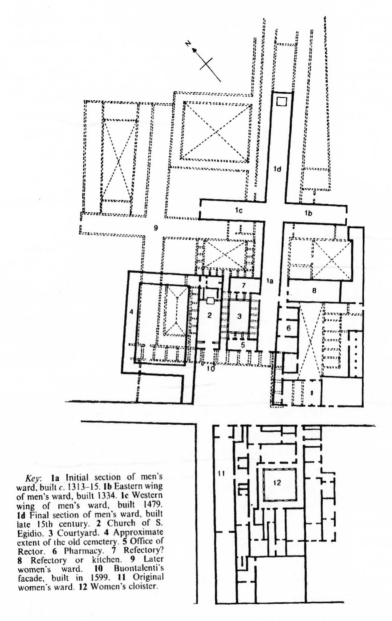

Key: **1a** Initial section of men's ward, built *c.* 1313–15. **1b** Eastern wing of men's ward, built 1334. **1c** Western wing of men's ward, built 1479. **1d** Final section of men's ward, built late 15th century. **2** Church of S. Egidio. **3** Courtyard. **4** Approximate extent of the old cemetery. **5** Office of Rector. **6** Pharmacy. **7** Refectory? **8** Refectory or kitchen. **9** Later women's ward. **10** Buontalenti's facade, built in 1599. **11** Original women's ward. **12** Women's cloister.

Fig. 21. Plan of the hospital of Sta Maria Nuova, Florence, in 1500 (p. 152). Opened in 1288, just outside the city walls, in the sixteenth century it was extended yet further by the construction of a new women's ward to the northwest. Drawn by Patrick Sweeney.

gious who cared for the inmates had no medical knowledge; St. Leonard's, York, had charters witnessed by *medici* (doctors) in the twelfth century, and in 1276 one of its sisters was described as a *medica*. Around 1400, John of Mirfield lived at St. Bartholomew's in London while composing his large *Breviary of Medicine*, which displays a substantial range of medical knowledge gained from practice as well as books. Other doctors are named as Wardens of hospitals, apparently enjoying the profits of office as recompense for services elsewhere as physicians to king or bishop. But medical men certainly attended the Paris Hôtel Dieu in 1231, and one can trace a gradual medicalisation, although still within a religious context, of the hospital of Sta Maria Nuova in Florence from its foundation in 1288 until the sixteenth century. From 12 beds for 'the sick and the poor' in 1288 this 'first hospital among Christians', as one Florentine proudly called it, expanded dramatically to a total of 250 for the 'sick poor' by 1500. By then stays by the able-bodied poor were discouraged, and about 3000 male and an unknown number of female patients were passing through its doors annually (with a cure rate, according to its records, of over 80 percent). It employed a physician and a surgeon by 1350, and had a medical staff of 10 doctors, a pharmacist, and several experienced assistants, including female surgeons, by 1500. Although catering largely for the poor, it had eight private rooms 'reserved for the sick of the higher classes'; it acted as a public dispensary, and even as a medical lending library. Its surgical clinic was open to outpatients with sores and minor illnesses, and its nurses visited the sick in private homes, even those of nobles and patricians. No wonder, then, that when Henry VII of England wished to build a great hospital in London, later the Savoy Hospital (under construction 1505–17), he sent to Florence for the statutes of Sta Maria.

The success of Sta Maria, or of its equivalents in Siena and Milan, can, in part, be attributed to the wealth of the northern Italian cities which enabled the injunctions of the statutes to be fulfilled. Elsewhere, as in Paris, we know of similarly detailed regulations for a hospital, but, equally, criticism of its failures, overcrowding, and medical deficiencies. The true picture is hard to see. Certainly, not everyone viewed these hospitals as death-traps; many elderly patients apparently lived for years as internal pensioners. The treatment provided, even if confined to warmth, food and shelter, helped to alleviate poverty and physical distress. The ban in many hospitals on sufferers from fever, plague or contagious diseases would have reduced cross-infection, and records of hospital epidemics are remarkably few. Hospitals catered mainly for those who lacked other means of support from their family and friends, and hospitals founded by trade guilds can be regarded as extending the mutual assistance of the workplace to those incapable of further work. Above all, there still remained the religious ethos, of Christian charity in the service of Christians. The statutes of Sta Maria organised not only warming the beds in winter, distributing chicken soup, making ward rounds, but also the receiving of communion and the summoning of foreign priests to attend to the spiritual needs of foreign pilgrims. It is the provision of religious care that above all unites the varied manifestations of the medieval hospital.

University medicine

The great age of the creation of hospitals, 1200–1350, coincides with the creation of the first universities in Italy, Spain, France, and England. The first university in a German-speaking region, that of Prague, was not founded until 1348, and the first in what is now Germany, Heidelberg, not until 1385. In Flanders, Scotland, and Scandinavia the fifteenth century saw the arrival of universities as the pinnacles of learning. Both hospital and university developed as a consequence of the increasing wealth of western Europe. The growth of towns led to a greater demand for services of all kinds, and the wealth generated was put to a variety of new purposes.

This is not to say that sophisticated medical teaching appeared only with the rise of the universities, far from it. Salerno was famous for medical instruction (above p. 139) centuries before the university or *studium generale* of Salerno was set up in 1280. The Englishman Alexander Neckham, writing in Paris in the 1180s, listed the medical texts necessary for a proper (and almost certainly idealised) education; and his contemporaries were complaining that their clerical students were being lured away from theology to the more lucrative pursuits of law and medicine, 50 years before a faculty of medicine was created within the university. Similarly, outsiders were studying medicine at Montpellier in 1137, long before its Lord granted formal permission for medical teaching, in 1180, or before the statutory creation of a 'united body (*universitas*) of medical teachers and students', in 1220, and of a *studium generale* of lawyers, doctors, and arts teachers in 1289. Medical

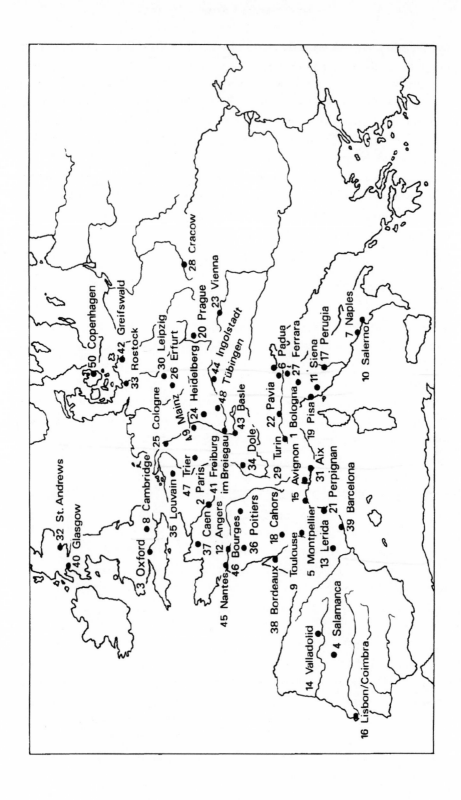

50 Copenhagen
42 Greifswald
33 Rostock
28 Cracow
30 Leipzig
26 Erfurt
23 Vienna
20 Prague
44 Ingolstadt
48 Tübingen
43 Basle
25 Cologne
24 Heidelberg
9 Mainz
6 Padua
22 Pavia
27 Ferrara
11 Siena
17 Perugia
7 Naples
10 Salerno
1 Bologna
19 Pisa
29 Turin
34 Dole
47 Trier
2 Paris
41 Freiburg im Breisgau
15 Avignon
1 Aix
31 Cahors
32 St. Andrews
40 Glasgow
8 Cambridge
3 Oxford
35 Louvain
37 Caen
12 Angers
46 Bourges
36 Poitiers
18 Cahors
9 Toulouse
5 Montpellier
13 Lerida
21 Perpignan
39 Barcelona
45 Nantes
38 Bordeaux
14 Valladolid
4 Salamanca
16 Lisbon/Coimbra

teaching interacted with other academic teaching, but its teachers did not immediately band themselves together as a faculty within a wider university. Indeed, it was precisely the success of the new universities in establishing themselves as the source of professional qualification in law and theology that encouraged already existing associations of doctors to join them and thereby secure (and enlarge) their own rights and privileges.

Historians have frequently distinguished the more clerically dominated universities of northern Europe, e.g. Oxford, where the faculty of theology took precedence, from the more secular ones of Montpellier and Italy, where arts and law were more important. They have also pointed to the varied organisation of medical instruction. At Paris and Oxford, membership of the medical faculty was restricted to teachers; at Montpellier the *universitas* of medicine contained both teachers and students; while at Bologna and Padua there co-existed within the faculty of arts and medicine both an organised student body and a doctoral college that included local doctors as well as professors. But these contrasts are less striking than the similarities.

Firstly, the medical doctorate, the MD, was a high qualification, obtained only after at least 10 years of study, and usually teaching. It was correspondingly expensive. Even the Bachelor of Medicine degree, MB, took several years of study, and required a preliminary training in arts.

Map 2. Map of European universities with medical teaching or degrees before 1480. (Based on H. Ridder-Symoens, *A History of the University in Europe*, Vol. I, Cambridge University Press, 1992, pp. 62–5.)

The Universities and foundation dates are as follows:

1 Bologna (founded *c.* 1180); 2 Paris (*c.* 1200); 3 Oxford (*c.* 1200); 4 Salamanca (*c.* 1218); 5 Montpellier (*c.* 1220); 6 Padua (1222); 7 Naples (1224); 8 Cambridge (*c.* 1225); 9 Toulouse (1229); 10 Salerno (1231/1280); 11 Siena (1246/1347); 12 Angers (*c.* 1250); 13 Lerida (1300); 14 Valladolid (*c.* 1300); 15 Avignon (1303); 16 Lisbon/Coimbra (1308); 17 Perugia (1308); 18 Cahors (1332); 19 Pisa (1343); 20 Prague (1347); 21 Perpignan (1356); 22 Pavia (1361/1412); 23 Vienna (1365); 24 Heidelberg (1385); 25 Cologne (1388); 26 Erfurt(1392); 27 Ferrara (1391/1430); 28 Cracow (1397); 29 Turin (1404); 30 Leipzig (1409); 31 Aix (1409); 32 St. Andrews (1411); 33 Rostock (1419); 34 Dole (1422); 35 Louvain (1425); 36 Poitiers (1431); 37 Caen (1432); 38 Bordeaux (1441); 39 Barcelona (1450); 40 Glasgow (1451); 41 Freiburg im Breisgau (1456); 42 Greifswald (1456); 43 Basle (1459); 44 Ingolstadt (1459/1472); 45 Nantes (1460); 46 Bourges (1464); 47 Trier (1473); 48 Tübingen (1476); 49 Mainz (1476); 50 Copenhagen (1479).

Note: Scottish and French universities, save for Paris and Montpellier, did not develop medical teaching until many years after their initial foundation, and then very sporadically. Medical teaching is documented for Salerno *c.* 1100, but the school was not part of a university until later; its existence in 1480 is problematic.

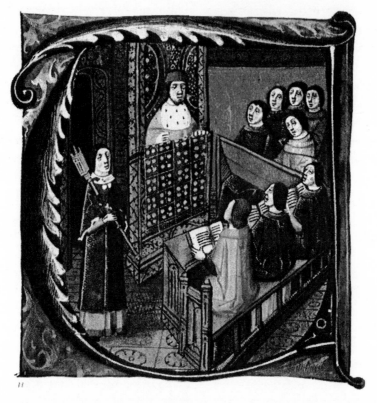

Fig. 22. A university lecture room. An initial from a beautifully illustrated manuscript of the works of Galen, written in Flanders *c.* 1460. (Dresden, Sächsische Landesbibliothek D b 92, fol. 503 v.)

Secondly, and partly because of the costs involved, the numbers of medical students were always small, both in themselves and in comparison to the total university student population. At Cologne only eight students out of 800 who registered between 1395 and 1445 studied medicine; at fifteenth-century Oxford one medical student graduated every two years, at Cambridge hardly two a decade. Even in Italy, Bologna granted 65 degrees in medicine and one in surgery between 1419 and 1434, Turin a mere 13 between 1426 and 1462. Padua was the exception: in 1450 nine medical or surgical degrees were awarded (out of 93 degrees in all), and medical students made up 10 per cent of the student population. Padua's medical faculty was unusually large, 16 in 1436; by contrast, Oxford had then just one MD resident and teaching.

Thirdly, the education provided closely resembled that given elsewhere in the university. It was based upon lectures on specific books,

156

usually parts of the *Articella* and Avicenna's *Canon*, supplemented by disputations on interesting problems and heavily influenced by the new Aristotelianism. All had studied, and in Italy many had taught, Aristotle, whose philosophy apparently explained the stability of the god-created universe, of which medicine was one part, and established the essential categories in which medicine was to be discussed. In Aristotelian terms, the aim of a medical education was knowledge, *scientia*, which was by definition certain, sure, and true, being logically derived from first principles, and which was taught in a logical progression, moving from universal causes to specific effects. Even when, from around 1315, the public dissection of a human corpse was gradually introduced into some university teaching, the professor of anatomy was less concerned to reveal the body for itself than to place what could be seen and what had been written about the body within the wider contexts of natural philosophy and therapeutic theory. A university-trained doctor thus gained knowledge that went beyond the individual body that he was to treat, back to irrefutable first principles, and to a complex of doctrine that was sustained by the rules of logic and, ultimately, by the tenets of theology. The medico-philosophical universe of Galen and Avicenna was compatible with that of great theologians like Albertus Magnus (1193–1280), who had much to say about medicine, and this apparently timeless compatibility itself served to guarantee the truths of Galenism.

It is easy to sneer at medieval learning, at professorial disputes about the definition of a drug's quantity, or whether a tumour indicated only a qualitative change within the body. One may deplore the proliferation of such questions as 'Can sleep be harmful ?', 'Does milk nourish the breasts?', and 'Does cold water help in tumours and pleurisy?'. But this is to miss the point of what was being taught. In order to interpret what was going on in the body one had first to understand what, in medieval terms, counted as fundamental knowledge; how matter came to be, how it changed, and the eternal laws it obeyed. One then saw how these were exemplified in Man, and thus learned the universal truths from which to resolve an individual case. The reputation of many Italian professors rested on their ability to reconcile these universal truths with their flourishing bedside practice. Ugo Benzi of Siena (1376–1439), no ivory-tower academic, was consulted by hundreds of patients, and his lectures on Avicenna's *Canon* attracted large numbers of students.

Teaching by commentary allowed for great flexibility. It involved a

157

variety of expositional skills – it is easy to forget how much the pyrotechnics of the lecturer may have been what attracted students – and professors could easily introduce new material, e.g. the new Galenic or Arabic material, or invoke wider considerations. The famous commentary on Galen's *Tegni* by Pietro Torrigiano (*fl.* 1317) was nick-named the '*Plusquam commentum* (*More than just a Commentary*)'.

A university medical education gave one access to the best patients. The new elites, who were increasingly trained themselves in the uni-versities as lawyers or theologians, favoured doctors who talked the same Aristotelian language. The Italian literary 'Dispute between the arts', in which doctors, lawyers, and orators asserted their own pre-eminence, depended on all these groups participating in the same social and intellectual world. If an MD involved a large investment in terms of time, books, loss of other earnings, and, finally, the degree fee, its potential profits were enormous. As the popular verse put it, 'Galen provides wealth, Justinian (i.e. a law degree) office'.

The claim of the graduate physician to cure rested on his under-standing of his patient's individual constitution and how it might be changed, for both good and ill. Familiarity with the patient, taking the pulse, examining urine and other excreta, and interpreting the patient's story (often told at a distance in a letter or by a friend or relative) would lead the doctor to an individual diagnosis and therapy. The more precise the advice, the greater the apparent expertise of the doctor. Likewise, a complex mixture of drugs, carefully chosen to obtain the exact grade of drug action, revealed both the doctor's accuracy of diag-nosis, and his ability to understand the often hidden workings of the natural world as expressed in its elements and qualities.

For this mathematics was needed, which, as taught in the university arts course, also involved an understanding of the workings of the heavens, 'astronomy', a term that also embraced astrology. This was a useful skill for doctors, who often took along to the bedside brief tables to help them calculate the position of the planets and their relationship to the body and its diseases. Medical astronomy had a long history. In its emphasis on the weather, the seasons, and certain mathematically related 'critical' days of an illness, it went back to the Hippocratic Corpus. Later Greek and particularly Arabic astronomer-physicians had developed these ideas further, which were repeated in such widely-cir-culated medieval tracts as William of England's *If One Cannot Inspect the Urine*, which explained how to judge disease from the stars and the signs of the zodiac without the need for uroscopy. Each planet, as it progresses through the heavens, exercises its influence on the body: it has its own diseases, and its own preferred parts of the body, and the learned physician should incorporate this knowledge into his therapy.

Medical astronomy took many forms. At one extreme, it involved very complex mathematical calculations of the interrelationship between planets and the manipulation of astrological tables; at the other, handy guides depicted visually to the illiterate the parts of the body and the diseases under the influence of the planets and the zodiac. Its practitioners were equally varied, from the Welsh priest-physician, Thomas Brown (*c.* 1395) to noted astronomers, like the Oxford physician Simon Bredon (*c.* 1310–72) and Giovanni Dondi (d. 1370), professor of medicine at Padua and designer of a celebrated astronomical clock. The medical professors of Louvain (Belgium) became rich in the fifteenth century by producing popular almanacs incorporating astrological and medical information. Few royal households lacked a physician-astrologer, like John of Bosnia (*fl.* 1450–84), who left the University of Valencia to serve the King of Anjou.

But astronomy had its dangerous side even for a doctor. John of Toledo (d. 1275) was imprisoned for astrology, necromancy, and alchemy, before being eventually released to become a Cardinal. Cecco d'Ascoli (1257–1327), poet, astrologer, and physician, was sentenced to death, while his contemporary, the professor and translator Pietro d'Abano, was pursued even in the grave, when the Venetian authorities ordered his body to be dug up and burnt. Such suspicions of doctors were not confined to Italy. The appointment of the Scot William Scheves as Archdeacon of St. Andrew's (Scotland) in 1472 was opposed by its reformist Archbishop on the grounds of his Louvain education in astrology and medicine. Undaunted, and supported by King James III and the Rector of St. Andrew's University, Scheves went off to Rome to complain, returning not as Archdeacon but as Archbishop.

Apothecaries and surgeons

Dietetics in accordance with the six non-naturals (p. 141) was the main therapeutic standby of the physician, supplemented by drugs and, occasionally, surgery. Most learned physicians had at least one pharmacopoeia, like the *Antidotary* of Nicolaus, *c.* 1150, widely available in Latin and in several vernacular versions, or the *Pandects* of Mattheus

Silvaticus (*c.* 1342), both more sophisticated in theory and broader in range than similar early medieval Latin tracts. But although they emphasised that the physician should make up his own drugs, and medieval miniaturists portrayed the doctor in his surgery surrounded by specimens of plants, it was often alleged that the average physician knew far less than a housewife (the lady of the manor was often literate enough to have her own notebook of remedies), and was at the mercy of the apothecary.

The word apothecary, 'storeman', seems to have been applied specifically to druggists first in the greatest of all medieval trading cities, Venice, where there were large stores, *apothecai,* housing drugs brought from the Greek and Muslim East. The relationship of apothecaries with those whom they supplied was generally easy. There might be occasional conflicts over University claims, recorded from 1271 onwards, to control apothecaries through an annual inspection, the use of a standard *Antidotary,* and, as at Heidelberg in 1471, an official list of drugs and official prices. In Cologne in 1470 a jar of theriac was burnt after being rejected by the university professors. But often physician, druggist, and spicer participated in the same Guild, as at Florence, to the disquiet of those who suspected a compact to make money, or, as the citizens of Leipzig complained in 1502, to foist worthless drugs on the general public.

Relations between doctors and surgeons are more problematic. Historians have often contrasted the pretensions, over-subtleties, and high fees of the one with the common-sense, altruism, and practicality of the other. The Later Middle Ages are depicted as an age of surgery, when, perhaps for the first time, the art of surgery became an independent and respected part of medicine.

There is some truth in this argument. Surgical writing from 1170 onwards shows a new sophistication and offers a substantially greater range of successful treatments: e.g. the operation to replace intestines protruding from a wound advocated by Roland of Parma (northern Italy, *c.* 1210) is neater than Galen's, and the techniques used by the English surgeon John of Arderne (*fl.* 1307–70) to cure an anal fistula are rightly praised. Hernias, wounds, nasal polyps, bladder-stone, and fractures had all been treated competently before 1200, and practical skills were not confined to surgeons. University statutes, particularly after 1320, frequently demanded a period of supervised practical training before a degree – how far these demands were met is another matter.

The exaltation of medieval surgery over physic may arise simply from a quirk of the evidence. The results of surgery are often perceptible, and thus much easier for later generations to appreciate. Teodorico Borgognoni's description of head wounds corresponds so closely to modern observation that one is confident that he knew what he was doing when cleaning a skull abrasion. The surgeon John Bradmore (d. 1412) tells how he removed an arrow from the head of the future Henry V in 1403 and foiled an attempted suicide in 1399 by washing a stab wound with wine (which reduced the possibility of sepsis) and then stitching the intestines and abdomen, and there is independent confirmation that both patients survived the operation. By contrast, even when a physician's patient lived for some years after treatment, doubt remains over the original diagnosis and efficacy of treatment. But although many purgatives and diuretics would not, in modern eyes, have contributed much to the cure of the disease, their immediate (and obvious) effects would have confirmed that their prescribers knew what they were doing. Nor should one forget that both Arderne and Henri de Mondeville (*fl.* 1310) asserted that they could do far more than most other surgeons, and that Bradmore's cure of Henry V followed on the failure of others. One cannot neglect the torments of those left for years with a suppurating wound after being cut for bladder-stone or the almost inevitable recurrence of an inguinal hernia. One can only shudder at the agonies of patients forcibly held (or chained) down while the surgeon plied the knife or the red-hot cautery, whose pain was only slightly dulled by draughts of opiated wine or by the soporific sponge. While surgeons rightly observed that wounds with a pure, white and odourless pus healed better than those with a watery, serous and evil-smelling one, they wrongly concluded that the former, 'laudable', pus was essential for all healing and that its flow should be promoted wherever possible. Surgery had its drawbacks as much as physic, and it was very much a treatment of last resort.

Nor was the intellectual gulf between surgeon and physician as wide as is often supposed. In Florence, alongside the semi-literate specialists in hernias, boils, eye diseases, fractures, and tooth-pulling, like Paolo di Ricco, 'blacksmith and doctor' (*fl.* 1422), and the appropriately named Domenico de Dentibus (Dominic Teeth, *fl.* 1352), can be set Giovanni di Bartolomeo, a bookless physician executed for heresy and necromancy in 1450. In the eyes of other surgeons, like Jacopo da Prato (*fl.* 1361), such men were all a threat to the good name of surgery. Jacopo, the

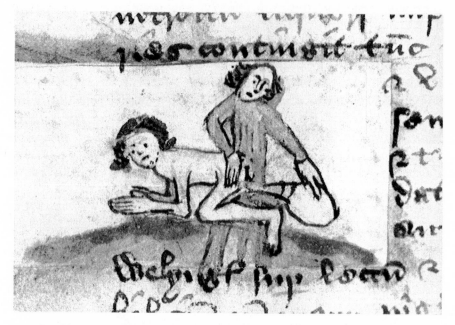

Fig. 23. A surgeon inserts a pipe attached to a pig's bladder to give a clyster or enema. A marginal drawing from a manuscript of the surgeon John of Arderne (1307–76). (The Wellcome Institute Library, London, WMS 550, fol. 193 v.)

author of *On Manual Operations*, taught surgery at the University of Florence. He was familiar with the works of Arabic surgeons and with Galen, like his contemporary in Avignon, Guy de Chauliac (1300–68), who in his great *Surgery* cited 38 works of Galen, some of them only recently translated. Even a barber-surgeon like Thomas Plawdon in London (d. 1413) might own a book, or books, on medicine and surgery that contained academic material.

Particularly in southern Europe, surgery was an acceptable skill for a physician to acquire. Frederick II, the ruler of Sicily and southern Italy, ordained in 1231 that a doctor could be licensed only after five years of medical study that had included surgery and had been validated by the teaching masters of Salerno. In northern Italy, writers such as Roger Frugardi (*fl.* 1170, author of a widely read *Surgery*), and Teodorico Borgognoni described operations performed by professors, doctors, and surgeons alike, and appealed to the *medici manuales*, doctors with manual skills. Surgical lectures in Italian universities were common, as were surgical degrees. In France Henri de Mondeville's audience in Paris and possibly Montpellier was not confined to surgeons. Henri may have been introduced to the new Italian surgery by Lanfranc of Milan, who lectured at Paris in 1285, or Guglielmo da Brescia (c. 1250–1326), who had studied and taught at Bologna before embarking on a lucrative clerical and medical career around Europe. In fifteenth-century Germany, leading physicians, often Italian-trained, like Peter of Ulm (c. 1390 to c. 1440), doctor to the Elector Palatine, did not fear to practise surgery. His Heidelberg colleague, Heinrich Münsinger (1397–1476), wrote a book on surgery incorporating therapies devised by both physicians and surgeons, and his own remedies circulated widely among surgeons and barbers, as well as physicians.

But elsewhere, the gulf between physician and surgeon was wider. Surgery was rarely included in the university curriculum outside Italy, and an Italian learned surgeon was warned that the French would treat him as shamefully as if he were a barber. Surgical practice in Northern Europe was largely organised on a guild basis, through a system of apprenticeship and examination by fellow guild members. In towns without a university, like London or, until 1457, Freiburg-im-Breisgau, the guild structure dominated medical life. In London, the Fellowship of Surgeons existed by 1368/9, and the much larger Company of Barbers was chartered in 1376. But the handful of university-trained physicians did not attempt to organise themselves until 1423, when a few physicians and surgeons, including the royal surgeon Thomas Morstede (d. 1450), successfully petitioned the Lord Mayor for a joint college 'for the better education and control of physicians and surgeons practising in the city and its liberties.' Of the life and activities of this association little is known. Its head, 'Master of the Mystery' or 'Rector of medical men', was Gilbert Kymer (c.1385–1463), Oxford don and court physician, who arbitrated in 1424 in a case of alleged improper treatment by surgeons. The Barbers, in their turn, had their rights to practise surgery confirmed by the Lord Mayor, despite Kymer's College, which then disappears from the records. Not until 1518 (p. 236) had the physicians any institutional means of enforcing their pretensions to control medical practice in London.

In Paris, by contrast, there was a three-cornered contest between physicians of the Faculty, the surgeons, organised into the College of St. Cosmas, and the barber-surgeons. The friendly relations between the first two in 1350 gradually turned to public hostility, even though the Faculty continued to offer lectures to master surgeons. Surgeons' complaints in 1499 that the members of Faculty were lecturing in French 'from Guy de Chauliac', not Latin, and that barbers were attending university dissections provide further evidence of a sensitivity to status, but may reveal little of the realities of medical life. More typical may have been English towns like Bristol or Norwich, where physicians, surgeons, and barbers joined together, or Cologne where graduate physicians could associate with 'empiric surgeons', provided they were good Christians. Admittedly, few medical guilds were as hospitable as that of Florence, which included all those with medical skills, from the Medici family's private physician to Monna Neccia, registered in 1359 as a ringworm doctor. Illiteracy was no bar, and the conditions for entry were lightly enforced – 'No one in the past has ever been refused', it was alleged in 1422. But tensions there were, for the begowned university professor was loth to attend, as Guild regulations demanded, a bone-setter's funeral, and there were several attempts to create a proper college, open only to graduates and with high entry fees, like that of Padua or, across the Alps, of Lyons, whose standards for entry were even higher than for a university degree.

These conflicts must be seen in a wider context of increased wealth, population, numbers of healers, and medical information. There was a new surgery as well as a new physic beginning in the twelfth century, and both socially and intellectually, leading physicians and surgeons in London or Paris had more in common with each other than with any of the host of barbers or other empirics. It was a Florentine physician, Niccolò Falcucci (d. 1412), who demanded the exclusion from surgical practice of empirics and wise-women, and who attributed even their lasting cures to luck. The rise of the universities shifted the definition of medicine towards a body of book-learning, an argument that increasingly appealed to surgeons who had read their Albucasis, their Roger, and their Guy de Chauliac. There thus arose an orthodoxy against which to measure the non-orthodox practitioner.

The professional pyramid

Learned physicians, the tiny apex of a broad pyramid, and learned surgeons constituted only a small fraction of those offering medical services. In 1435, seventeen London surgeons petitioned for the confirmation of the privileges of the Fellowship of Surgeons, a number not reached again for a century. At York one physician and eighteen barbers attended its 7500 inhabitants in 1381. Below the barbers could be found a multitude of healers, some combining medical assistance in addition to another occupation, some, especially women, dispensing home-medicines to their neighbours. To Florence between 1380 and 1446 flocked graduates of Bologna or Padua, eye-doctors from Cortona, bone-setters from Rome, and whole families of experts from upland Italy in eye-diseases, bladder-stone, hernias, and urino-genital problems. In the countryside, where graduate physicians were far fewer, one might choose between the lady of the manor (with her own network of friends with similar interests), the local priest, herbalists, midwives, and purveyors of traditional 'folkloric' remedies. Nor were country folk simply left to magic, sorcery, and charlatanry. Even remote Spanish villages tried to discover the competence of a healer, and were suspicious of travelling quacks and magicians. Indeed, medical magic is mentioned more often in connection with large towns and royal courts than with the countryside. Five 'sorcerers' were allowed to attempt to cure Charles VI of France in 1403, but when they failed, they were burnt at the stake. Michel de Discipatis, a former Dominican monk with many patients at Chambéry (France), the capital of Savoy, was luckier. In 1417, he escaped with life imprisonment after being accused of apostasy, sorcery, astrology, and illegal medical practice.

This variety of healers was matched by a variety of attempts at regulation. Sometimes the decision was left to a university Faculty, a local College of physicians, or a body of medical (and often surgical) experts set up by the ruler. In the Kingdom of Sicily the royal physician took charge of official licensing, assisted by a small committee. Ecclesiastical authorities, whose administrative system went down to parish level, might also be involved, especially in controlling midwives (p. 171). How effective such control was is debatable. The frequency and ferocity with which irregular practitioners, throughout Europe, were hauled through the law-courts shows that not everyone was willing to trust to the often expensive hands of physicians, surgeons, and other guild members. Successful regulation of medical practice may in fact reveal more about the power of a ruler, a medical association, or a city council to enforce its will on other members of the community than about the quality of healing available. In a small town like Freiburg-im-Breisgau, the authorities could easily ensure in 1457 that 'surgeons, barbers, physicians, apothecaries, rootcutters, and empirics' plied their skills only after approval by the medical Faculty of the new university. In Vienna, where in 1454 a mere 11 MDs served a population of 50,000, such a task was vain and unending.

The increasing size of towns and sophistication of civic organisation explains the development of a system of physicians paid by the community in return for medical services. Although such doctors had been known in Antiquity (pp. 38, 45), a link with their medieval successors is at best indirect. The earliest known public contracts come from two rich northern Italian cities, Reggio in 1211 and its neighbour Bologna in 1214, where Ugo Borgognoni of Lucca was granted (officially at his own request) citizenship for his family and a stipend in money and property. His contract is typical of many later contracts in three ways. Firstly, it imposed a residence requirement on what the town hoped was a competent healer whether physician or surgeon – and Ugo stayed for over 40 years. Secondly, it struck a balance between the doctor's private and public duties. Ugo's primary service to Bologna lasted six or eight months, extendable in time of conflict, and he could (and did) take non-Bolognese patients who paid appropriately. Finally, there was a flexible level of fees for citizens; the poor paid nothing (a reward in heaven, said the council at Urbino, being a more than adequate recompense for the doctor), the rich a cartload of wood or hay. Sometimes a city council fixed maxima for visits or drugs, and often distinguished between treating citizens inside or outside the city walls, and between treatment and consultation. In Venice, a civic doctor's consultations were free, even to nobles if they came themselves to the surgery (an important qualification in a status-conscious society). But non-citizens were generally excluded from any free treatment, and non-civic doctors made their usual charges.

Frequently the civic doctor offered public advice, especially on plague, and delivered his opinion at inquests or police investigations. He might be obliged to attend the municipal hospital, or treat injuries resulting from official punishment or torture. At least two civic doctors in Venice, both famous as teachers elsewhere, contracted to take pupils along with them on their rounds. It is equally important to state what these civic appointees did not do: oversee the public health arrangements of the community, have the right to check on pharmacists, or pursue charlatans. That was left to lay magistrates, although civic doctors might well be summoned to advise a Health Board or accompany an official to inspect a town hospital or a druggist's stock.

This system of publicly hired physicians and surgeons spread relatively quickly in Italy and beyond. By 1300, they were found in all the larger towns of northern Italy (e.g. Perugia, 1222) and in several smaller; by 1400 the system was almost universal in the market towns of Italy and important outposts of the Venetian empire, and had been adopted also in the larger towns of Provence, Aragon, and Valencia (Spain). By 1500 civic doctors were appointed even in Italian towns with hardly a thousand inhabitants (e.g. Sacile, northern Italy), and in northern France, Flanders, and many large German towns. They did not, however, as yet cross the Channel.

The system had its drawbacks. Penny-pinching councils liked value for money; a young graduate or an older man apparently down on his luck were common options, but subsequent experience might reveal their incompetence. A legal contract did not prevent a man from moving on – an investment in a prospective civic doctor by paying his university fees was wasted if he preferred a career as a professor or papal physician. In times of plague, not every civic doctor remained at his post, and a community might find itself without medical advice just when it was most needed. Salaries were expensive – in 1324, the Grand Council of Venice, alarmed at the costs of its 31 civic doctors and surgeons, determined on a reduction by not filling some vacancies, and by paying new appointees less. In 1416, the council of Udine (northern Italy) appointed the same man to serve as both town doctor and schoolmaster. In the face of claims that an abundance of doctors would enhance a city's prestige and population, others were more sceptical. A city like Milan or Florence had enough rich citizens to attract competent doctors and, in exchange for tax breaks, these plutocratic practitioners, it was thought, would easily be persuaded to help the poor for nothing. Larger Italian cities in the fifteenth century gradually reduced the number of civic doctors, and even smaller ones considered alternatives. In 1451 Udine suspended the salaries of two of its three civic doctors and devoted the money saved to a worthier cause – the erection of a municipal bell-tower.

The increasing numbers of civic doctors, as of all providers of health, must be seen against a wider context – the burgeoning of towns and cities from around 1100, a demographic and economic process interrupted only by the arrival of the Black Death, and the increasing wealth of some of their citizens created a new market for medical care, at all levels. Attempts to regulate this market were made by the authorities, national, ecclesiastical, university, and local, using a variety of often overlapping and competing strategies that involved both lay and professional expertise. But neither medical nor lay authority had the power (or the punishments) to secure obedience to their regulations. Patient preference for a bone-setter, herbalist or wise-woman could defy even a tight guild-based system, and was not necessarily foolish. Evidence from Spain for the period 1300–50 shows how, as ever more healers, university-trained or not, offered their services, patients, even if coming gradually to prefer the evidence of a medical degree, nevertheless retained control over their choice of adviser. Solid experience and local familiarity counted for much, and, for the rest, peasants and townsfolk alike displayed a proper healthy scepticism.

Women's problems, women's healers

It is a commonplace that in the Middle Ages women's illnesses were women's business. True, the process of childbirth was largely left to women – the mother is pictured with midwives, friends, and neighbours, and a Flemish husband was even fined for hiding behind a staircase to eavesdrop on his wife in labour. From 1400 onwards, midwives were being paid by some town councils to act in a variety of cases involving female physiology, obstetrics, and infant care. They tested for virginity or impotence, and certified the deaths of infants. Some obstetrical texts were directed specifically to women, occasionally modifying the language of a learned and gender-neutral text to fit a feminine audience.

But such female-oriented texts are the exception. Although empirical knowledge of childbirth remained largely women's knowledge, and manual vaginal exploration was carried out by women, most medical compendia contained long sections on obstetrics, and most gynaecological treatises were written by and for male practitioners. An English 'woman's guide to health' formed part of a surgical compilation aimed at and owned by a male practitioner, and another version of the same text circulated along with the *Medical Compendium* of Gilbert the Englishman (*c.* 1240) and texts on blood-letting, prognostics, and buboes. A few illustrations (admittedly in non-medical tracts) show a doctor present at birth as adviser to the midwife in a difficult case and occasionally delivering the baby himself.

But even if most obstetrical care was in the hands of women and many midwives were literate, to assert that women's illnesses were treated by women is exaggerated. Case histories by male healers show them treating men and women alike, even if direct physical examination was very rare. Palpating the stomach, taking the pulse, inspecting urine were independent of gender, and woman was considered subject to the same overall constraints of nature as man. Various ethical injunctions, from the Hippocratic *Oath* on, presupposed that a doctor would treat female patients, for both their reproductive and their general health. Claims that women were ashamed to show diseases of their private parts to doctors or that male doctors bungled their treatment of women do not suggest a rigid division of the sexes. These demands for an acknowledgment of a superior feminine competence brought European fame to their presumed author, 'Trotula', a woman of Salerno. Nevertheless, although a respected female practitioner, Trota, lived before 1150 in Salerno, 'Trotula's' book itself is a composite work mainly written by men. Neither the rhetoric of a woman's medicine for women nor monastic moralists' denunciations of young monks led astray by female patients may correspond to actual practice.

Certainly medical writers themselves did not hesitate to discuss gynaecological problems, or counsel both sexes for sexual disorders – love-madness was taken seriously as an emotional problem with physical consequences – and bowdlerisation is strikingly rare. Gynaecological information and details of the sexual organs circulated widely, albeit often in Latin. While clerics thundered in sermons against abortion and contraception, even for health reasons, medical writers regularly advised on such matters. Bernard of Gordon was almost alone in omitting abortifacients and contraceptives and in allowing coitus only for the sake of offspring, a commonplace among theologians. Indeed, far from remaining silent, medical authors often produced long lists of suitable therapeutic agents for increasing sexual pleasure and potency (for sexual activity was, in medical eyes, necessary for maintaining a balance of humours, and female orgasm essential for conception, at least of male children). Sometimes overt contradictions appear within the teachings of a single author. Albertus Magnus in *On Plants* listed the substances used by doctors, exorcists, and magicians to prevent conception or cause abortion (e.g. the pear), acts which he condemned in his theological writings. The *Treasury of the Poor*, ascribed to Peter of Spain, the later Pope John XXI, listed 34 prescriptions for aphrodisiacs, 26 for contraceptives, and 56 to ensure fertility. Others were recommended 'to bring about menstruation', and potentially an abortion. Even if there existed networks of information among women on the efficacy of various herbs, the same information was publicly retailed by male authors and teachers. Not every theologian, however, considered contraception homicide, and abortion under 40 days (when, on some arguments, the foetus became ensouled) was treated leniently. In 1409 Adelheid of Stuttgart was simply sent back across the Rhine from Sélestat (Alsace) and barred from the city for three years after being convicted of procuring abortions for many respectable women.

Adelheid may have treated only women, but other female healers dealt also with male patients. English records show a few women called 'leech' or '*medica*' – Euphemia, abbess of Wherwell, Hampshire (d. 1257), administered to her fellow nuns 'all the necessities of life, for sickness and for health', and had an infirmary built on the most hygienic of plans. At the hospital of St. Leonard's, York, one sister, Ann, was described in 1276 as a *medica*. 'Women of Salerno', as well as Trota, are occasionally mentioned in the male Salernitan medical literature, and not just for their recipes, and a few women healers were accepted into the Florentine medical guild. The medical writings of Hildegard of Bingen (Germany, 1098–1197) are in their learning and practicality the equal of any by her male contemporaries. In Spain, Bevenguda of Valencia was commended by the king in 1394 for 'treating and curing many men and children of both sexes of serious conditions and illnesses'. In the kingdom of Naples between 1273 and 1410 at least 23 women were licensed by the authorities to practise surgery in their own region, 11 without restriction on the sex of their patients. A few female surgeons are known from other parts of Europe, where they learned their craft as apprentices to father or husband, taking over from them when they died.

The number of known female practitioners is small, one or two per cent of all practitioners, and may be distorted by biases inherent in the sources. University-trained physicians, possessors of wealth sufficient to make a will, and guild officials are far better represented in surviving documents than women (of all classes). Furthermore, medical historians have tended to marginalise lesser healers as empirics, charlatans, wise-women, or midwives, terms which have led to an underestimate of the role (and abilities) of women healers. Nonetheless, although some women knew as much and practised in the same way as men, they were increasingly excluded in the late Middle Ages, caught in the middle of conflicts provoked by the increasing professionalisation of medicine. The statute of 1271 which subordinated French surgeons, apothecaries, and herbalists to the physicians of the Paris Faculty, confining them to their own specialities, made no distinction between male and female. But in 1322, the prosecutor of a female unlicensed healer, Jacoba Félicie, and several other male healers, appealed to it as if it specifically banned women. Her claim that she should be allowed to practise since she would not threaten women's modesty, was dismissed as worthless and frivolous. A similar process can be seen in Spain. By 1299, medical practice was occasionally restricted to those who had 'learned the science of medicine'; all others, male or female, Christian, Jew or Muslim, were indiscriminately banned. Thirty years later, legal prohibitions were being aimed directly at women – they were to confine themselves to treating women and children, and their treatments were carefully specified. The example of Bevenguda, (p. 170), however, cautions against overestimating the effectiveness of these restrictions. In England, a petition to Parliament in 1421 to ban women from practising physic under pain of long imprisonment and a hefty fine received a lukewarm response, but elsewhere the restriction of medical and surgical practice to graduates or guild members further confined women healers to the home or midwifery.

Attempts to control midwifery, however, come remarkably late. The first known order, from Brussels, dates from 1424, but regulations are rare until the next century. In Brussels, the town authorities (who had already employed midwives for some decades) established a board of five 'chief midwives', the town physician, and the priest of St. Gudula to approve all midwives. Their criteria were based on moral considerations – although the chief midwives might be thought good judges of a woman's practical competence. The order's preamble hints at a further reason, for it talks of dangerous birthing practices, and the possibility of a child dying unbaptised, and hence not going to Heaven, because of a midwife's ignorance.

By the end of the century midwives were coming under increasing suspicion of witchcraft. A papal Bull of 1484 drew attention to the attacks of witches on the reproductive functions and fertility of men and women, an area of special interest to midwives. Two years later, in their widely influential *Malleus maleficarum* (*Hammer of Witches*), Henricus Institoris and Jacob Sprenger accused midwives of a variety of crimes – killing a child in the womb or shortly after birth, eating a child in a witches' congress, and offering a new-born child to the devil in a blasphemous parody of baptism. They brought forward alleged examples of witch midwives, mainly from the area of the Upper Rhine, and similar outrages were later reported from Italy, Spain, France, and Belgium, reflecting in exaggerated form concerns long expressed by bishops and local synods about midwives' baptisms. How far such reactions represented reality or the fears of the group least in touch with midwives, ecclesiastical bureaucrats, is an open question. In a society familiar with the tale of the Venomous Virgin, who meant death to any man who slept with her, and which believed that post-menopausal women infected small children with a glance and that a pubic hair of a woman mixed with menses and placed in a dung-heap engendered poisonous snakes, all those who came into contact professionally with women's sexual organs were doubly suspect. But the rhetoric of witchcraft was used far less against midwives than against wise-women and empirics who employed chants, charms, and prayers. These were often far more marginal than the midwife, who, as the Flanders evidence shows, was as conscious of her own moral and social status as any town councillor.

The midwife's view, however, is largely absent from the enormous medieval literature on gynaecology. Its authors drew on a variety of traditions – Aristotle (directly and in Arabic dress), Galen, Soranus (at least in outline in a Latin tract ascribed to Muscio), and the Bible – which together showed that men and women had the same physiology, but in superior and inferior versions. Female organs of generation resembled those of men, but in reverse; the womb was a penis inverted and stuck inside the body. The female body displayed more of the fleshy, oozing, physicality of labile matter than the male. It was more unformed, with openings and leakages: the regular copious outflow of blood in menstruation corresponded to the irregular nosebleeds and haemorrhoids in an adult male, and both had the same natural explanation.

On the topic of generation, doctors, philosophers, and theologians each had their own standpoints and definitions, e.g. of the time when the soul entered the foetus. Here Galen's tripartite soul came into apparent conflict with Aristotle and Christianity. Some philosophers argued that from conception the embryo had the power of sensation and nutrition, to which was later added that of rationality. Others thought this damaged the unity of the Christian soul, and posited that the newly arrived rational soul, itself already endowed by

172

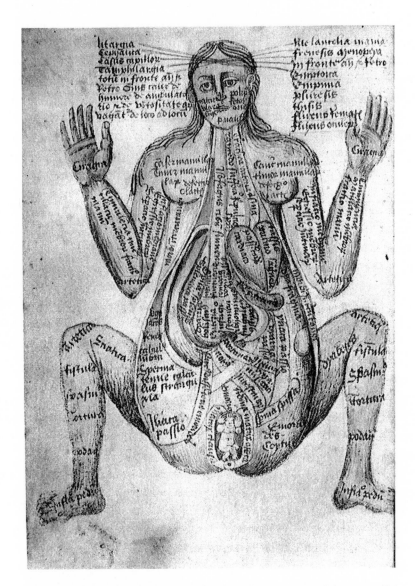

Fig. 24. The diseases of women. One of a series of pictures appended to a so-called *Anatomy of Galen* (in fact a medieval *Anatomy of the Pig*), in an illuminated manuscript in Middle English. (The Wellcome Institute Library, London, WMS 290, fol. 52 v.)

God with all its powers, replaced the matter-created sensitive and vegetative forms. Others, like Albertus Magnus, imagined the soul as developing partly from natural generation and partly from Divine intervention, an unsuccessful attempt to reconcile all sides. Almost everyone, however, agreed that the embryo must be formed (at between 30 and 45 days in boys, later in girls) before the rational soul was infused into it to give movement (a time-scale which cannot be identified with quickening).

Similar subtleties were employed to decide the role of male and female in generation, where Aristotle's division into male form and female matter was opposed to Galen's theory that both male and female sperm were essential for generation and that menstrual blood provided the matter on which both sperms were nourished. Some authors thought the ovaries the equivalent of male testicles as the production centres of sperm, or, more Aristotelian, mere counterweights to open passages for male sperm to enter. Albertus Magnus argued that they produced only 'a moisture that fomented the desire to receive the male seed'. Other writers united within the same concept of fluid three, to our eyes distinct, processes – ovulation, cervical secretion, and vaginal lubrication.

Whatever conclusion was reached might have enormous consequences. It mattered to theologians how the Virgin Mary conceived Christ: was it out of menstrual blood, or was menstrual blood what remained after the creation of a special blood, well digested, cleaned, and purified, that went into the formation of any embryo? Doctors might reject such subtleties, but they needed to know how to promote conception among the childless, and how the physiological process of generation affected health, both mental and physical.

Another quasi-medical question which preoccupied moralists and medical men for centuries was why a woman, who, as Aristotle and Galen agreed, was colder and moister, should nonetheless feel a more burning sexual desire than a man. To this problem, whose reality was considered self-evident, new answers were constantly propounded. One Salernitan writer thought in terms of the natural world – damp wood takes a long time to catch fire, but burns for longer. Constantine the African, in his *Pantegni*, suggested that the woman derived a double pleasure from both emitting and receiving seed. Aristotelians like Albertus Magnus argued that woman was so moist, so lustful, and, at the same time, so passive, that she could never be satisfied. By 1400 the argument had moved on: woman's pleasure was greater in quantity but less in quality than man's. Such responses take us into a range of misogynistic abuse that characterised all women as naturally flawed, unstable, and crooked in judgment. The best response to this anti-feminism,

174

that of Hildegard of Bingen, was based on the same physical, moral, and psychological data. The qualities that Albertus considered the causes of female instability appeared to Hildegard far more positive. Not only did they fit woman for child-bearing, but they made her passions milder, and hence she was unlikely to fall into the (typically male) errors of desire, fear, or shame. But in a masculine world of medical and philosophical theory, this feminine conclusion was met only with silence.

The medieval body

It would be facile to claim that many of these gynaecological problems noted in the previous section could have been solved if only medieval medical men had had a better knowledge of the body or favoured the perceptible evidence of anatomy over that of texts and logic. Such a claim underestimates the difficulties involved in obtaining such evidence and the constraints, both internal and external, on its interpretation. It also misrepresents the variety of ways in which later medieval society perceived and explained the human body.

From 1200 onwards, the human body became more and more a part of theological discourse. While some still considered it a mere prison or tool for the soul (the most common attitude among the early Church), others increasingly emphasised the soul's embodiment within the here and now. The physicality of Christ was stressed in works of art and accounts of visions. The consecrated bread on the altar, Christ's body, miraculously turned to bleeding flesh in the mouth of the recipient at mass. The power of a saint was associated with physical relics, and possession of an arm, or even a tooth, protected against evil. Pious fraud or theft supplemented the trade in relics – Bishop Hugh of Lincoln (c. 1140–1200), accused of biting off a piece of the bone of Mary Magdalene while venerating it at Fécamp (northern France), argued that if he could touch Christ's body in the Mass, he could certainly chew the Magdalene's arm. The *Golden Legend*, the most popular collection of lives of the saints, added gruesome details of physical mutilation to the stories of martyrdom that had been the stuff of pious instruction since at least the fourth century. Such saints as escaped death for their faith might be noted for their patience in illness, mental as well as physical. Descriptions of mystical experience took on physical form. Ecstatic delight, sensations of Christ the heavenly lover, to say nothing of mystical lactations, bleedings, and the reception of the stigmata (the marks of

Christ's wounds), most notably by St. Francis of Assisi (1182–1226), first appear or are more often recorded from the twelfth century on. The doctrine of the physical resurrection of the body at the Last Judgment was also reemphasised. Theologians were convinced that the body, whether turned to dust or eaten by wild beasts, would then be restored to pristine wholeness, and they discussed, often using the latest medical theories, precisely how this physical regeneration would occur.

In such discussions theological considerations took precedence. The attack on the Cathar heretics, with their strong antitheses between good and evil, body and soul, helped to propagate the new Christian physicality, as did the Aristotelianism of the universities, with its belief in humanity as composed of both form and matter. Yet medical ideas also played a part, not least because many of the theologians concerned with these new ideas on the religious body also wrote on natural philosophy, medicine, and even gynaecology. They were familiar with the notion, deriving ultimately from Galen, that body and soul were closely linked, and with theories of generation and nutrition that involved the transformation of matter. Those who compared the blood flowing from the wounds of martyrs with milk, for instance, knew that in medical theory both were explicable in the same way.

Scholars were also familiar with the Aristotelian ladder of nature, with rational Man at its summit, and with the consequences of this doctrine, that in its material aspects the human body could be described and explained like that of a pig. On a continuum between animals and talking birds, were the *Cynocephali* (dog-headed men living, according to various map-makers, in India, Africa, Finland, or slightly below Paradise), and persons born with aquiline noses. All were governed by the same natural principles.

Given this belief in the unity of creation – and leaving aside the even more important problem of access to human corpses – it is easy to see why the earliest recorded medieval anatomies, at Salerno and Bologna, took place on animals, and why the practice continued; how the body works may be better demonstrated on an analogous animal than on man, and surgical skills sharpened on less hazardous subjects than patients. It is the introduction of specifically human anatomy that requires explanation, not the persistent use of animal analogies, or the two and a half centuries it took for human dissection to become common in European university teaching.

The first recorded public human dissection, of an executed criminal, was performed around 1315 by Mondino de' Liuzzi in Bologna, although others before him may have used human material, e.g. a skull or bones. In 1308 the Venetian Senate gave permission for an annual dissection. But permission is not the same as action, nor was the example of the northern Italians followed quickly elsewhere. In Spain, the first public dissection is recorded at Lerida in 1391; in the German regions, at Vienna in 1404. Yet these were isolated examples, and anatomy teaching using a human corpse did not become standard practice until the middle years of the sixteenth century. Even when university statutes prescribed regular annual anatomies, the difficulty of finding a suitable corpse meant that years might pass between anatomies, which, when they occurred, were usually of men, who were far more likely than women to be executed as criminals or heretics. The occasional anatomy of a woman attracted large numbers of spectators by its rarity and the titillating prospect of the revelation of the hidden secrets of woman. Perhaps, thought the Vienna medical faculty, anatomies should only take place behind closed doors and with a very restricted audience.

Three factors contributed to the development of human anatomy from 1315. The first was the new Galenism, even if very little of Galen's own anatomical writing was available in Latin (p. 144). Mondino knew only *On the Use of Parts of the Body*, in a vastly abridged translation entitled *De juvamentis membrorum*, and the complete version by Niccolò da Reggio, finished in 1317, was rarely copied because of its size. But it was Galen's example, not his books, that provided the spur. Details of his discoveries were available through the Arabic compendia, and the new translations conveyed his injunctions to practise anatomy. Galen, everyone knew, had dissected animals, but he had also inspected the human body. The new Galenism thus provided an example to imitate, as well as a framework for the investigation of the human body that went beyond the recitation of the names and numbers of parts as found in Isidore of Seville or in Avicenna's *Canon*. In its Aristotelian emphasis on function and purpose, the new Galenist anatomy relegated to secondary status such questions as the number of bones in the body (variously calculated as 203, 229, 241, and 248, with further qualifications depending on what was defined as a bone).

Religious developments also influenced the introduction of human anatomy. From 1200 on, the bodies of those dying abroad, especially

177

on the Crusades, were being cut or boiled so that the heart or bones could be brought home for burial, a procedure condemned by Pope Boniface VIII in 1300. However, the proliferation of reliquaries (consecrated receptacles containing a part of the body of a saint or a relative) suggests that this ban was ineffective.

Even more important, autopsies involving the cutting of a corpse became common in Italian, French, and German towns from about 1250. Town surgeons were called in to investigate woundings and murder, and to suggest a cause of death. How large the step was from this to a university anatomy of an executed criminal is debatable. Certainly, the condemned criminal had forfeited civic rights, and, in some eyes, any future place in heaven, and the theological concern with the resurrection of a Christian body, whole and intact, did not always extend to that of the sinner, which artists depicted at the Last Judgment as a mass of jumbled or incomplete limbs destined for Hell. If civil authorities could mutilate and dismember those who had broken the law, why not a university medical teacher, with consequent benefit to medical knowledge? Provided the dissected bits of the corpse were kept together and given Christian burial, religious proprieties were satisfied.

A public dissection was at once spectacle, ceremony, and instruction. The motives of the audience, sometimes numbering over 50, might range from prurience to professional interest. The dissection was held in a church, a hall, or sometimes in a temporary booth, usually in winter when the cold weather delayed putrefaction, a hazard that Mondino's order of dissection, the lower abdomen, the thorax, and the skull – was avowedly devised to reduce. The religious setting was not the only quasi-ceremonial element. There was a complex ritual at an anatomy, in which begowned members of the medical faculty and students gathered about the corpse. A senior student in full academic robes read from an anatomical text, while a surgeon dissected the body, and the professor pointed out significant features. In some later illustrations, the contrast between dissector and the physician-expositor on his high throne is sharpened by the abolition (or marginalisation) of the third figure; others omit the reader. Common to all is a sense of ceremony, for civil, religious, and university authorities agreed that the corpse should be accorded due reverence, and this highlight of a medical year (or decade) was attended with as much pageantry as the taking of a doctoral degree. Together the ritual solemnity, the demands of statutes, the educational aims, and the linkage of the transient body to the more permanent words of a text within the institutional framework of the university made socially and morally acceptable what was an inherently objectionable activity.

Although Mondino himself cut up the corpse, and expected his medical reader to do likewise, by 1400 the actual dissection was accompanied by a commentary on his book. It told the audience what they should see before them, whether in the corpse or in drawings and specifically prepared bones and muscles, no bad thing when even those standing by the body could not easily make out the fine details. Mondino's book was also concerned with more than description – questions of function and purpose were as important as those of site, size, or shape. Hence the custom arose of at least dual participation in an anatomy, a dissector who concentrated on the actual cutting, and an expositor who considered wider and more controversial questions. It may be no coincidence that artists drew the audience arguing among themselves, even as they viewed the corpse. The visual evidence of the body supplemented the doctrines of the text, which provided the basis for a broad discussion of form and function that went far beyond mere description.

A belief in the overriding descriptive power of images has bedevilled many modern discussions of medical illustration. The medieval copyists of crudely drawn bones and arteries are contrasted with the new scientific artist, Leonardo da Vinci (1452–1519), who carried out his own dissections and went to the Florentine hospitals in search of potential subjects to draw. His remarkably accurate drawings of the eye, muscles, and bones are rightly admired, especially when juxtaposed to the often fanciful illuminations in medieval manuscripts. But Leonardo too followed tradition occasionally. He believed in a five-lobed liver and in a direct connection between the spinal cord and the spermatic ducts (for many thought that semen was produced from the pneuma contained in the spine). His concentration on a geometrical universe led him equally into error, however fruitful his hypotheses. But Leonardo was not the only artist of his day to be interested in dissection, or to draw human figures accurately. The painters of scenes of medical activity in fifteenth-century manuscripts display a new realism, and some certainly made anatomical drawings from life. To ascribe the visual crudity of medieval anatomical images to an absence of artists skilled in representing reality is certainly misplaced for fifteenth-century Italy, France, and Flanders.

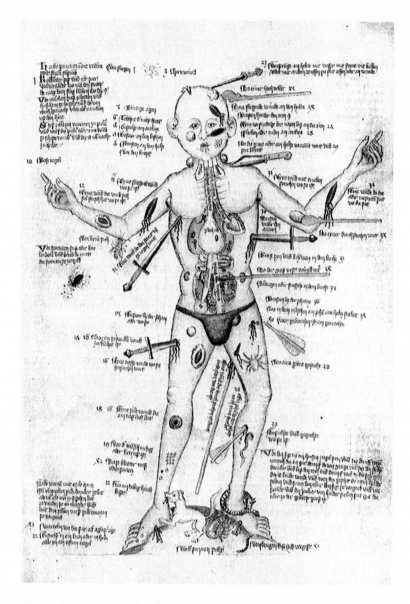

Fig. 25. 'Wound Man'. This illustration, in a Ms. written around 1460 in Erfurt, Central Germany, is keyed to a text on the opposite page detailing the likelihood of survival from each injury. (The Wellcome Institute Library, London, WMS 49, fol. 34 v.)

One way out of this problem is to deny the supremacy of image as description, and to argue that illustrations served to represent not so much what was before the artist's eye as the general truths of reason in visual form. In many manuscripts their prime function was mnemonic, not descriptive. Just as a calendar provided the travelling doctor with a handy reference to good or bad days for bleeding or purging, so maps of the veins in the body reminded him where to bleed. By reducing several hundred pages of text to a visual pattern, these images had the merit of portability and brevity. Illustrations of the brain similarly corresponded to the chambers described by philosophers and theologians, not to those in an actual skull, because they were used to support philosophical theories, not to overthrow them. The gruesome picture of 'wound man', hurt by everything from snake bites and cudgellings to wasp stings and 'bad spots', was a visual guide not to injuries as such, but to the prospects of treatment, being occasionally keyed to a text that indicated which wounds were generally fatal and which not.

Pictures also cost money. Beautiful illuminated medical manuscripts, such as the Florentine Nicetas codex of surgery (written in Constantinople c. 900) or the Bodleian Apuleius herbal (Bury St. Edmund's, c. 1120), were luxury items, carefully preserved and rarely used in daily practice – the average herbal or surgical text had few, if any, illustrations. The scenes of medical life that adorn the opening of each book in the Dresden Galen (painted in Flanders around 1460) reveal the wealth of the original owner more than details of contemporary practice. Only the very wealthy could afford such books, and hence pictures of caesarian section adorn moralising tales of Julius Caesar more often than a surgical handbook. Illustrations of the emperor Nero dissecting his mother (a medieval exaggeration of a classical story) demonstrate filial depravity, not medical anatomy, in books destined for a princely library.

At best, medical manuscripts have only a handful of drawings, most coming from the (relatively wealthier) fourteenth and fifteenth centuries. The most common illustrations show urine glasses, or a male figure marked with points for blood-letting or with the signs of the zodiac. They are sometimes found together with the so-called 'five- (correctly nine-) picture series', schematic representations of the five systems of the arteries, veins, bones, nerves, and muscles, together with the genitalia; the stomach, liver, and viscera; the womb, usually with one or two foetuses inside; and the brain and eyes. Where and when this series was formed is controversial, but an origin in late-antique Alexandrian Galenism would also explain the diffusion of the same images in the Middle Eastern world, particularly in Persia (p. 121).

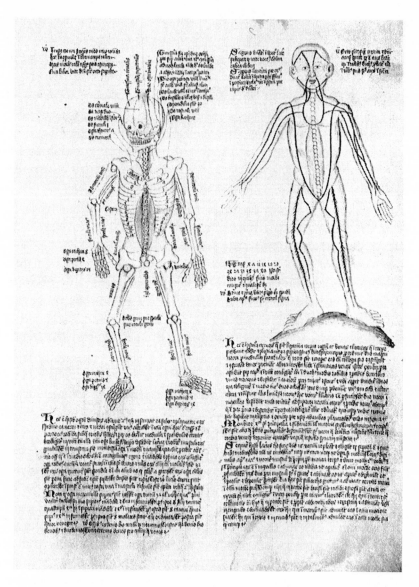

Fig. 26. 'Bone Man' and 'Nerve Man', two of the 'nine-picture series'. These illustrations often accompany a short summary of Galenic anatomy from Late Antiquity (The Wellcome Institute Library, London, WMS 49, fol. 37 r.)

These illustrations reinforced the verbal message, or recalled to mind the standard conclusions of learned physic and medical astrology. As such, these images were a success, for they survived into the age of print, wound-men in particular appearing in sixteenth-century surgical and theological texts. They presented the body as a teaching-aid, neatly labelled and connected to the world of the stars and of the patient. Like Mondino's verbal account, they offered an insight into and beyond the body, into the universal and not simply the individual, and located it within a variety of contexts, medical, philosophical, astrological, and philosophical. They diverge from modern anatomy not only in their anatomical errors – e.g. a seven-boned sternum, a brain with separate chambers for each faculty, a stomach as a round cooking-pot – but, more significantly, in their whole intellectual universe. To make sense of their images one must make sense of their contexts.

Some medieval diseases

In 1396, Francesco Datini of Florence consulted several doctors about his wife Margherita's double tertian fever. They prescribed a highly effective remedy, – three sage leaves, picked and eaten after saying three Ave Marias and three Paternosters. In 1397 her attacks returned with renewed violence. She suffered also from colds, headaches, indigestion, and the mysterious 'mal di madre' (the mother's disease), which she treated with a prayer to St. Elizabeth worn as an amulet. She lived in constant fear of the plague, which could strike suddenly by day or night; her small nephew, Nanni, had in 1383 died within 36 hours of catching it. Although friends recommended draughts of theriac, a mighty and complex antidote prepared in public in a great cauldron under the supervision of the medical professors of Florence, Margherita and Francesco were less enthusiastic. In their view, flight, repentance, and faith in God formed the best prophylaxis. They may have been right. Both lived into old age – Francesco died in 1410 aged 75, a martyr to bladder and kidney disorders, and Margherita in 1423 aged 65.

This glimpse of a Florentine couple's health reveals several significant features of medieval therapeutics, not least their self-diagnoses, and their ability to use the same language and categories of illness as their various medical advisers, whose remedies extended from pills to charms, or simply gloomy resignation. Their names for diseases were sometimes learned, sometimes popular. Some diseases are identifiable (e.g. bladder-stone); others present only vague symptoms. The 'mal di madre' may be colic or more closely related to some inflammation of the womb (the 'mother'). Its name proclaimed its relationship to women and to the womb, just as, elsewhere, scrofula became the 'royal disease' because English and French kings 'touched' for it. But 'royal disease' also denoted other completely unrelated diseases (jaundice, leprosy, a wasting disease, and even, in Anglo-Saxon England, spasm of the sinews and swelling of the feet), to the consequent confusion of later writers. Above all the Datini family feared the plague, which from 1348 onwards had regularly devastated Florence. Because they were wealthy, Francesco and Margherita were less likely to catch the plague, which raged in the poorer areas of the city, or diseases such as smallpox, tuberculosis, typhus, measles, and meningitis which spread quickly in the crowded tenements. They had no tiny babies to die of the diarrhoeas, the *bachi* (worms) and the *pondi* (heavinesses), or the convulsions that carried off many young children every summer. The Florentine *Books of the Dead* show a veritable annual massacre of the innocents from infectious diseases, with summer far more dangerous than the damp chills of winter. Malnutrition, less of a problem to the rich Datinis, also contributed to the annual harvest of death. Few men or women would have lived beyond 35, even in the somewhat healthier countryside.

The rest of this section focuses on three conditions, madness, leprosy, and plague, which have been considered quintessentially medieval and reveal the variety of medieval ideas on causation and therapy.

MADNESS

Of all the conditions described by medieval writers, madness is the most complex. Doctors, following Galenic precedent, distinguished four main categories, frenzy, mania, melancholy, and lethargy, each resulting from a particular humoral imbalance. This was sometimes attributed to a change of atmosphere – the influence of the moon (true lunacy) – but more often to the effect of a particular mental condition, 'passion'. Their learned clients shared their belief. When Master Lorenzo di Sassoli described to Francesco Datini in 1404 how best to maintain his health, he dealt fully with the emotions. He was pleased that Francesco occasionally became angry and shouted, for this encouraged his natural heat; a sad and worried Francesco portended physical illness, for mental trouble, 'more than anything else, destroys our body'. Moderation, even in worry, was his advice; general peace of mind would prevent even physical anguish.

Against this psychosomatic approach of the doctors, familiar with the emotions as one of the crucial non-naturals (p. 141), can be set an approach based on theological or moral considerations. Madness here was linked to possession, usually by devils constantly on the look-out for victims. Sometimes they were invited in by a sort of pact; more often they took advantage of individual sinfulness – e.g. a dancing girl's distraction of a crowd listening to a preacher – to gain possession. Sometimes an inadvertent curse on an unruly child allowed a demon in, or one might be unwittingly deceived by a devil in disguise. Henry the vintner, according to Caesarius of Heisterbach (1180–1240), was seduced by a beautiful woman, who carried him off into the air and deposited him in front of a monastery, madly crawling on all fours. Weak in body and spirit, he died within a year. Those, of either sex, who were raped or had lost their virginity illicitly were often deemed mad, an alternative explanation for what would otherwise have been considered a cause of deep dishonour, since all sexual activity by the sane was assumed to be voluntary. Madness was also ascribed to the effects of sorcery, particularly by one's enemies, an explanation which reduced any personal stigma of insanity. But from the twelfth century on, madness became increasingly moralised. Infidels, atheists, and Jews were viewed as potentially mad, and literary and theological texts frequently depicted the consequence of immorality in terms of madness. In contrast to Dr. Lorenzo, St. Thomas Aquinas (1225–74) exploited a Galenic physiology to explain precisely why the sins of passion, e.g. anger, brought about madness and loss of reason. On his schema, madness was largely one's own responsibility, the result of erroneous belief and an immoral life-style.

Others viewed madness more positively. Divine madness had led David to compose the psalms, one of which, Psalm 52 ('The fool hath said...'), was frequently illuminated with an initial letter showing a mad figure. Prophecy was also described, depending on one's theological standpoint, as a holy, God-sent madness or as demoniac possession. The scriptural 'Blessed are the poor in heart' was interpreted to refer to the simple-minded, to whom, as another Gospel text put it, things might be 'revealed beyond the understanding of the wise'. Many authors exalted the village idiot, singing cheerfully, if tunelessly, to the glory of God; in fact, as well as in the word's etymology, the cretin thus represented the true Christian. From the twelfth century onwards, monastic writers also stressed a holy folly, a love of God beyond all human understanding and far surpassing the human love-madness of troubadours and poets. The search for God, and its resolution through mystic grace, would lead to a divine madness, in which one might retrieve through divine ecstasy a pristine purity and wholeness lost with the Fall of Adam.

These diverse views of madness were balanced by an equal variety of suggested cures. Some involved medical intervention, bleeding and drugs thought to calm the mind or evacuate bad humours. Alongside a long-term gentle psychotherapy of soothing words and pleasant surroundings, doctors recommended short-term shocks – sudden shouts and even stuffing the head of a frenetic into the lung of a recently killed cow to frighten him or her back to normality. But most doctors preferred the longer approach, hoping that by regulating the whole lifestyle the mad could be restored to sanity. For those ostensibly possessed by demons, religious therapies were advised. Biographers of saints tell how they cured the possessed they met on their travels, and reports of healings at their shrines are even more numerous. Over 80 saints are recorded in France between 1200 and 1400 as performing such miracles, from St. Adelphus of Metz to St. Wulfran of Sens. Thirty five can be considered specialists in mental disorders, like St. Willibrord, whose shrine at Echternach (Luxemburg) was often visited by epileptics. Three shrines, in particular, had a more than regional reputation for treating madness – that of St. Mathurin at Larchant, St. Acairius at Haspres, and St. Dymphna at Geel, all in northern France and Flanders. Here medical and religious therapies co-existed – bathing and special foods alongside the intervention of the saint. At Geel, in the thirteenth century, a large hospice was built to accommodate the mentally ill, but it could not cope with the large numbers who came on pilgrimage and who wished to stay near the shrine. Many were thus lodged, under the supervision of the church, in houses in the village. From this developed a special 'family colony', in which the mentally ill were (and, after seven centuries, still are) looked after within the community.

Almost unique in more recent times, Geel was not unusual in the Middle Ages. Although there are stories of the mentally ill chained up in a locked room at home or in prison – in fifteenth-century Nuremberg families could hire a cell in the town gaol – and although, in the fourteenth century, 'Mad towers' were built (e.g. at Caen in France, or Lübeck in Germany) to keep the dangerously mad isolated in a sort of earthly Purgatory, most of the insane were kept at home, in their own villages. The same law codes which defined the incapacity of the insane also expected them to be cared for within their own communities, where the fear of their madness was reduced by familiarity. The trend towards incarceration is counterbalanced by one which sought to integrate the mad – as holy fool, as an object of special divine care, or even as the ultimate paradox, a court fool. Modern anthropologists also see the Feast of Fools as a way in which medieval society tried to accommodate mental disorder by taming it through a reversal of normality and a universal adoption of madness. How far it succeeded is unclear, but there is no doubt that late-medieval society had developed a variety of strategies for coping, few of which demanded incarceration or withdrawal from the family environment.

If variety characterises medieval approaches to madness, attitudes to leprosy (Hansen's disease) were very different. Its physical manifestations, scaly flesh, collapsed tissues, the loss of extremities, and the degeneration of bones, suggested a veritable living death. Medical advice concentrated on prophylaxis or amelioration in the initial stages, for, once leprosy had taken hold, there was no effective cure.

Medical diagnosis was hampered by two problems. Firstly, there was no reliable classification of skin diseases; scales and pustules were only symptoms, an indication of more serious humoral changes which, according to medical theorists, constituted the disease. Thus the same symptom could indicate several diseases, and, conversely, what modern physicians consider separate diseases came within the same medieval description of leprosy. Not every medieval leper suffered from Hansen's disease. Secondly, the various methods of translation, and ignorance of the Greek or Arabic originals, meant that the Latin word *lepra* (scale) might apply to different disorders even within the same book. Those who attempted to give an account of leprosy that included all previous examples of *lepra* thus compounded the difficulties of making sense of this disease.

Some medieval physicians were aware of these confusions, and tried hard to distinguish leprosy from other similar conditions, not least because of the terrible consequences of a wrong diagnosis. They inspected blood, to see whether any of it adhered to a smooth bowl; if it did, then leprosy was confirmed. Although the coagulation of blood is a good diagnostic, the subtleties of minute observation in a modern blood test were hardly possible in 1300, and this test was one among an increasing variety of very un-modern procedures, all of which were considered valid by medieval practitioners.

Leprosy, once diagnosed, meant almost inevitable isolation from the community. Lepers were given special clothing, a bell or rattle to warn others of their approach, and gloves. The disease was thought extremely contagious (although the risk of contagion is very slight), and even the presence of lepers loitering near a church or on a bridge was regarded as extremely dangerous, for they might infect the ambient air. The favoured solution, from 1100 onwards, was isolation in a leper house outside the town, and without any medical assistance, save the provision of food and shelter. It involved doctors, civic officials (Florence had an official 'responsible for expelling the infected'), and, not least, the Church.

The injunction in Leviticus 13.46 that the 'unclean' should dwell alone outside the camp, and other biblical examples of expulsion and isolation, provided a method of action and its justification. In 1179 the Lateran Council ordered all lepers to be cut off from society, with their own churches and burial places. Religious rites accompanied the formal abandonment of the leper. Sometimes a priest symbolically threw earth over the leper standing in a grave, chanted the psalms for the dead, or handed over materials for a coffin. The spouse of a leper might even remarry in his (rarely her) lifetime. Although the Gospel healings of lepers were not forgotten, remarkably few leprosy cures are recorded among the miracles of medieval saints, except for St. Lazarus, who gave his name to an isolation hospital, a lazaretto. The Church's only consolation lay in interpreting the leper's suffering as a literally earthly Purgatory which brought a swift reward in Heaven, where, as Luke 16.19–25 had foretold, the leper rested on Abraham's bosom in Paradise. God, said Guy de Chauliac, loved the leper above all creation; and, said others, once the leprosy had been shown to a priest, the leper gained immediate health, forgiveness, and sure salvation.

Leprosy was an exemplary disease in other ways. More than most biblical diseases it was associated with sin. Miriam, who lied about her brother Moses (Numbers 12); Naaman the Syrian and Gehazi, Elisha's grasping servant (II Kings 5); and even the lepers of the Gospel miracles were all thought to have brought on their own leprosy by their misdeeds or infidelity. Medieval sermonisers linked leprosy especially with the sin of lust, which in turn confirmed the belief that it was spread venereally. The friction of intercourse opened up the body to receive the noxious effluvia of an infected partner – a theory revived in renaissance discussions of the new venereal disease, syphilis (p. 218). Leprosy was a renowned (if unquantifiable) hazard not only for those who frequented brothels, like the students in the popular medieval tale of the Venomous Virgin. In *The Testament of Cresseid* by Robert Henryson (*fl.* 1470–1500), Cresseid was punished in this way by God for her pride and lust. Leprosy was thus caused by sin as well as contagion.

Medieval leprosy also raises a demographic problem. The twelfth and thirteenth centuries saw a massive increase in the number of hospitals built to house lepers. Small in size, rarely with more than a dozen inmates, they were ubiquitous in Western Europe. France by 1226 had around 2000; in England around 130 were founded between 1150 and 1250, and a further 70 in the next hundred years; leper hospitals stood outside all the major Italian towns by 1300. Yet by 1350 they were in decline; new foundations were few (only 12 in England after 1350) and inmate numbers dwindled. Some houses fell into ruins, others were diverted to other purposes. In England, the hospital at Stourbridge, just outside Cambridge, founded around 1150, had been dissolved by 1350; that of St. Nicholas, Royston, some 15 miles south, had by 1359 become a chapel at which mass was said for the souls of its patrons and benefactors. The reasons for this steep decline are much disputed. Some have argued that it was the horror of leprosy, not its actual prevalence, that created the boom, and that sober calculation of the reality gradually prevailed. But it is difficult to believe that hard-nosed Italian town councillors or impecunious Englishmen expended large sums of money on merely fashionable causes (although fashions in charity cannot be denied). Nor can the Black Death have been entirely responsible for the decline in the numbers of lepers (although, physically weakened, they may well have been particularly susceptible to the plague) for numbers were falling well before 1348, and the foundation of a new leper hospital just outside Cambridge in 1361 shows that there, at least, leprosy continued to be considered a problem. Other explanations in terms of more accurate methods of diagnosis, climatic changes or an altered pattern in the actual behaviour of the disease itself, particularly in its relationship with tuberculosis, although suggestive, are far from proven. Yet, even if the disease affected fewer people, its image remained to terrify and to torment.

PLAGUE

The great plague of 1347–51, later known as the Black Death, is the most famous of all epidemics. Its course can be tracked from Central

189

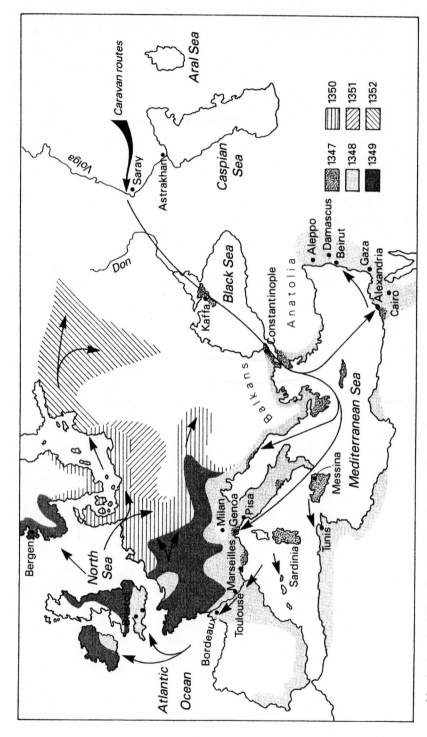

Map 3. Map of the Black Death in Europe.

Asia, via the shores of the Crimea, to Sicily, Genoa, and the rest of Europe, as well as through the Islamic world, month by month, if not day by day (see Map 3). Its epidemiological consequences are also clear. Plague, largely absent from Europe for 800 years, now became endemic for the next three or four centuries. Although population loss varied from place to place, and a general demographic decline can be traced from 1314–15 onwards, this epidemic killed around 25 per cent of the population of Europe. In the 50 years after 1350, the average life-span may have shrunk to a mere 20 years. Many villages were deserted, while even large towns contracted greatly – between 1338 and 1427 the population of Florence dropped by almost three-quarters. The economic impact is harder to quantify; wages generally rose as fewer workers were available, but the economic downturn visible in the 1350s was already beginning before 1347. But it would be wrong to overemphasise the direct consequences of the Black Death, or to view it as a single apocalyptic turning-point in European history. Rather it is the accumulation of frequent, regional epidemics that distinguishes the period following the Black Death from what had gone before. A Europe relatively free from even regional epidemics now became home to plagues and pestilences. Instead of sporadic, local incidences of epidemic disease, however terrible their effects, like the 'plague' on humans and beasts that followed the great flood of Rome in 1231, now whole regions suffered immense, sudden, and repeated catastrophes.

To identify pre-modern plagues is not easy, and the Black Death is no exception. Modern diagnostic criteria are either irrelevant, inapplicable, or too specific for the evidence available. The descriptive categories of ancient and modern physicians rarely coincide, and the pattern of a disease in a virgin population may differ considerably from that in a region where it is endemic. Death records often hide several diseases within the same set of statistics. Although most scholars believe that the Black Death was bubonic plague, the result of the transmission of the bacillus *Yersinia pestis* from animals, especially rats, to humans by means of fleas (notably *Xenopsylla cheopsis*), not all the features of the disease as seen in modern Manchuria or India correspond to those the medieval chroniclers described. The sudden, swift onset of the disease and death, and a pattern of speedy distribution might suggest that there was also direct human to human transmission, in the form of pneumonic plague, spread by droplet infection, and even of septicaemic plague, where the human flea, *Pulex irritans*, acted as vector.

Nonetheless, although epidemiological puzzles still remain, sixteenth-century writers on plague, whose accounts agree more closely with modern descriptions of bubonic plague, were sure that the disease they were describing in their own day had ravaged two hundred years previously.

The arrival of AIDS in the 1980s has given Western scholars a glimpse of the fear induced by the arrival of the Black Death, so movingly described by its contemporary Boccaccio in his *Decameron* and by many less famous local chroniclers. But even AIDS, with its slow and insidious transmission, cannot convey the feeling, familiar from letters and official pronouncements, of terrified apprehension as news arrived of the plague drawing ever closer, and, still more, when recurrences were announced in nearby towns. Nothing like this had been known before, but in one sense this was not an unknown disease, for it fitted neatly into the categories used to define, explain, and act against epidemic disease. Doctors, officials, clerics, and laymen all had their own ways of combating (or, at least, explicating) the disease, and all were adept at finding reasons for justifying what little success they had and for explaining away their failures.

To set these groups and their preferred strategies against one another, to play off religion against medicine, contagionists against miasmatists, professionals against laymen, and even doctors against surgeons, is easy, for authors or preachers often derided as ineffective the proposals of others. But all operated with the same scheme of explanation, and differed more on the appropriate place for intervention (and who might intervene) than on the theory. They invoked a hierarchy of causes, of which some applied to other diseases, e.g. leprosy, and others related specifically to 'plagues' or, as medieval physicians defined it, 'the series of changes that produced in many individuals conditions of illness leading to death'.

At the top of the hierarchy was God, who in His wisdom sent plague to punish mankind for its sins. In this case, as the Medical Faculty at Paris declared in 1348, one could only turn in humility to Him – but it might still be unwise to neglect medical advice. Below God were the 'natural causes', changes in the atmosphere that turned the air hot, sticky, and putrid. These changes might be the result of planetary positions; for instance, the conjunction of Saturn, Mars, and Jupiter on March 20, 1345. Alternatively, this celestial influence might derive from some 'hidden property', working like poison in the air. The air might become putrid through earthly causes – nasty vapours ('miasms') from stagnant pools, decaying corpses, caverns, dung, or the exhalations of sufferers themselves – and might have been deliberately poisoned by outsiders – Jews, Muslims, lepers, and the like. Only a change in the air could explain why the disease spread quickly and persons remote from one another fell ill in the same way. Some doctors, and many laymen, also referred to contagion as a factor in the spread of the disease. But their concept of contagion was not as specific nor the same as that of modern bacteriologists – medieval contagious diseases included asthma, phthisis, pneumonia, leprosy, scabies, pleurisy, colds, frenzy, lethargy, vitiligo, and ophthalmia. Nor was a theory of contagion necessarily opposed to one of miasmas; many late-medieval writers slipped easily from one to the other. The Venetian authorities in 1300 decided to remove lepers from the city because their contagious breath was polluting the air. Plague, it was almost universally accepted, could be spread by direct contact, contagion in the strict sense, but that was only one way. Even those who strongly advocated quarantines and the banning of potential plague-carriers believed that the air was the most effective bearer of contagion, and that their proposed measures also improved most effectively the quality of the atmosphere. The removal of bad smells went hand in hand with the removal of plague sufferers.

But the mere existence of plague did not entail that everyone would fall victim to it. A few writers, relying on some recondite Galenic passages, suggested that one could become ill with plague only if one actually received a seed of the disease and one's physical constitution was already fertile ground for it. But most authors concentrated on what might be termed individual receptivity, the ultimate determinant of plague. If the body was strong enough to withstand morbid changes, no illness resulted; if not, then one would be ill, and possibly die.

Where and how one acted depended on one's perception of the importance of the various stages of this hierarchy. If God alone was the cause, then only religious manifestations would be effective – individual acts of contrition, attendance at Mass, or public confessions, processions, and fastings. The so-called Flagellants, men, and some women, who, particularly in Central Europe from 1348, publicly beat themselves, hoped by their mutual scourgings and denunciations of sinners and Jews to deflect the wrath of God. Others, even among the ecclesiastical authorities, saw these processions as a serious threat to the established order. Pope Clement VI prohibited Flagellant pilgrimages, and the Bishop of Breslau had one of their leaders burnt alive.

Physicians called in to attend the sick or to advise lay officials stressed the proper treatment of the individual. They also had the astronomical skill to decipher the heavens, to foretell when the planetary conditions might change, for better or worse, and to suggest which areas might be less susceptible. If they could not alter the stars, they could read their message. Their therapies depended on the assumption that plague involved some aerial putrefaction, i.e. an excess of heat and moisture in the air. If one could not reduce one's intake of air – by slimming, for instance – then one should endeavour by 'diet' (i.e. controlled lifestyle) to reduce the body's own heat and moisture. Those who were already naturally hot and moist were most at risk – young, fat, pregnant, and libidinous women in steamy cities (e.g. Paris) were thought unlikely to survive. One could also attempt to change one's micro-environment by lighting fires, fumigating rooms, or applying closely to the nose a pomander, whose fragrant odours were believed to dry the deadly air. (Possibly, like mothballs, their smell might have deterred any infected fleas.) Finally, if, as many physicians thought, the air was in some sense poisoned, then one might take theriac, a complex antidote to poison, made and prescribed for centuries by the most learned of physicians.

But physicians, however well-intentioned, did not have the power to effect any public-health measures. They could advise, but they could not command. That was the responsibility of the magistrate, who took as precedent the rules for dealing with sufferers from another contagious disease, leprosy. Only a magistrate had the means to intervene at a social level, and the effectiveness of his intervention was also an index of his or his office's power. In Venice a committee of three nobles was established against the Black Death. They laid down rules for burial, released some debtors from the overcrowded gaols, allowed surgeons to practise medicine, and banned from entering the city all persons who were or appeared to be ill. Those who were caught were jailed for 40 days. In Milan, the council sealed up the occupants of the first three houses affected and left them to die. In Florence a committee of eight assumed almost dictatorial powers. However, their sensible plans to clear the streets of rotting rubbish and dung – a solution welcomed by doctors – came to little as few citizens were left for the task. Besides, the common imposition of regulations that demanded the killing of dogs (and cats) as dirty animals also helped keep the plague endemic by removing the very animals that might have reduced the rat population. In Pistoia (Italy), the town council published nine pages of regulations, banning all incomers (including their own citizens who happened to be away) and the entry of linen and woollen goods; they tightened the rules for the food market and placed a limit on the numbers of attenders at funerals. But elsewhere little was (or could be) done. In London, the city council had tried in 1344 to clean up its filthy streets, but once the plague struck, even these regulations were ineffective. The complaint of King Edward III in 1349, that masses of foetid dung lay in the streets 'in this time of infectious disease', was met with the response that there were now no men to remove it. Even the burial of corpses was almost impossible.

The reactions of ordinary citizens in 1348 can only be imagined. Boccaccio, writing of his own experiences in Florence, described a variety of responses, from flight (on the whole possible only for the rich) to a complete breakdown of all moral self-regulation. For every one who turned to religion or tried to help others, another embarked on a final glorious carousel in the face of certain death. Others turned to magic and sorcery or sought for scapegoats – the rich, the government, and especially the Jews, who were massacred in large numbers from Aragon to Poland.

Responses to the Black Death were both complementary and, less often, contradictory. They were complementary in that they enabled different sections of society to focus on strategies for survival with which they were familiar, had worked in the past, and corresponded to their own abilities to intervene. The (later) Datini letters and the Venetian archives amply show how one group or one community could adopt all these strategies at once in a coherent defence against the plague. There is no sense that one strategy was necessarily always better than another. The fact that Boccaccio regarded all medical intervention as useless or some considered the doctors' prescriptions to strengthen the body and astronomical explanations mere mumbo-jumbo, did not stop medieval patients or civic authorities from employing doctors or seeking exactly the same advice and reassurance from them in subsequent plagues. From the thirteenth century on, confraternities, groups of religiously-minded laymen (and occasionally women) concerned with the care of the sick, the burial of the dead, and the relief of poverty, complemented the work of physicians and civic officials in looking after plague victims. This was a religious and a popular response, and demonstrated civic solidarity in a time of grave crisis.

Conflict between these interpretations and responses arose only when one of them was followed to the exclusion of all others. Doctors and officials usually agreed, but increasingly from the fifteenth century onwards, strong differences emerged between secular and religious approaches to plague. It was hard to reconcile a physician's view that the city of Pisa was more exposed to plague as a coastal city to which people travelled constantly by sea from all over the world with one that related susceptibility only to declining standards of public morality and irreligion. In Brescia (Italy) in 1469 the civic authorities deliberated carefully before allowing the Corpus Christi procession to go ahead, despite the danger of congregating in large numbers, since it might induce God to end the plague. Others, particularly the Venetian Health Board, had less faith in divine intervention. A preacher at St. Mark's in 1497, while allowing that the Board had been wise in their own eyes to close churches for fear of plague, nevertheless warned them that such action would not assuage the wrath of God. Only the sweeping away of sin – the abolition of blasphemy, the closure of 'the schools of sodomy, the nunneries of prostitution', and the abandonment of usury and false justice – would bring an end to the disaster.

This conflict of ideas also reflects a conflict of authority. The growth of civic, lay administration in Europe, and the increasing power of secular government now permitted action to be taken over large areas of civic life independently of, and occasionally in opposition to, the Church. This is particularly visible in the development of Health Boards in fifteenth-century Italy.

Already in 1348 some Italian towns had established temporary committees to co-ordinate public health measures against the plague. Following the precedents for action against lepers, they removed the sick to isolation hospitals or the increasingly underused leper-houses outside the town (hence 'Lazaretto' came to mean a plague hospital) or banned persons or goods from entering or leaving a town. Gradually even small communities throughout Italy adopted similar measures. In 1377 the republic of Ragusa (now Dubrovnik, Croatia), enacted a period of quarantine (30 days, increased in 1397 to 40) on a nearby island for everyone coming from plague-infected areas. Marseilles did likewise in 1383; Venice banned all refugees from plague in 1400, and imposed quarantine measures in 1423; Pisa followed suit in 1464,

Genoa in 1467. Doctors alone could not have done this, for these measures, which cost money and affected the lives of all citizens directly and indirectly, required the administrative and financial co-operation of government.

Before 1400, Health Boards composed of lay officials, although with medical advisers, were temporary affairs, dealing with a specific epidemic. In the Duchy of Milan, however, a permanent magistracy 'for the preservation of health' in the city of Milan itself was established early in the fifteenth century. In 1450, the single commissioner headed a staff of: one physician, one surgeon, one notary, one barber, two horsemen, three footmen, one officer in charge of the Bills of Mortality, one carter, and two gravediggers. But other towns in the Duchy, like Pavia or Cremona, continued for another century to appoint plague commissioners as and when plague arrived. Few Italian cities followed Milan's example immediately; Venice appointed a permanent Commission of Public Health, consisting of three noblemen, only in 1486; Florence a similar commission of five in 1527, both with their own staffs. Northern European towns, smaller, less prosperous, and with weaker administrations, lagged behind Italy by more than a century – London and the rest of Britain by even more.

With permanency came opportunities for expansion. Bills of Mortality were initiated in Milan in 1452, listing names and causes of death, and putting under civic control details that had formerly concerned only individuals or the Church. The system, however, was not Milanese in origin. In Florence, the officials of the Grain Office, responsible for the food supply and for enforcing legislation on personal consumption, had from the 1380s recorded deaths, and the costs of funerals, weddings, and banquets. The Florentine gravediggers kept their own lists of deaths; those of the Guild of Physicians and Apothecaries, which supervised gravediggers, survive from 1450 onwards, and existed earlier. Other Tuscan towns, like Arezzo and Siena, kept municipal records of deaths from the 1370s on, and by 1500 required all deaths to be certified by a qualified physician.

Health Boards also extended the practices of quarantining and shutting borders and town gates for fear of an epidemic. Health passes were introduced around 1480, a procedure that foreigners considered merely another excuse for Italians to extract money. Public health in its widest aspects, from the quality of meat, wine, and fish in the local market and the cleanliness of streets, via hospitals and cemeteries, to the control of physicians, beggars, prostitutes, and Jews, all might fall under the remit of the Health Board. Its enormous powers even extended to the execution of those who violated plague orders, and its information networks stretched far beyond the city walls. Not surprisingly, some resented these all-embracing, intrusive, and expensive powers. By 1500, once plague had been officially declared present, economic disaster was almost inevitable. Trade was suspended, travel interrupted, suspected sufferers and their households taken to the lazaretto for at least a month (if they survived incarceration alongside others with the plague). Amid this economic misery, extra money had to be found to pay for doctors, food, beds, and treatment for those in the lazaretto, the fumigation (and occasional destruction) of infected houses, and all the essential administrative paraphernalia. It was a courageous physician who announced the presence of plague, rather than an 'epidemic fever', and a lucky official whose financial and administrative decisions satisfied all members of the community.

Doctors and surgeons treated and prescribed for individuals and regulated their humours; city authorities took responsibility for cleaning the air and removing the pestilential contagion; the Church confessed penitents and prayed for divine mercy. Together, they hoped to ward off the most terrifying of all diseases, but at a cost. Reflecting on the huge expenditures on plague relief and on the thousands who died when, Health Boards notwithstanding, plague came to Venice, Milan, or Genoa, historians debate whether the effort was worthwhile. If nothing had been done, would the mortality have been still higher? Or, since some towns escaped infection, should one accept with many contemporaries that the failure of plague to take hold or spread outside the poorer areas to which it was increasingly confined proved that a successful defence against plague could be mounted? Whatever the answer, one should at least take note of the variety of ways in which all levels of society coped with epidemic disease. Plague, unlike gout or tuberculosis, was a complex problem that involved both individuals and the community in a complex series of responses.

The missing century

The fifteenth century in European medicine has rarely enjoyed a good press, even when scholars have deigned to notice it. This is partly the result of chance, for it occupies an ambiguous position between the

Middle Ages and the Renaissance, between an age of manuscript and one of print. At a time when Italian men of letters, 'humanists', were rediscovering the Latin literary classics of Antiquity, and, from the 1420s, the Greek, Italian medical men appear locked in a medieval past. Save for Celsus, whose *On Medicine* was found in Siena in 1426, no ancient medical author or treatise reappeared in an accessible form until the 1490s, and the impact of Greek, so overwhelming from 1525 to 1550, was scarcely felt except within a very tiny circle of mainly northern Italians in the 1490s. Not surprisingly, the medical humanists and translators of the 1520s, confident in their recovery of the Greek Galen and Hippocrates, damned the works of their immediate predecessors as dark and confused, written in barbarous Latin full of Arabisms and in an old-fashioned script, and showing in their contents the lamentable results of centuries of misunderstanding and misplaced schematism.

To the prejudices of the next generation have been added modern assumptions about the Renaissance and, above all, the new medicine and science that allegedly replaced the learning of the book with that of experience, and enabled medicine at last to progress. The fact that most writings of the fifteenth century remain in manuscript, or that those books of medicine and science printed before 1500 are more likely to contain works from the twelfth century or earlier than from the fifteenth, is not interpreted as a consequence of a book-trade seeking solid profit in standard authors and medical set-texts, but as a judgment on the quality of that medical learning. Disciplinary boundaries have also hindered any proper appreciation. Those who study Renaissance art and literature concentrate first on Italy from 1350 onwards before passing to Northern Europe only at the beginning of the sixteenth century. Fifteenth-century medicine, which even in Italy displays few links with the artistic and literary revival of the classics, thus appears irrelevant – although one can hardly think of the development of plague controls (pp. 196–8), outside the context of the development of Italian renaissance states – or left to medievalists. Yet even here, an Italocentric bias (and Latinate training) among medical and scientific historians has largely excluded anything that lies off the route that links Oxford and Paris with Montpellier and northern Italy. The Rhine, the Pyrenees, and the Austrian Alps are bigger barriers to scholarly understanding today than they were in reality then.

But a crude survey of the medical world of the fifteenth century that concentrates only on Italy or novelties is doubly unfair, for it minimises changes taking place within the standard framework of medicine and takes as its definition of progress one laid down by the opponents of medieval medicine. Where enough material survives and has been properly studied, historians have discovered a vigorous medical culture. The lectures on medicine at the University of Naples in 1440, still largely interpreting the texts of the *Articella*, ranged widely over the whole of medicine and were not confined to verbal exposition. The university authorities at Bologna and Padua were well aware of the need to keep attracting students, and there is little indication here of a dull repetition of outdated lectures. The medical men at the court of the Tyrol (Austria) in the second half of the century indulged in lively debates on a variety of topics, explained what they were doing to those who knew only German, and shared in a wide range of other cultural activities, from poetry and history to alchemy. Among them was Ulrich Ellenbog (*c*. 1435–99), who wrote arguably the earliest tract on occupational diseases, *Von den giftigen besen Tempffen und Reuchen* (*On Poisonous, Bad Vapours and Fumes*), in 1473 for the goldsmiths of Augsburg, and who owned a major library of theological, philosophical, literary, and medical texts. At Vienna, the complicated medical astrology developed by its medical professors from the 1450s onwards helped to renew interest in mathematics in general.

The apparently standard and largely unaltered form of university statutes across Europe did not preclude any change within medicine, let alone in surgery, generally taught outside the universities. Surgeons frequently announced improvements in techniques, new drugs were beginning to arrive at the end of the century from India and Africa, and physicians reported their own novel cures for others to follow them. University lecturers did not, on the whole, simply parrot the words of their predecessors, and at Vienna, Cologne, and Erfurt, there is evidence that they responded to what students (or the governing authorities) wanted. Yet this did not entail the rejection of what had gone before. The Aristotelian and Galenic systems together had an undeniable stability, as well as a flexibility that allowed for change and disagreement in particulars without necessarily damaging the whole. (And, it might be added, alternatives to these systems were, at this date, equally open to attack.)

Technical advances in surgery, e.g. the introduction of the suture-ligature (passing a suture under a blood vessel before it is tied) in order to stop bleeding, by Leonardo di Bertipaglia (*c*. 1380–1465), were easily assimilated within the traditional framework of surgery. Other develop-

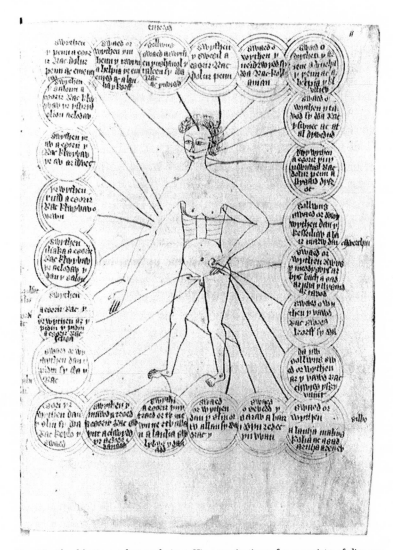

Fig. 27. Blood-letting, advocated since Hippocratic times for a variety of diseases, was performed by all types of practitioners, physicians, surgeons, barber-surgeons, and the ubiquitous barbers, and many manuals gave advice on do-it-yourself bleeding. Illustrations showing planetary determinants, or, as here, the results of bleeding at a particular site, are common in medieval manuscripts. This manuscript was written in 1488–89 in Welsh by the poet Gutun Owain, perhaps for the abbey of Valle Crucis (N.E. Wales); similar recommendations were available throughout Europe in Latin and other languages. (Ms. Mostyn 88, p. 11. By courtesy of the National Library of Wales.)

ments in surgery and physic were rather changes in classification, the reordering of material derived from both past writings and present experience. Whether one treated pleurisy with phlebotomy involved

201

complicated calculations of the causes of the disease and the possible response of the patient. The treatment of gunshot wounds also invited similar classificatory alternatives. A surgeon who defined a gunshot wound as laceration coupled with bruising, applied a gentle, cooling treatment; the view that prevailed at the end of the century, that it involved some poisoning, demanded as a consequence the standard therapy for poisoned wounds, burning with hot oil to eliminate the poison.

Two features are typical of fifteenth-century learned medicine. The first is a growing rejection of authorities, in part the result of the perceived difficulty of reconciling texts whose vocabulary was often imprecise and unclear. Jacques Despars (c. 1380–1458), a leading Parisian professor, concluded that one could no longer talk properly about 'cerebral faculties' because of disagreements over the ways in which these words were applied. His contemporary at Pavia, Antonio Guaineri (d. 1448), dismissed a century and a half's learned discussion that had pitted authority against authority on the workings of drugs in pleurisy with these words: 'Let us leave these good fellows in Paradise, where all disputes subside'. The long-lived professor of practical medicine at Bologna, Giovanni Garzoni (1419–1505) scandalised some by his insistence that Galen was far less useful for medicine than Hippocrates.

This new reserve towards authority accompanied a rejection of scholastic theory in favour of an emphasis on practice. Fifteenth-century commentators on Avicenna or Galen rarely involved themselves in the logical disputations common a century before or in the theoretical questions that were to divide the next. Leonardo di Bertipaglia in his commentary on Avicenna's *Canon*, Book 4 was much less concerned with the underlying theory of head-wounds than the humanist surgeon Berengario da Carpi in his short work *On Skull Fractures* (Bologna, 1518). This concern with practice, with what worked, encompassed debates on the propriety and effectiveness of alchemy, astrology, and even magic in treating disease. Some physicians rejected all these arts but others were prepared to accept them after they had been given a sanitised explanation: to say that a drug worked with an occult (or hidden) property was not thereby to become a sorcerer, but simply using Aristotelian language to describe effects not otherwise explicable in precise terms.

Pragmatism reigned, and arguably the fifteenth century shows the revival of practical medicine at the expense of theory. The literary monuments of the century are the books of *practica*, and, in particular, the volumes of case-histories produced by Italian professors. From Ugo Benzi (1376–1439), Antonio Cermisone (d. 1441), and Bartolommeo da Montagnana (d. 1452) at Padua, to Gianmatteo Ferrari (d. 1472) at Pavia, and Baverio de' Bonetti (d. 1480) at Bologna, one can trace an Italian tradition of producing case-histories to accompany lectures on the standard texts. Leonardo da Bertipaglia's lectures on Avicenna consist largely of a brief explanation of the text, followed by indications for practice (sometimes illustrated from his own patients) and a list of drugs and plasters. Montagnana's 350 *Consilia* (*Case-histories*) constituted, according to the preface, a 'marvellous guide to practice', while an editor of Cermisone's *Consilia* (publishing a mere fraction of what survives today in manuscript) claimed in 1476 that all medicine could be better taught through such case-histories than through lectures. At Padua and elsewhere in Italy students indeed had both – that, among other things, was what was keeping northern Italy a Mecca for medical students. Bedside consultations, possibly ward-rounds, autopsies, and a regular programme of dissection gave to an Italian medical education an increasingly practical emphasis. The notebook of John Argentine (*c.* 1442–1508), who studied in Italy and ended his life as Provost of King's College, Cambridge, is concerned entirely with therapy, carefully listing a variety of diseases and their treatments.

The literary productions of the medical professors at the German universities during this period are equally concentrated on medical practice – plague tractates, health guides, recipe collections, and *consilia* – and, to judge from surviving manuscripts, their advice was eagerly accepted by colleagues, surgeons, barbers, and patients. One of the most widely circulated books in all Germany was *A Very Useful Little Book on Distillations* ascribed to Michael Puff von Schrick, a member of the medical faculty at Vienna from 1433 until his death in 1473. In it some 82 herbal distillations were described, along with directions for their manufacture and use. Its kernel was a genuine tract by Puff, written in 1455 and revised in 1466, supplemented by three other short tracts on herbal waters. It was a national best-seller, going through 38 printed editions between 1476 and 1601, to say nothing of at least 14 surviving copies in manuscript. Here medical learning and theoretical knowledge were united with popular healing and practical information.

It is thus ironic that from the 1490s onwards the medical humanists, the standard-bearers of the medical Renaissance, should have concentrated once more on theory, on the meaning of words and the citation of authorities, and on a revival of Galenism. Their predecessors had been aware of the crisis of authority, and the problems involved in reconciling text with text, but they could neither appreciate the extent of their own difficulties (for they knew little, if any, Greek or Arabic) nor resolve them. Their concentration on practical experience obscured, but it did not alter, the underlying theoretical conflict. The arrival of the new Greek Galen in 1525, larger and more splendid than before, provided the key to unlock the future. Others, however, still preferred the solidity (a favoured term) of medieval practical medicine.

The Later Middle Ages mark the beginnings of a medicalisation of European society. Institutions gradually replace informality, regulations supplant neighbourly advice. In AD 1000 doctors were few in number, confined largely to court or monastery; by 1500, they were common throughout the urban civilisation of western Europe, and faced competition from other organised practitioners – surgeons, barber-surgeons, barbers, and apothecaries. The squabbles over professional hierarchy are but one feature of a growth in medical power which assigned more and more areas of life to medical control; autopsies, sometimes held under the watchful eye of a professor, supplemented or replaced the opinions of a local jury; midwives joined worthy matrons in pronouncing on impotence or loss of virginity; health officials, not just one's neighbours, told one where to throw one's rubbish. The Church still claimed an oversight over all Christian life, and still had its own methods for the relief of suffering. But, increasingly, these were becoming secondary, accepted as an occasional miracle, derided as superstitious magic, or reduced to a caring role, while physicians and other medical professionals did the job of curing. These moves towards a more medicalised society involved, if not a new medical effectiveness against disease (which is hard to determine), at least the belief that practitioners of medicine and surgery had something to offer their patients. The plurality of approaches to health of the Early Middle Ages was supplemented in some regions by a more formal hierarchy that separated professional from lay, surgeon from barber, and doctor from quack. From birth to death, from being delivered by the hands of a civic midwife to dying in a hospital – and even beyond, if one was dissected at a public anatomy display – medicine, legally defined and legally organised, gained a hold in the Later Middle Ages that it had previously lacked or lost. If the roots of the Western tradition of medical ideas go back to Classical Antiquity, those of its institutions indubitably have their origin in the Middle Ages.

Chronological table for chapter 6

Year	Medical and scientific events	Year	Contemporary events
		1492	Christopher Columbus crosses Atlantic and lands on West Indian island
1495	French army of Charles VIII, infected by syphilis during seige of Naples, then spreads it to other parts of Europe on way back to France		
1497	Hieronymus Brunschwig's *Chirurgia*		
		1498	Vasco da Gama sails to India via Cape of Good Hope
		1500	Pedro Cabral lands on the coast of Brazil
1512–13	Portuguese reach the Moluccas, the Spice Islands		
		1516	Death of Hieronymus Bosch, Flemish painter
		1517	Martin Luther's 95 Theses nailed to door of castle church at Wittenberg – beginning of Protestant Reformation
1519	Thomas Linacre's translation of Galen's *Method of Healing* Death of Leonardo da Vinci		
		1519–22	Magellan's expedition circumnavigates the world

Year	Medical and scientific events	Year	Contemporary events
		1520	Hernando Cortez leads Spanish takeover of Aztec Empire
1521	Berengario da Carpi's *Commentary on the Anatomy of Mondino*		
1525	Complete works of Galen first printed in Greek	1525	Francis I of France captured at battle of Pavia
1526	First Greek edition of Hippocratic corpus		League of Cognac set up
1527	University of Marburg founded by Philip, landgrave of Hesse		
1530	Girolamo Fracastoro's *Syphilis Sive de Morbo Gallico* Otto Brunfel's *Herbarum Vivae Eicones*		
1531	Galen's *On Anatomical Procedures* translated by Guinther von Andernach		
		1532	Suleiman the Magnificent, the Ottoman ruler, besieges Vienna
		1533	Francisco Pizarro puts Inca Emperor Atahualpa to death
		1536	Death of Desiderius Erasmus, Dutch humanist John Calvin's *Institutes of the Christian Religion*
1541	Death of Paracelsus		
1543	Andreas Vesalius' *De Humani Corporis Fabrica* Nicholas Copernicus' *De Revolutionibus Orbium Coelestium*		
1544	Pier Andrea Mattioli's *Commentaries on Dioscorides' Materia Medica*		
1544–45	Botanical gardens created in Pisa and Padua		

Year	Medical and scientific events	Year	Contemporary events
		1545	Council of Trent, which initiates Catholic Counter-Reformation, begins its meetings
		1547	Ivan IV ('The Terrible') crowned Czar of all the Russias
1551	First volume of Conrad Gesner's *Historia Animalium*		
		1553	Michael Servetus burned at the stake in Geneva
		1558	Elizabeth I becomes Queen of England
1559	Realdo Colombo's *De Re Anatomica*		Treaty of Cateau-Cambrésis
		1560	The English language *Geneva Bible* completed
1563	Garcia D'Orta's *Coloquios dos Simples e Drogas... da India*		
1565	First part of Nicolas Monardes' *Dos Libros...*, on American medical drugs		
1571	Peter Severinus' *Idea Medicinae Philosophicae* and Guinther von Andernach's *De Medicina Veteri et Nova*		Battle of Lepanto, destruction of Turkish fleet by European Holy League
		1572	Saint Bartholomew's Day Massacre in France
1575	Leiden University in Holland is founded		
		1578	Francis Drake on voyage round the world
		1584	Sir Walter Raleigh discovers 'Virginia' William of Orange assassinated
1585	Foundation of the University of Edinburgh		

209

Year	Medical and scientific events	Year	Contemporary events
		1588	Spanish Armada defeated
1589	Galileo Galilei professor of Mathematics at Pisa		
c. 1590	Dutch spectacle makers Hans Lippershey and Zacharias Jansen invent microscope		
1590	Death of French surgeon Ambroise Paré		
1597	Andreas Libavius' *Alchemia* (one of the first chemistry text-books)		
1600	William Gilbert's *On the Magnet*		
		1601	English Poor Law system established
		1602	Shakespeare's *Hamlet*
1603	Accademia dei Lincei, informal scientific society, founded		Elizabeth I dies, succeeded by James VI of Scotland and I of England. Hereditary shogunate rules Japan until 1867
1604	Hieronymus Fabricius ab Aquapendente's *On the Formation of the Fetus*		
1605	Francis Bacon's *The Advancement of Learning*		Gunpowder plot
		1605–15	Miguel de Cervantes' *Don Quixote*
		1607	Jamestown, Virginia, established
1608	Hans Lippershey invents telescope		
1609	Johann Kepler's *New Astronomy*		
1610	Galileo's *Sidereal Messenger* (describing the moons of Jupiter seen by the telescope)		
		1611	Authorised, 'King James', version of the Bible
1614	John Napier invents logarithms		

Year	Medical and scientific events	Year	Contemporary events
		1618	Thirty Years War (1618–1648)
1620	Francis Bacon's *Novum Organum*		Pilgrim Fathers leave in Mayflower to found Plymouth Colony, New England
1621	Robert Burton's *The Anatomy of Melancholy*		
		1625	James I of England dies
1628	William Harvey's *Exercitatio Anatomica de Motu Cordis et Sanguinis in Animalibus*		
		1630	Building of Taj Mahal in India began by Shah Jehan
1632	Galileo Galilei's *Dialogue on the Two Chief Systems of the World*		
1637	René Descartes' *Discourse on Method*		
1638	Galileo Galilei's *Discourses on Two New Sciences*		
		1642	Beginning of English Civil War. Abel Tasman discovers Tasmania and New Zealand
1643	Evangelista Torricelli invents barometer		
		1644	End of Ming dynasty and beginning of Manchu dynasty in China Quakers founded by George Fox
1647	Blaise Pascal experiments to show existence of vacuum		
		1649	Charles I executed
1651	William Harvey's *Exercitationes De Generatione Animalium*		

Year	Medical and scientific events	Year	Contemporary events
1651	Otto von Guericke invents air-pump		Thomas Hobbes' *Leviathan*
1652	The Dane Thomas Bartholin demonstrates lymphatic system in humans		
1653	Francis Glisson's *Anatomia Hepatis* gives a detailed anatomy of the liver		
1655	Christian Huygens designs first pendulum-clock		
1657	First fountain pen made in Paris. Leopoldo de Medici founds the Accademia del Cimento in Florence, the first formal scientific institution		
		1658	Aurangzeb, Moghul Emperor, begins his rule over India
1660	Royal Society founded		Restoration of Charles II to English throne
1661	Robert Boyle's *The Sceptical Chemist*		
1663	Marcello Malpighi's *De Pulmonibus*		
1664	Thomas Willis' *Cerebri Anatome*		
1665	Robert Hooke's *Micrographia*		Death of Philip IV of Spain
1666	Académie Royale des Sciences founded		Great Fire of London
1668	Newton builds first reflecting telescope		
1669	Richard Lower's *Tractatus de Corde*		
1672	Thomas Willis' *De Anima Brutorum*		
1673	Marcello Malpighi's *De Formatione Pulli*		
		1674	John III Sobieski King of Poland
1675	Nicholas Lemery's *Cours de Chemie*		
1676	Edmé Mariotte's *Essai sur la Nature de l'air*		
1680–1	Alfonso Borelli's *De Motu Animalium*		

Year	Medical and scientific events	Year	Contemporary events
		1682	Peter I becomes Czar of Russia
		1685	Revocation of Edict of Nantes
1686	1st volume of John Ray's *Historia Plantarum*		
1687	Isaac Newton's *Philosophiae Naturalis Principia Mathematica*		
		1688	'Glorious Revolution' in England. James II deposed
1689	Death of Thomas Sydenham		
1693	Foundation of University of Halle		

6 Medicine in Early Modern Europe, 1500–1700

ANDREW WEAR

Disease and society

THE DEMOGRAPHIC BACKGROUND

In 1650 the puritan preacher Isaac Ambrose pointed out the nearness of death in daily life: 'We live and yet whilst we speak this word, perhaps we die. Is this a land of the living or a region of the dead?' Ambrose's message was more convincing in demographic terms than it would be nowadays in a Western developed country. Today, we expect death in old age, but in the sixteenth and the seventeenth centuries, as in previous centuries, the young were expected to die as well as the old.

Although the civil registration of births, marriages, and deaths was not begun in most European countries until the nineteenth century, the demographic facts of life and death are available for early-modern Europe because parish churches in some countries were ordered to keep a register of births, marriages, and deaths. Historical demographers have used these parish data to recreate the demographic regime of early modern Europe.

Infant mortality, the number of live births dying in the first year of life, is a sensitive indicator of the health of a population, for it reflects the quality of health care services and the general environmental hygienic and nutritional status of infants and hence of the population in general. Today in Western Europe an infant mortality rate of around 9 per 1000 live births is the expected norm. In early modern England infant mortality was by comparison extremely high, around 150–200 per 1000 live births, and varying according to locality and country. For instance, the low-lying marshy areas of southern and eastern England, where 'agues' or malarial fevers were endemic together with water-borne diseases like dysentery and typhus, had infant mortality rates as high as 250–300 per 1000. Generally, however, towns and cities were less healthy than the countryside.

Other countries often had higher rates of infant mortality than England: France before 1750 had over 200 per 1000, Denmark 206 per 1000 (1645–99), Geneva 296 per 1000 (1580–1739). Eight German parishes for the period before 1750 had a mean of 154 per 1000, but with a wide variation ranging from 90 per 1000 to 250 per 1000. Such variation was the norm across Europe. Historical demographers have shown that death was not ever present throughout Europe. For instance, the English parish of Hartland in northwest Devon enjoyed a very favourable mortality level. High infant mortality significantly reduces overall life expectation, but at Hartland in the seventeenth and eighteenth centuries infant mortality was comparatively favourable, below 100 per 1000 live births. Its population of between 1000 and 1500 had an expectation of life at birth of 55 years or more for the whole of the period from 1558 to 1837, levels not achieved until 1920 in England as a whole. The scattered nature of Hartland's population housed in widely spaced farmsteads, the isolation of the place, bounded as it was on two sides by the sea and lacking highways, helped to keep infection away, while the large ratio of farmland to population would have produced good nutritional levels. Breast-feeding that lasted over a year with consequent longer birth intervals may also help to explain Hartland's low infant mortality.

Social conditions as well as geographical environments caused ill health and death. This was most dramatically seen in the man-made environment of cities where crowding and unsanitary conditions meant unhealthy places. In London, deaths exceeded births, and its population could not have been self-sustaining, let alone have increased from 120,000 in 1550 to 490,000 by 1700, had it not been for an influx of incomers from the countryside. This was realised by the first student of population demography as well as by modern demographers. John Graunt (1620–74), a haberdasher who became a Fellow of the Royal Society, in his *Natural and Political Observations.... upon the Bills of Mortality* (1662), followed the numerate philosophy of the 'new science' (p. 340). His book was based on a quantitative analysis of the weekly bills of mortality compiled by London's parish clerks that set out the numbers and causes of death in each parish. Graunt noted that between 1603 and 1644 burials exceeded christenings and concluded:

> From this single Observation it will follow, that London should have decreased in its People; the contrary whereof we see by its daily increases of Buildings upon new Foundations, and by turning

of great Palacious Houses into small Tenements. It is therefore certain, that London is supplied with People from out of the Country, whereby not only to supply the overplus differences of Burials above mentioned, but likewise to increase its Inhabitants according to the said increase of housing.

Within cities, wealth often determined healthy and unhealthy areas. For example, 60 per cent of households in the London parish of St. Peter Cornhill in the 1638 parish tithe census were 'substantial' (living in property worth a rent of £20 or above) while the parish of Allhallows London Wall was one of the poorest in London with only three per cent of its households listed as substantial. In St. Peter Cornhill in the period 1580–1650 out of a thousand live births 631 would survive to the age of 15, but only 508 did so in Allhallows London Wall. In Geneva in the seventeenth century, infant mortality among the 'grande bourgeoisie' was 208 per 1000 whilst for the 'lesser' bourgeoisie it was 358 per 1000. Social inequalities led to large health inequalities.

THE DISEASES OF SIXTEENTH- AND SEVENTEENTH-CENTURY EUROPE

It is clear that, despite differences, the young of all classes were at great risk of death. The expectation of life at birth in early modern England was usually between 30 to 40 years. If someone survived to the age of 20 they could expect nearly 40 more years of life. The great killers of the young were infectious diseases, which today in developed countries are often preventable or curable. Smallpox, plague, dysentery, tuberculosis, diphtheria, scarlet fever, whooping cough, influenza, pneumonia, and other infectious diseases helped to kill between 40 to 50 per cent of Europe's children by the age of 15.

It is nearly impossible to give accurate figures of the causes of death, let alone of morbidity, the incidence of particular diseases within a population. Causes of death were not usually registered, and when they were, as in northern Italian cities and in the bills of mortality of the London parishes, it is difficult to translate them with any certainty into modern categories. In London the 'searchers of the dead', usually old women employed by the parish, certified cause of death using categories based on symptoms as much as on disease categories. Terms such as 'aged', 'bloody flux', 'ague and fever', 'surfet', and 'suddenly' used by the searchers of the dead were clear enough to contemporaries, but appear vague in terms of modern medicine. Many deaths from heart attacks or strokes may have been confused or labelled 'struck suddenly', and many cancers would have been missed.

New diseases also hit Europe, although none had as great an effect on European mortality as did plague. There was the short-lived and mysterious 'English Sweat' which appeared in 1485 and disappeared after 1551. It took an epidemic form, reappearing in 1508, 1517, 1528 and 1551, and travelling to Europe in 1529–30. Death came suddenly, after a short attack of intensive sweating and in some cases discoloration of the skin. The disease was most probably influenza.

Typhus, like syphilis, entered Europe at the end of the fifteenth century, probably via soldiers coming back to Spain from Cyprus. It was a disease of armies, prisons ('gaol fever'), hospitals, and also of crowded slums where infected lice (as we know today) could easily move from person to person. The poor suffered most from typhus, but the numbers of deaths are hard to quantify. Unless they occurred in closed institutions such as prisons or in armies (as in 1526 when the French were forced to break off the siege of Naples because of typhus), deaths from typhus were difficult to pin-point.

Syphilis had a tremendous cultural and psychological impact. It spread through Europe at the end of the fifteenth century and was at the time thought to have been brought back by Columbus' sailors from the New World (p. 225). In the early years of the epidemic, its symptoms were especially dramatic. Ulrich von Hutten (1488–1523), an itinerant German scholar, doctor, and adventurer who suffered from syphilis himself (p. 308), described the horror of the new disease. The physicians,

> cared not even to behold it; so much less at the first to touch the infected; for truly when it first begun, it was so horrible to behold. They had boils that stood out like acorns, from whence issued such filthy stinking matter, that whosoever came within the scent, believed himself infected. The colour of these was a dark green, and the very aspect as shocking as the pain itself, which yet was as if the sick had lain upon a fire.

By the end of the sixteenth century the more fulminant and extreme forms of syphilis were receding as milder and more chronic forms became dominant. But the stigma of syphilis remained and its associations with immorality, crime, and poverty led medical practitioners of all sorts to advertise the private and confidential nature of their cures. Sometimes they encouraged their patients in the belief that the well-to-do and the respectable could catch syphilis without sexual intercourse (as the surgeon William Clowes wrote), or that many non-venereal conditions could mimic syphilis. The 'searchers of the dead' in London often deliberately failed to record syphilis as a cause of death. The moral and social stigma connected with the disease thus led to deception all round.

Although learned medical writers often found a 'new disease' to have been described by the ancients, both learned and popular culture believed in the possibility of new diseases. The plague pandemic of 1347–51, syphilis, the English sweat, tarantism (epidemic dancing mania seen especially in Italy and believed both to be caused by the bite of a spider and to cure it) numerous instances of 'new' fevers and the identification of rickets as a new disease by Glisson, Bate, and Regemorter in *A Treatise of the Rickets* (1651) all confirmed the belief that new diseases could come from God, the stars, or nature herself, and created a sense of uncertainty and terror of the unknown.

Also terrifying were periods of extremely high mortality. The existence of infectious disease such as plague and smallpox that took an epidemic form meant that different localities at different times could experience sharp rises in their death rates. These short-term mortality crises produced not only demographic but also social and cultural devastation. Some places might escape for long periods of time, while others could suffer successive crises. Demographers have disagreed over the definition of a short-term mortality crisis. But if crisis mortality is defined as an average yearly mortality at least 10 per cent above the expected trend, or as at least a 25 per cent rise in the monthly total of deaths above the trend (in practice it could sometimes reach above 100 per cent), then England suffered 37 years of crisis mortality between 1541 and 1750.

FAMINE

In the minds of many contemporaries such crises were caused by the 'three arrows of God' – war, famine and pestilence. Famine years occurred in continental Europe regularly up to the mid-eighteenth century and then tapered off, first in France, then in Germany and central Europe. England was more fortunate. In the late sixteenth century crises of subsistence affected parts of the North of England and a few isolated spots in the South, but after the mid-seventeenth century such crises were absent from England. The move from dependence on one grain crop, the increase in spring-sown crops such as oats and barley to complement winter sowing, and the establishment of a large unitary market for grain helped to eradicate famine in England. This, taken together with England's more favourable mortality figures, confirms the widespread perception of the time that England was healthier than the rest of Europe.

Demographers suspect the existence of famine when a sharp increase in the price of grain, usually following a crop failure, is associated with a rise in mortality. As well as causing large-scale deaths especially among children and the elderly, famine produced great social disruption. The crowds of poor fleeing famine often helped to spread typhus. The movement of grain to famine areas may also have brought with it rodents carrying plague. Plague followed famine in many parts of Europe in 1596–98 (though not in England) and depressed Europe's population both numerically and psychologically (the crisis of the 1590s brought to an end the strong population growth of the sixteenth century – the population of Europe just before the Black Death was around 90 million, in 1400 it was 65 million, in 1500 it was 84 million, in 1600 it was 111 million, and in 1700 it was 125 million; from the 1590s to 1700 Europe's rate of population growth declined).

Famine caused death by starvation, and low levels of nutrition have been thought to increase susceptibility to infection and to render some infections fatal which might otherwise be innocuous. Chronic protein deficiency in young children may have produced low intelligence as occurs in Third World countries today. But given the lack of historical records this remains conjectural. What is also difficult to discern is the level of regular as opposed to extraordinary starvation. The poor were often found starved to death in the streets in times of plenty, but such background levels of famine mortality go undetected by demographers. Culturally, however, starvation was engrained in the popular mind. The common prayer was 'from war, plague and hunger, deliver us O Lord'. St. Basil in the fourth century had written of starvation as a disease. Certainly its effects and its outcomes were the same as other diseases and indeed some physicians in the sixteenth century sought herbs that, like the manna that came from Heaven, would satisfy and cure hunger.

PLAGUE

Another arrow of God, plague, finally disappeared from Western Europe in the eighteenth century. Before then it continued to wreak havoc in epidemic form as it had done since the pandemic of 1347–51. Its visitation upon a place produced very high mortality. Around a fifth of London's population died in each of the plague outbreaks of 1563,

1603, 1625, 1665 (fewer in 1578, 1593, 1638). Felix Platter (1536–1614) the town physician of Basle in Switzerland, collected some of the first detailed statistics of plague mortality. Between 1609 and 1611 in Basle, 6408 caught plague, of whom 3968 died, a case fatality rate of 61.9 per cent. The population of Basle has been estimated at 15,000, so in one and a half years around 42 per cent of the population had suffered from plague and 26 per cent had died of it. In 1630–31, Venice lost over 30 per cent of its people, while the combination of plague and starvation in 1656 in Genoa led, in the estimate of contemporaries, to the death of three quarters of its population. The village of Eyam in Derbyshire, England, suffered a 40 per cent mortality in 1666 when, in a famous incident, it agreed to quarantine itself and not allow any inhabitant out of the village.

Secular and religious approaches to the plague continued to exist side by side in the sixteenth century. In the very severe plague outbreaks of the 1570s the Archbishop of Milan, Carlo Borromeo, had insisted on penitential processions and public prayers and emphasised that health officials should not stop church services or public processions. Compromise was possible: when Borromeo headed a procession through Milan in 1576 holding before him a holy relic – one of the nails of the Cross – all the women and children stayed at home by order of the health magistracy or health board (on the development of which, see p. 196). Other religious measures appeared to pose no threat to health, as when towns promised to build votive churches in return for the ending of plague (as with Palladio's Redentore in Venice). Even the Papal States had their own health magistracies. The church accepted that God often worked through natural means, and both the church and the health magistrates co-operated on such issues as the charitable relief of the plague victims.

The measures of the Italian health magistracies were emulated by other countries. France in the fifteenth century and Scotland and Russia by the early sixteenth century were setting up in their cities and surrounding areas *cordons sanitaires*, providing isolation facilities, controlling trade goods, and issuing health passes. England acted later. Here, there was no national policy on plague before 1518 when a Royal Proclamation decreed that those infected identify themselves by carrying a white stick and that infected houses be marked for 40 days by bundles of straw hanging from their windows. In the 1530s and 1540s individual towns such as Shrewsbury, York, Nottingham, Durham, and Newcastle isolated plague victims by keeping them in

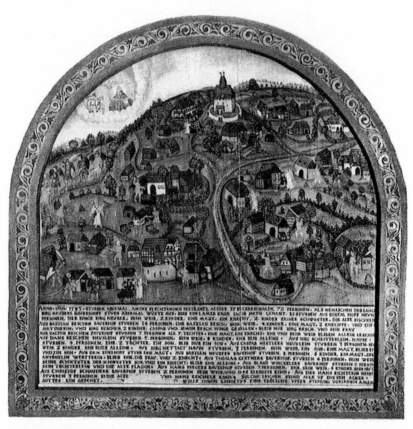

Fig. 28. The plague striking the village of Ruckerswalde in Saxony in 1583. The angels of God with swords raised visit the houses of the village. The painting in the village church is notable for giving the number of dead and listing in each household how many died and who survived.

temporary hospitals, huts, or cabins outside the city walls or bounds, as had been the practice with lepers in the Middle Ages.

A uniform plague policy across England was put in place in 1578 when the Privy Council set out its Plague Orders, which remained basically unchanged until 1666. The administration of the Orders fell not on physicians but, as in Italy, was devolved into the legal sphere, to the justices of the peace, who were the local representatives of the Crown. The English measures were similar to those on the continent. The policy of shutting up both ill and healthy in infected houses for six weeks was not new, but its harsh enforcement did not allow for visits to the sick as in the Netherlands. What was new was the financing of the plague measures, especially for the support of those quarantined in their homes and for the payment of guards, from a rate or local tax on

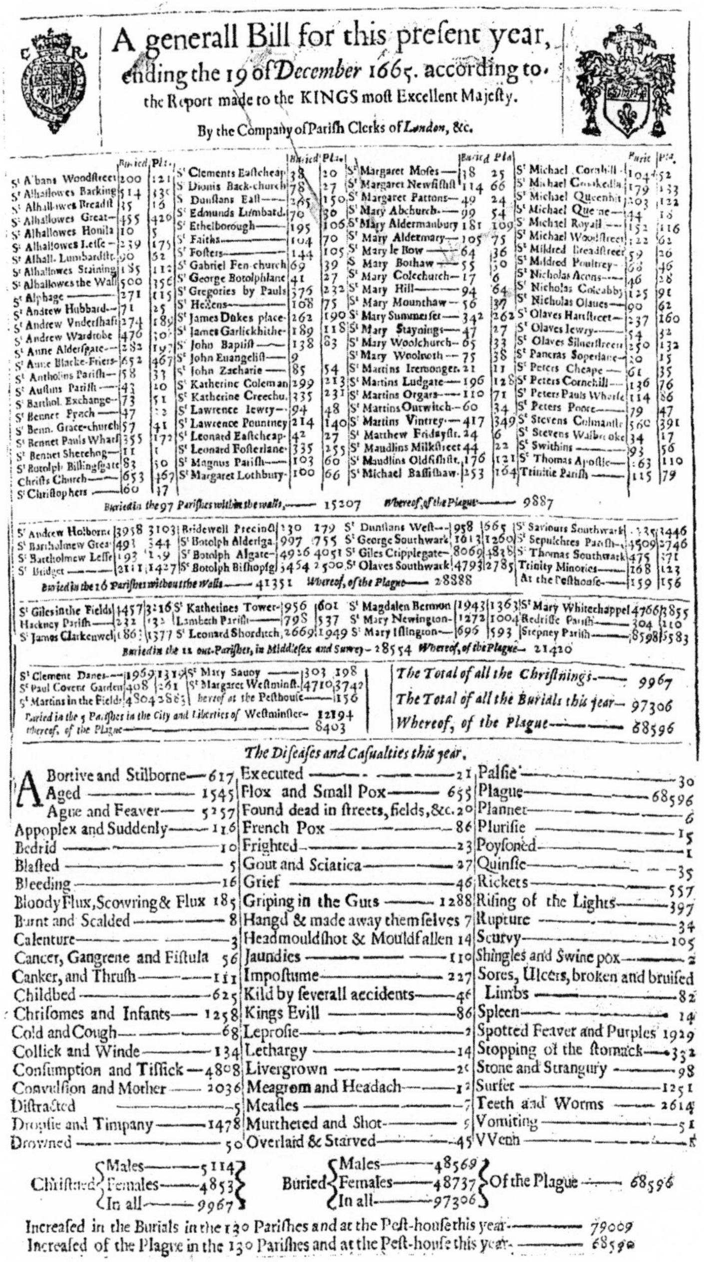

A generall Bill for this present year, ending the 19 of *December* 1665. according to the Report made to the KINGS most Excellent Majesty.

By the Company of Parish Clerks of *London*, &c.

	Buried	Pl.		Buried	Pl.		Buried	Pl.		Buried	Pl.
St Albans Woodstreet	200	121	St Clements Eastcheap	38	20	St Margaret Moses	38	25	St Michael Cornhill	104	52
St Alhallowes Barking	514	330	St Dionis Back-church	78	27	St Margaret Newfishst	114	66	St Michael Crookedla.	179	133
St Alhallowes Breadst	35	16	St Dunstans East	265	150	St Margaret Pattons	49	24	St Michael Queenhit	203	122
St Alhallowes Great	455	420	St Edmunds Lumbard.	70	30	St Mary Abchurch	99	54	St Michael Quene	44	18
St Alhallowes Honila	10	5	St Ethelborough	195	106	St Mary Aldermanbury	181	109	St Michael Royall	152	116
St Alhallowes Lesse	239	175	St Faiths	104	70	St Mary Aldermary	105	75	St Michael Woodstreet	122	62
St Alhall. Lumbardstr.	90	52	St Fosters	144	105	St Mary le Bow	64	36	St Mildred Breadstreet	59	26
St Alhallowes Staining	185	112	St Gabriel Fen-church	69	39	St Mary Bothaw	55	30	St Mildred Poultrey	68	46
St Alhallowes the Wall	500	356	St George Botolphlane	41	27	St Mary Colechurch	17	6	St Nicholas Acons	46	28
St Alphage	271	115	St Gregories by Pauls	376	232	St Mary Hill	94	64	St Nicholas Coleabby	125	91
St Andrew Hubbard	71	25	St Hellens	108	75	St Mary Mounthaw	56	37	St Nicholas Olaves	90	62
St Andrew Vndershaft	274	189	St James Dukes place	262	190	St Mary Summerset	342	262	St Olaves Hartstreet	237	160
St Andrew Wardrobe	476	308	St James Garlickhithe	189	118	St Mary Staynings	47	27	St Olaves Iewry	54	32
St Anne Aldersgate	282	197	St John Baptist	138	83	St Mary Woolchurch	65	33	St Olaves Silverstreet	250	132
St Anne Blacke-Friers	652	467	St John Euangelist	9		St Mary Woolnoth	75	38	St Pancras Soperlane	30	15
St Antholins Parish	58	33	St John Zacharie	85	54	St Martins Iremonger.	21	11	St Peters Cheape	61	35
St Austins Parish	43	20	St Katherine Coleman	299	213	St Martins Ludgate	196	128	St Peters Cornhill	136	76
St Barthol. Exchange	73	51	St Katherine Creechu.	335	231	St Martins Orgars	110	71	St Peters Pauls Wharfe	114	86
St Bennet Fynch	47	22	St Lawrence Iewry	94	48	St Martins Outwitch	60	34	St Peters Poore	79	47
St Benn. Grace-church	57	41	St Lawrence Pountney	214	140	St Martins Vintrey	417	349	St Stevens Colmanstr	560	391
St Bennet Pauls Wharf	355	172	St Leonard Eastcheap	42	27	St Matthew Fridaystr.	24	6	St Stevens Walbrooke	34	17
St Bennet Sherehog	11	1	St Leonard Fosterlane	335	255	St Maudlins Milkstreet	44	22	St Swithins	93	56
St Botolph Billingsgate	83	50	St Magnus Parish	103	60	St Maudlins Oldfishstr.	176	121	St Thomas Apostle	163	110
Christs Church	653	467	St Margaret Lothbury	100	66	St Michael Bassishaw	253	164	Trinitie Parish	115	79
St Christophers	60	47									

Buried in the 97 Parishes within the walls, — 15207 *Whereof, of the Plague* — 9887

St Andrew Holborne	3958	3103	Bridewell Precinct	230	179	St Dunstans West	958	665	St Saviours Southwark	4235	3446
St Bartholmew Great	493	344	St Botolph Aldersga.	997	755	St George Southwark	1613	1260	St Sepulchres Parish	4509	2746
St Bartholmew Lesse	193	139	St Botolph Algate	4926	4051	St Giles Cripplegate	8069	4838	St Thomas Southwark	475	371
St Bridget	2111	1427	St Botolph Bishopsg.	3454	2500	St Olaves Southwark	4793	2785	Trinity Minories	168	123
									At the Pesthouse	159	156

Buried in the 16 Parishes without the Walls — 41351 *Whereof, of the Plague* — 28888

St Giles in the Fields	4457	3216	St Katherines Tower	956	601	St Magdalen Bermon	1943	1363	St Mary Whitechappel	4766	3855
Hackney Parish	232	132	Lambeth Parish	798	537	St Mary Newington	1272	1004	Redriffe Parish	304	210
St James Clarkenwel	1863	1377	St Leonard Shorditch	2669	1949	St Mary Islington	696	593	Stepney Parish	8598	6583

Buried in the 12 out-Parishes, in Middlesex and Surrey — 28554 *Whereof, of the Plague* — 21420

St Clement Danes	1969	1319	St Mary Sauoy	303	198
St Paul Covent Garden	408	261	St Margaret Westminst.	4710	3742
St Martins in the Fields	4804	2883	*hereof at the Pesthouse*		156

Buried in the 5 Parishes in the City and Liberties of Westminster — 12194
Whereof, of the Plague — 8403

The Total of all the Christnings — 9967
The Total of all the Burials this year — 97306
Whereof, of the Plague — 68596

The Diseases and Casualties this year.

Abortive and Stilborne	617	Executed	21	Palsie	30
Aged	1545	Flox and Small Pox	655	Plague	68596
Ague and Feaver	5257	Found dead in streets, fields, &c.	20	Planner	6
Appoplex and Suddenly	116	French Pox	86	Plurisie	15
Bedrid	10	Frighted	23	Poysoned	1
Blasted	5	Gout and Sciatica	27	Quinsie	35
Bleeding	16	Grief	46	Rickets	557
Bloody Flux, Scowring & Flux	185	Griping in the Guts	1288	Rising of the Lights	397
Burnt and Scalded	8	Hangd & made away themselves	7	Rupture	34
Calenture	3	Headmouldshot & Mouldfallen	14	Scurvy	105
Cancer, Gangrene and Fistula	56	Jaundies	110	Shingles and Swine pox	2
Canker, and Thrush	111	Impostume	227	Sores, Ulcers, broken and bruised Limbs	82
Childbed	625	Kild by severall accidents	46	Spleen	14
Chrisomes and Infants	1258	Kings Evill	86	Spotted Feaver and Purples	1929
Cold and Cough	68	Leprosie	2	Stopping of the stomack	332
Collick and Winde	134	Lethargy	14	Stone and Strangury	98
Consumption and Tissick	4808	Livergrown	20	Surfet	1251
Convulsion and Mother	2036	Meagrom and Headach	12	Teeth and Worms	2614
Distracted	5	Measles	7	Vomiting	51
Dropsie and Timpany	1478	Murthered and Shot	9	Wen	8
Drowned	50	Overlaid & Starved	45		

Christned: Males — 5114, Females — 4853, In all — 9967
Buried: Males — 48569, Females — 48737, In all — 97306
Of the Plague — 68596

Increased in the Burials in the 130 Parishes and at the Pest-house this year — 79009
Increased of the Plague in the 130 Parishes and at the Pest-house this year — 68590

Fig. 29. A summary from the bills of mortality of the deaths in London parishes. The plague was responsible for the majority of deaths. Printed in *London's Dreadfull Visitation: or, a Collection of all the Bills of Mortality for this Present Year* (London, 1665). (The Wellcome Institute Library, London. L352.)

houses, organised by the justices of the peace. The combination of a central government order with a locally collected tax was new to Europe and also characterised the English Poor Laws of the sixteenth and early seventeenth centuries.

The English Plague Orders set out special prayers to God to be said in churches to assuage His punishment. As in the rest of Europe, the state shared the view that plague was a punishment for the sins of the community as a whole. But the scope for conflict between religious and public health measures was less in Protestant countries, for the Reformation had abolished prayers to saints, and the procession of a saint's relics through a city was condemned as superstitious idolatry.

Plague left England after 1670, and Europe in the next century. Various reasons have been given for this such as the replacement of the sedentary house or black rat (*Rattus rattus*) by the less domestic field or brown rat (*Rattus norvegicus*) in the eighteenth century. But plague was disappearing earlier. Most generally accepted is the view that the local and then the national *cordons sanitaires* did finally work. England avoided plague by rigorous quarantine measures introduced in 1655, when plague threatened from the Netherlands, and again in 1709–13 and 1720–22, when it could have entered from the Baltic ports and Marseilles respectively.

Apart from outbreaks in Palermo in 1743 and Cadiz in 1800 (and Russia in 1770–71), Western Europe was free from plague. It constantly threatened, however, from the Ottoman Empire in the Balkans and Asia Minor, where plague was rife. It was kept at bay by the eastern border barrier erected by the Hapsburg Empire, which utilised *Bauernsoldaten* (peasants who were offered land in return for a five month stint of border duty) to watch over the 1900 kilometres of the frontier. The plague decrees, *Pestpatente*, of 1728, 1737, and 1770 set up a frontier force of 4000 men in normal times, and 7000 when plague was notified in any part of the Ottoman Empire. Plague measures such as quarantine and disinfection of goods, animals, and people had clearly become effective by the eighteenth century, for the few outbreaks that occurred in Europe were effectively limited in their spread (as in Marseilles). When in 1840 the Ottoman government took action along European lines to contain plague, it was quickly successful.

Plague was probably the only disease successfully eliminated in the period, and it was an administrative rather than a medical success. In fact in the early modern period, medicine did little or nothing to improve the survival chances of Europe's population. Infant mortality remained high, and if plague and famine slowly disappeared and short-term mortality crises retreated into folklore, other diseases such as smallpox, typhus, and probably tuberculosis ensured that the overall death rate in Europe remained the same as before. The changes in medical theory and therapeutics from which so much was hoped made no impression on the statistical picture. An individual who had malaria may have been helped by the use of cinchona bark (quinine), which was imported from Peru in the seventeenth century, but it still remained as true in 1700 as in 1500 that no one could confidently expect to live to old age.

EUROPEANS ABROAD 1492–1800

The voyages of discovery at the end of the fifteenth and in the sixteenth centuries began the process of European settlement abroad. First in America, and then in the Pacific in the eighteenth century, Europeans produced by their mere presence profound demographic effects. Europeans also theorised about the healthiness of their new environments, adapted to new climates, and brought with them as part of their 'cultural baggage' the medical care systems of their home countries.

Demographically, Europeans represented disaster to the peoples they encountered. When the Spanish came to America their diseases destroyed the Native American Indians. The Old World (Europe, India, Asia) disease mix had over time left a population with a degree of immunity to most infectious diseases. America, however, had been isolated from the European disease environment. Diseases like smallpox, measles, diphtheria, chickenpox, mumps, plague, influenza, scarlet fever, amoebic dysentery, and malaria appear to have been absent from America. The coming of Europeans to America began a very unequal disease exchange. Whether syphilis came from America to Europe is debated by historians. It may have been present in the Mediterranean regions in an endemic, non-venereal form which could have mutated into a sexually transmitted disease. Again, yaws, which is caused by an organism indistinguishable from that which produces syphilis, was present in the Old World and could have changed into venereal syphilis. A non-venereal form of syphilis was present in America, and there is also a very small amount of skeletal evidence for venereal syphilis, but located away from the areas of European settlement. If syphilis came from America where it was present, it may have undergone a transformation in Europe from a non-venereal into a venereal form. Its impact upon mortality was not great, and Europe received no other disease from America. But a whole series of European diseases hit the Native Americans. These produced 'virgin soil epidemics' with extremely high mortality rates due to their lack of previous exposure. The size of the Native American population at the time of Columbus' first voyage in 1492 has been variously estimated as between 50 and 100 million. Disease brought in by Europeans and then by African slaves reduced the population by 90 per cent. Some parts, such as the Caribbean, suffered a total loss of population.

Smallpox and measles were probably the greatest killers. Either can kill between one-third and one-half of a non-immune population. In 1518–19 the Caribbean Indians were devastated by smallpox, which then travelled to Mexico and thence to Peru, clearing the way for the Spaniards to take the Aztec and Inca empires (but see the article by Francis Brooks in 'Bibliography' for a contrary view). In North America in the next century, John Winthrop, the governor of Massachusetts, acknowledged in his puritan way the providential hand of God when he wrote (in 1634), 'For the natives, they are near all dead of Small Pox, so as the Lord hath cleared our title to what we possess'. There were constant reports of epidemics hitting Native Americans in the sixteenth and seventeenth centuries. Often they cannot be identified, but the diseases listed above could have been responsible.

Some diseases came to America from Africa. Yellow fever and the falciparum form of malaria did not exist in Europe. Vivax malaria, the milder type of malaria, came from Europe, but falciparum malaria and yellow fever were introduced through the slave trade. As the Native Americans died out and were also not deemed strong enough to work the sugar cane fields of the West Indies, slaves began to be imported from Africa, especially from West Africa. They brought with them falciparum malaria, and, in the water casks of the slave ships, the mosquito that carried yellow fever. The first outbreak of yellow fever in America was probably in Boston in 1693. (Yellow fever typically hit ports, as the *Aedes aegypti* mosquito, which spread it, had a short range and kept near to water; people soon learned to escape by moving inland for a while.)

Falciparum malaria, to which some slaves had a degree of genetic immunity through the sickle-cell trait (they also had some immunity to yellow fever), debilitated and killed whites in the hotter parts of America. Whites were thus being exposed to some of the disease environments of West Africa, which until the later nineteenth century was often literally 'the white man's grave'. The result of the opening of the slave trade meant that the disease exchange had become three-way.

A similar chain of events unfolded when the South Pacific was explored following the voyages of Samuel Wallis (1766–68), Louis-Antoine de Bougainville (1766–69), and James Cook (1768–70, 1772–75, 1776–80). Virgin soil epidemics, especially of measles, decimated the inhabitants of the Pacific Islands and the Maoris in New Zealand (the latter were also killed by slower acting tuberculosis). The population of islands like Tahiti, which had been viewed by European explorers in the eighteenth century as an arcadian paradise peopled by noble savages, went into rapid decline. This was brought about by a combination of newly imported diseases (such as syphilis), and the impact of an industrial civilisation upon Stone Age societies whose resistance to alcohol, to the sale of guns, and to missionaries was as low as their resistance to European diseases. Tahiti's population declined from approximately 40,000 in 1769 to around 9000 by 1830, while the Maori population fell from an estimated 150,000–180,000 in 1814–15 to 56,049 by the time of the census of 1857–58. Such figures led Charles Darwin to write in the *Descent of Man* (1871),

> When civilised nations came into contact with barbarians the struggle is short, except when a deadly climate gives its aid to the native race... New diseases and vices have in some cases proved highly destructive; and it appears that a new disease often causes much death, until those who are most susceptible to its destructive influences are gradually worked out, and so it may be with the evil effects from spirituous liquors.....

The demographic destruction caused by Europeans and their diseases fed the sense of racial superiority felt by Europeans with consequences that are still present today.

SCURVY

One disease did, however, especially affect the ships' crews which set out from Europe. Scurvy (which today we know is caused by a lack of vitamin C) killed crews on long sea voyages. It was encountered on land during sieges and famines and from the 1520s 'land scurvy' had been counted as one of the 'new diseases'. However, it showed itself most spectacularly at sea, not so much in the relatively short voyage from Europe to America, but in circumnavigations of the world, in trans-Pacific voyages and in long naval blockades with no fresh supplies of food.

The numbers that fell victim to scurvy could be enormous. George Anson's circumnavigation of the globe was ordered by the British Admiralty in 1740 to break the Spanish monopoly in the Pacific and to capture the Spanish treasure ship sailing between Mexico and the Philippines. Out of the 1955 men that set out, 320 had died from fevers and dysentery and 997 from scurvy by the time Anson returned to England in 1744, as against only four in enemy action.

The use of lemons as a cure for scurvy was known to the Spaniards in the early sixteenth century, and Sir Richard Hawkins used oranges and lemons when his crew fell ill with scurvy during his 1593 voyage to the Pacific against the Spanish. He wrote:

> That which I have seene most fruitfull for this sickness, is sowre Oranges and Lemmons, and a water.... called Doctor Stevens water.....[which] gave health to those that used it. The Oyle of Vitry [sulphuric acid] is beneficiall for this disease... But the principall [cure] of all is the Ayre of the Land; for the Sea is naturall for Fishes and the Land for men.

But it was difficult to get universal agreement that lemons and oranges cured scurvy. There were no clinical trials in the sixteenth and seventeenth centuries. The very nature of medicine at this time worked against any consensus. Hawkins and others used many 'specific' remedies like oranges or Dr. Stevens' water; which one worked was difficult to disentangle, especially if new foods, like fruits, were taken on board every time a ship made land, as commonly happened. Moreover, Galenic theory structured around the 'six non-naturals' (p. 141) taught that different aspects of life-style and the environment could cause disease, a widespread belief shared by seamen from Hawkins' time to that of Captain Cook in the later eighteenth century.

Even though medical theories changed in the seventeenth and eighteenth centuries, the multifactorial nature of medicine did not. Nor did the lack of any means of achieving consensus (a notorious fact of medical life for much of the eighteenth century and before). The use of oranges and lemons for scurvy kept on being rediscovered and lost. The Dutch East India Company perhaps kept faith longest with citrus fruits. Throughout the seventeenth century they ensured supplies by planting orchards in Mauritius and St. Helena, and then at the Cape of Good Hope, where they were reported in 1661 to have 1000 citrus fruit

trees. Like others, however, they also used a variety of different remedies.

It was James Lind (1716–91), the Edinburgh naval surgeon, who
demonstrated that oranges and lemons, and not other remedies, could
cure scurvy. He did this by dividing 12 sailors suffering from scurvy
into six groups of two and, for fourteen days, giving them one of six
common treatments for scurvy. Even though the treatment of two
oranges and one lemon a day per man lasted for only six days due to a
lack of supplies, Lind reported in his *Treatise of the Scurvy* (1753) that
the oranges and lemons had cured the men, while of the other treatments only cider had had some partial effect.

Lind's results were not taken up immediately, partly because he
decided to evaporate lemon juice into 'rob of lemon' by heating it for
easier storage on board ship, so rendering it ineffective (heat destroys
vitamin C), partly also because Lind was not a strong advocate of his
own ideas. Moreover, when he became physician to the Royal Naval
Hospital at Haslar, Lind was not able to reproduce his previous experimental results showing the efficacy of oranges and lemons. The search
for a cure continued. Captain Cook on his first Pacific voyage of
1768–70 tried a variety of remedies including sauerkraut, onions, salep
(a powder made from dried orchids used to thicken soups), and malt
wort as well as oranges and lemons. However, Cook, like Lind and most
sea captains and surgeons, believed that attention to diet, cleanliness,
and morale was a necessary complement to any specific cures.

It was only when Gilbert Blane, a naval physician with the right
naval connections, and a believer in the efficacy of oranges and lemons,
was appointed a Commissioner of the Board of Sick and Wounded
Sailors (the Navy's health and welfare directorate) in 1795 that lemon
juice became standard fare in the Navy. As a result, the death rate from
scurvy was dramatically reduced. This was one of the few successes of
medicine before the advent of 'scientific medicine' in the late nineteenth
century (and it was a success based on experience rather than understanding, as it was not until the early twentieth century with the discovery of vitamins that scurvy was seen as a deficiency disease). Blane's
administrative skill and the Navy's ability to get crews to down three-
quarters of an ounce of lemon juice a day helped as much as medical
expertise (this was a time when the Navy was moving from eighteenth-
century paternalism to an impersonal nineteenth-century organisation,
like the new prisons and factories, where disciplined uniformity was all).

ACCLIMATISATION OF EUROPEANS ABROAD

For Europeans the key to living abroad was climate and acclimatisation. Many illnesses in foreign parts, it was thought, were due to a change of air (or climate). The air into which a person was born naturally suited their humoral constitution. A foreign climate would often threaten the newly arrived settler, for their constitution, it was believed, could not cope with the climate. The solution was a period of 'seasoning', which would allow the body to adjust to the new environment (and when work was supposed to be limited and diet carefully monitored).

When the English settled in hot places, like North and South Carolina in America in the seventeenth and eighteenth centuries, they adjusted their life-styles. The death rate was much higher than in Old England or New England and, as the saying had it, 'Carolina is in the spring a paradise, in the summer a hell, and in the autumn a hospital'. Heat was perceived as a killer. Houses were moved to higher ground, away from the coast, which it was believed was not only mortally hot but had dangerous vapours. Clothes no longer followed English fashions but became lighter, and houses were designed to maximise coolness and ventilation rather than, as in the old country, to retain heat.

The theory of acclimatisation remained current until the end of the nineteenth century when the organisms causing diseases like malaria were discovered. Some of the environmental measures that resulted from the theory did in fact reduce the death rate. Army hill stations in India could be healthier than those on the coast. Positive results were also produced by other hygienic measures such as good ventilation and the provision of fresh water. These were derived, like the belief that climate caused disease, from classical ideas of health and the environment.

White settlers in foreign parts adapted their life-styles, but they retained their 'cultural baggage' when it came to their systems of medical care. The Spaniards, for instance, had much more central authority in medicine (as they did in government) than the English. In Spain the tribunal of the Protomedicato (first established on a secure basis in 1477 and named after the King's physician who sat on it) was usually composed of two physicians and two surgeons who examined and licensed physicians, surgeons, and some types of empirics, and supervised apothecaries and the quality of their wares. In New Spain (Mexico), Spanish institutions were quickly set up. Mexico City appointed a *pro-*

tomedico to examine practitioners in 1525. And in 1570 the Spanish Crown appointed Francisco Hernandez as *protomedico* to regulate medicine in the whole of New Spain. The lack of educated physicians put a practical limit on the *protomedicato's* powers (there was a need to accept empirics and 'curanderos', traditional healers), but a key part of the Spanish medical system had been transplanted across the Atlantic.

Similarly, Catholic Spain possessed many church-run hospitals which were founded for philanthropic and therapeutic purposes. In 1521 Cortes had built the first hospital in Mexico City for the Indian and Spanish poor. By the end of the seventeenth century there were over 150 hospitals in New Spain. They were seen by the religious orders as a means of converting Indians to Christianity (the existence of town hospitals helped to bring the Indians into the towns where it was easier to convert in large numbers).

In education also the Spaniards imitated their home country. The universities of Mexico City and Lima in Peru were founded in 1551, and Mexico had a chair of medicine in 1578 and Lima in 1621. Medical books were being printed in the sixteenth and seventeenth century in the Spanish American territories.

Similarly, Old England provided the model for New England. There was no licensing of medical practitioners in New England; it only existed in England for London through the College of Physicians (p. 236) and it was not very effective. There were very few university trained physicians in New England and the informal system of medical care characteristic of England and centred on family, neighbours, skilled women, and clergymen was also developed in America. There were some paid practitioners in New England but the distinction between physicians, surgeons, and apothecaries that existed in England were elided by the New England 'doctor' who combined all three jobs, and who would be trained by apprenticeship.

England had few hospitals up to the end of the seventeenth century. New England had none. The first was the Pennsylvania Hospital founded in 1751. The first medical faculty was that of the College of Philadelphia, set up in 1765. Only in 1783 did Harvard create its Medical School, nearly 150 years after its foundation. The New England colonies took the deregulated, informal non-institutional English system to an extreme. And indeed, for most of the eighteenth century an English American physician could only become learned in medicine by travelling to Europe and, especially, to Edinburgh.

THE WORLD OF THE SICK

Patients and practitioners Most well-to-do people were ill at home. This meant that the sick (or their relatives) were far more in control of events around the sick bed than if they had been in an institution like a hospital, where not only treatment but their daily routine would have been out of their control. From home they could decide on what type of medical practitioner to pay for from the huge variety that existed in the medical market-place (wise-women, astrologers, herbalists, uroscopists, empirics, apothecaries, barber-surgeons, physicians, or specialists like tooth-drawers and lithotomists). Or they could rely on their immediate family, especially the female members, who would have had medical skills handed down from mother to daughter, by word of mouth and perhaps in a book that included medical remedies alongside food recipes, and voluntary help was also available from neighbours, clergymen and their wives, or from gentlewomen who treated the poor of their area as an act of charity, but who also gave their expertise to the more respectable sick.

University-trained physicians tended to be in urban areas where patients had enough money to pay the high fees that they charged. As in the Middle Ages, some towns and cities hired learned physicians as town physicians so as to have some medical expertise available. The coverage of town physicians was uneven across Europe and much depended on local initiatives. Towns and cities like Basle and Zurich in Switzerland, Amsterdam and Delft in the Netherlands, and for a time Berlin at the end of the sixteenth century appointed town physicians who provided medical help for the sick poor, gave advice on plague, and helped to oversee the regulation of medical practice in the town.

In Italy the *medici condotti* (town physicians) were no longer given contracts by the larger towns and cities, which probably felt they had enough learned physicians in private practice. But smaller towns such as Burano, Feltre, and Rovigo in the Venetian territories with populations of under 5000 still continued to pay physicians to treat their inhabitants free of charge. The Venetian and Tuscan countryside was well supplied with doctors and surgeons through the *condotta* system (in 1630, in the latter, there was more than one physician and more than one surgeon for 10,000 people; in cities like Milan, Florence, and Venice there were between four to six physicians per 10,000 population).

In Spanish cities in the second half of the sixteenth century there were similarly four to five learned doctors per 10,000 population. In England,

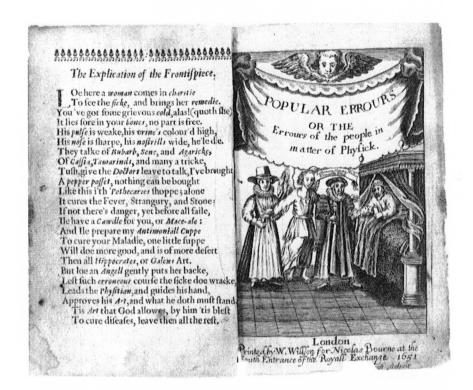

Fig. 30. Attack on charitable women treating the sick. In the picture and poem Christianity, in the shape of an angel, pushes back the woman and gives the physician the right to treat the sickman. From the frontispiece of James Primrose, *Popular Errours or the Errours of the People in matter of Physick* (London, 1651). (The Wellcome Institute Library, London. L7147.)

London was a strong magnet for the learned physicians. In 1600, with a population of 200,000, London had fifty physicians affiliated to the College of Physicians of London, which represents a ratio of 2.5 per 10,000. There were in addition, 100 surgeons and 100 apothecaries and a further 250 mainly unlicensed practioners (not including nurses and midwives) who made a living in London. The ratio of practitioners to population appears very favourable if these practitioners are taken into account: 25 per 10,000 or one for every 400 of London's inhabitants.

Apothecaries and surgeons often gave medical advice and treatment despite the protests of the physicians, and being cheaper, they were used by a wider section of the population. However, in the countryside such 'regular' practitioners were often not available. Ralph Josselin, a seventeenth-century English clergyman, inspected his own urine, read one or two medical books and largely treated himself with the herbal remedies which his wife made up or which Lady Honeywood, the wife of a local notable, advised; only very rarely did he write to physicians to send a medical opinion by letter. The question of the geographical availability of medical help and expertise cannot be answered using twentieth-century criteria such as the number of licensed physicians or nurses in a given population. Self- and family-medication and recourse to a variety of 'irregular' practitioners and healers was the norm in country areas and often in towns and cities.

Women were especially important in early modern medicine. They not only cared for their sick relatives, as is often the case today, but also treated both serious and minor illnesses. Women were also in charge of birth. Across sixteenth-century Europe the birth chamber was peopled by women. The 'gossips', who were usually relatives and neighbours and gave encouragement to the mother to be, and the midwife (a mother herself and trained by apprenticeship) dominated proceedings. Men were usually absent from the birth chamber, except for the relatively rare and dreaded occasion when a male surgeon was called in to use his instruments to break up and bring out a dead foetus from the womb. All the expertise was usually home-grown, learned from experience and from other women in a domestic setting. Midwives in Paris did begin to get some formal training at the Hôtel Dieu, the great hospital of Paris, from 1631, and in Amsterdam midwives had to attend lectures on anatomy and the theory of obstetrics after 1679. German cities such as Nuremberg (1417), Frankfurt (1456), Munich (1480), and Stuttgart (1489) had employed midwives and had their proficiency examined by physicians and their morals attested to by respectable, well-to-do women – the 'honourable' or 'sworn women'. (Morality was deemed important as a midwife might have to administer emergency baptism and was duty bound to report cases of infanticide and to question unmarried women in the middle of labour as to the identity of the father; in England when a midwife received a licence to practise from her local bishop (which was not absolutely necessary) it certified not only her skill but also her character.) City-employed midwives also appeared in early seventeenth-century Holland. However, it is difficult to see midwives under the authority of physicians, for most were in private practice and had decided for themselves when they were skilled enough to practise. They, therefore, constitute a relatively autonomous female craft which integrated well with the all-female occasion of the birth. It was in late seventeenth-century England that

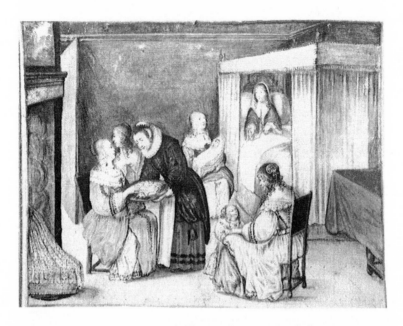

Fig. 31. A birthroom in seventeenth-century Holland; the maid giving sweetmeats to the gossips emphasises the social nature of the occasion. (Anonymous Dutch painting, The Wellcome Institute Library, London. L19348.)

the 'man-midwife' began to take over from women midwives, especially in difficult deliveries (p. 430); in much of the rest of Europe the man-midwife came much later on the scene.

As in previous centuries attempts at licensing and regulating medical practice were patchy and varied widely in effectiveness. The institutions set up in the Middle Ages (p. 164) continued to give a sense of communal identity to physicians, apothecaries, and surgeons, and they also often tried to police medical practice. City colleges of physicians and guilds of apothecaries and surgeons were common in France, Germany, Italy, the Netherlands, and England. Their attempts at regulation were supported by governments and city councils, but also at times frustrated by them. It was common for travelling mountebanks to set up a stage in a town, where they would attract a crowd by providing entertainment with clowns, beautiful dancing girls, conjuring tricks, music, and perhaps a monkey or two. In the process they would advertise and sell their cure-all remedies, sometimes swallowing poison and then taking their panacea to demonstrate its effectiveness. Despite the complaints of the learned physicians, the mountebanks, empirics, herbalists, and other unlearned practitioners continued largely untroubled from prosecution and were sometimes given recognition by the authorities. The health magistracy in Venice licensed the sale of empirics' remedies. In 1586 Cesare Corvini of Ancona demonstrated the effect of his remedies to the *provedditori* in the Health Office, and Scoto of Mantua, who travelled to London and performed conjuring tricks before Queen Elizabeth I, persuaded the Venetian health officials to note down the virtues of his famous therapeutic oil. The London College of Physicians, founded in 1518 by the Crown on the model of the Italian City College of Physicians, claimed to regulate the activities of the London apothecaries and the surgeons, and to have the right of licensing and regulating medical practice in London and seven miles around. But the government often protected those the College officials sought to prosecute. Queen Elizabeth and her ministers intervened regularly on behalf of favoured healers. In 1581 Sir Francis Walsingham, Secretrary of State to Elizabeth, wrote on behalf of Margaret Kennix:

> Whereas heretofore by her Majesties commandment upon the pityful complaint of Margaret Kennix I wrote unto Dr Symmondes [the former President of the College]... signifying how that it was her Highness pleasure that the poore wooman shoold be permitted by you quietly to practise and mynister to the curing of diseases and woundes, by the meanes of certain Simples [herbal remedies], in the applieing whereof it seemeth God hath given her an especial knowledge, to the benefit of the poorer sort, and cheefly for the better maintenance of her impotent husband, and charge of Family, who wholy depend of the exercise of her skill; forasmuch as now I am enformed, she is restrained either by you, or some other of your College, contrary to her Majesties pleasure, to practise any longer her said manner of ministring of Simples, as she hath done, whereby her undoing is like to ensure, unles she maie be permitted to continue the use of her knowledge in that behalfe. I shall therefore desire you forthwith to take order amongst your selves for the readmitting of her into the quiet exercise of her small Talent, least by the renewing of her complaint to her Majesty through your hard dealing towards her, you procure further inconvenience thereby to your selfe.

Royal courts in the German States and in France as well as in England often favoured and supported empirics and fashionable healers. The learned physicians, therefore, were not able to exert enough influence with governments to achieve effective regulation over medicine. In fact, the London College of Physicians had its powers to regulate and licence practitioners regularly challenged in the seventeenth century, and it was in disarray in the later parts of the century with the decline of Galenic medicine in the face of new chemical and mechanical approaches (pp. 317–25, 340–61). It lost further power when in the Rose case (1702–4) the House of Lords (sitting as England's supreme court) decided that apothecaries could in effect practise medicine, something that the physicians had always opposed.

In one area there was a new link between the State and medicine, which added to the recognition by governments of the status and value of learned physicians and surgeons. From the thirteenth century in Spain and Italy, surgeons especially were called to give evidence as expert witnesses as to the cause of suspicious or violent deaths. In cases of wounding they had to certify if the wound would have, or had, caused death. In Catholic countries where Roman Law (Civil Law) and Church Law (Canon Law) were applied, surgeons and physicians often testified on issues that lay on the boundary between medicine and the law. The Emperor Charles V (r. 1519–55) enacted in his legal code of 1533 (the *Constitutio Criminalis Carolina*, which he wished to apply to all the territories of the Empire), that in all cases of suspected murder surgeons had to be consulted. In 1536 France followed suit. By the mid-sixteenth century disputed points of medical evidence were being sent by the courts in the German states and in parts of Italy to university medical faculties to be resolved. In England it was not until the nineteenth century that the medical expert emerged, though surgeons did give evidence in murder trials from the mid-seventeenth century.

Forensic medicine slowly developed a literature of its own. Ambroise Paré (1510–90) in his *Traite des rapports* (*Treatise on Reports*) of 1575, dealt with how a surgeon should write reports on different types of wounds, infanticide, death by lightning, the signs of wounding or of hanging done upon a dead or living man, suffocation, and the proofs of virginity. Another forensic treatise, much larger in scope, was written by Paulus Zacchias (1584–1659), the personal physician to Popes Innocent X and Alexander VII and *Protomedicus* to the Papal State. His seven volume *Quaestiones Medico-Legales* (*Medico-Legal Questions*; 1621–35) dealt with topics where medical knowledge could inform Canon Law on such issues as the viability of the foetus, the causes of foetal death, types of madness, poisoning, impotence, malingering, torture, witchcraft, miracles, virginity, and types of wounds. However, despite the development of forensic medicine, it provided medicine with only a small additional degree of recognition and authority by the State.

Early modern Europe was not strongly 'medicalised'. Patients and other lay people as well as medical practitioners treated the most serious illnesses (if not surgical conditions). Everyone could give advice, the bedside was a public place where relatives, friends, and onlookers could criticise the practitioner and offer alternative treatments or advice on where to find a better practitioner (a state of affairs which the learned physicians bitterly deplored). There was also diversity and a lack of uniformity in patients' beliefs as to the cause of illness. God, witchcraft, the stars, as well as natural reasons, were all involved. Remedies could be equally varied: prayer, exorcism, magical words and objects as well as herbs, minerals and animal material, and procedures such as bleeding and purging. Patients often brought into play more than one explanation (for instance, both God and natural causes as the reason for their illness) and would feel free to use a variety of practitioners.

Also the boundaries between learned and popular medicine were porous and blurred. Learned physicians and surgeons borrowed and used popular remedies from wise-women and lay people, as they had in the Classical period and in the Middle Ages. At the same time learned medicine was popularised in a number of vernacular books written by physicians and laymen such as Sir Thomas Elyot (1499–1546), whose *Castell of Health* (1539) was one of the most popular and frequently reprinted guides to health and was based on his reading of Greek and Arab authors. Educated lay people, moreover, often understood the language of learned medicine as they shared a common educational basis with physicians. And physicians, if they wanted to keep their patients in what was a competitive market, would comply with the expectations of their clients as to treatments – many of which, like purging or the use of herbal remedies, were a normal part of lay or self-medication. This led to a more equal patient–doctor relationship than is usually the case today, for medical knowledge, terminology, and treatments were not so esoteric that they put the patient at a disadvantage.

No one group of medical practitioners developed a monopoly of practice, and the classical and medieval tradition of different kinds of medical practitioners continued into the sixteenth and seventeenth centuries. The lack of any general consensus on what was the best type of medical practitioner, and the lack of effective licensing (even in Spain, where the tribunal of the 'Protomedicato' examined and licensed practitioners on a nation-wide basis, licensing was not universal) ensured that lay people not only had choice but also a sense of independence when it came to deciding how they were to be treated. The patient had more power than today in the patient–doctor relationship.

There was a strong belief that medical expertise did not lie only among the learned. In the description of Florence's premier hospital, Sta Maria Nuova (pp. 151–2), sent around 1500 to Henry VII of England to help him in the planning of what became the Savoy hospital, the skills of the unlearned women treating women patients are fulsomely praised:

> The women include several skilled in surgery, for experience is mistress of all things. These have many remarkable cures to their credit and are even more trusted than the men.

Medical skill could also, as in Margaret Kennix's case (p. 236), be given by God. The English statute of 1542–43, which allowed unlearned practitioners to practise, in a limited way, supported charitable medicine learned of God:

> divers [several] honest persons, as well men as women, whom God hath embued with the knowledge of the nature, kind and operation of certain herbs, roots and waters, and the using and ministering of them to such as been pained with customable diseases... the said persons have not taken anything for their pains or cunning [skill] but have ministered to poor people only for neighbourhood and God's sake, and of pity and charity...

The sense of medical expertise among lay people was also part and parcel of the self-sufficiency that was the norm for many in the sixteenth and seventeenth centuries. Before the 'commercial revolution' of the eighteenth century when the selling of goods and services became widespread, most well-to-do households baked their own bread, brewed their own beer, made hams and sausages from the pig that they reared and slaughtered, and dried and distilled their own herbs to use as cordials and medicines. Making do with one's own resources was part of the household economy of the period and applied to medical care and treatment as to much else. Where medical expertise was on sale, especially expensive medical expertise provided by learned physicians, was in the cities and towns, where also other services and goods were sold and where clients were present in sufficient numbers and with enough money.

It is difficult to over-emphasise self-help or family help. But people also went to healers and they bought the remedies of travelling empirics and herbalists and the services of wise-women, midwives, apothecaries, surgeons, and perhaps physicians, just as they bought cloth and other goods from travelling peddlers. They had wide choice, and the only limitation was that of money.

Clergymen often treated illness in their neighbourhood. They might do so as an act of charity and in imitation of the example of Christ, the divine physician, who cured both the body and the soul. Often, especially in the countryside, they could be the only people with access to medical books and with the ability to read them. Protestant reformers in England during the Civil War period of the 1640s hoped to reorganise medical provision and to create a nationwide health service centred around clergymen who would act as physicians, their learning and sense of charity making them, in the eyes of the reformers, eminently qualified for such a role. In Lutheran Denmark in the early seventeenth century, ministers were encouraged to study some basic medicine.

However, specifically religious causes and cures for sickness had existed for centuries. Both Catholics and Protestants thought of illness as a God-sent punishment for sin or as a trial of one's faith (as in the case of Job). In the Catholic Church, prayers to the saints and the Virgin Mary, as well as to God, pilgrimages to miraculous shrines, the giving of votive offerings, the use of the sacraments, and the anointing of the sick with holy oil were all used as religious cures. In the Protestant churches prayers to the saints and the Virgin Mary were seen as superstitious, and the sick were urged to communicate by prayer directly with God without the mediation of the church. For Calvin (1509–64) the age of miracles was past and there was no real miracle in the sacraments; the communion wine did not actually turn to Christ's blood nor bread into his flesh. Likewise Calvin's interpretation of the passage in Mark 6. 12–13 where the apostles anointed the sick with oil and healed them was that the oil nowadays had no miraculous power.

Both Catholics and Protestants continued to seek from religion cures for illness. Christianity, after all, was a healing religion. Christ had healed the sick, the lame, and the blind, and he could cure body as well as soul. If Protestants no longer believed in miracles from oils or sacraments and rejected the services of priest or minister in their pleas for divine aid, they still, like Catholics, believed that God could directly, of his own power, effect cures. Indeed, the Calvinist sense of providence, that God decided on everything that happened to a person, served to make many Protestants feel that illness along with other misfortunes was sent by God in response to their actions. Meditation on one's sins would reveal why God had sent illness, and knowledge of what particular sin had caused God's punishment was the pre-condition for true repentance.

Governments supported the belief that illness could be caused by God. The ideology of states was often expressed in religious terms: wars were fought in the name of religion, the secular authorities provided their services to burn heretics, censorship was often religious, and church courts policed personal morals. The nations and city states of Europe were Christian, even though of different varieties after the Reformation. Communal diseases and disorders like plague and famine, as already discussed, led to the the ordering of communal religious responses, processions of holy relics through cities and towns in Catholic countries, days of prayer and humiliation in Protestant ones. The religious ethos of the period meant that naturalistic medicine could not have a monopoly on healing.

DEATH

In one area of life, medicine was excluded and religion dominated. Physicians were absent from a dying person's bedside. It was considered unethical to take money when cure was impossible. But even more important was the cultural nature of dying. It was a religious event; the transition from this short life to another life of eternal heaven or everlasting hell. How a person died was important, for it could determine whether they went to heaven or hell. From medieval times a genre of books, the *Ars Moriendi* (*Art of Dying*), had taught people how to die. A calm and rational demeanour was necessary while forgiving one's enemies and seeking forgiveness from others. For Catholics it was vitally important to make a last confession and to take the sacraments and so die without sin (a point of view derided by Protestants). The fear, often expressed, of dying suddenly without confession was thus the very real fear that unconfessed and unforgiven sins would lead to damnation in the afterlife (hence the practice of taking confessions before a battle). Protestants did agree with Catholics that the dying person should show a willingness to die, an eagerness to go to the next life. Although Protestants believed that one should live a good life every day, rather than on one's dying day, they believed with Catholics that the time of dying was one of special peril to Christians. This was when the Devil's temptations were at their greatest, and when the Devil and God fought for the soul of the dying. Hence the need to compose one's mind, to be rational, and to meditate earnestly and eagerly upon the world to come, so keeping the wiles of the Devil at bay.

In this scene doctors had no role to play. It is not until the later eighteenth century that doctors begin to 'manage' death by the use of opiates. In that more secular time the patient could be stupefied, as a rational mind was no longer needed to meet the trial of dying.

Descriptions of death-bed scenes come from the literate, and there is often a sense of idealisation about them. But that should not lead us to dismiss them as unrealistic, for the need to die well was such that English parishes paid 'watchers of the dying' to keep the dying-poor company through the night, and the hospital of Sta Maria Nuova in Florence made sure that 'when a patient is close to death, we place before him an image of Christ on the cross, and a nurse watches over him, never leaving him and reading him the Creed, the Lord's Passion and other holy texts'.

Religious explanations for plague, and for madness in the form of possession (madness is discussed in Chapter 7, pp. 425–9) and the religious emphasis on dying well gradually declined in intensity after *c.* 1660. The new age of reason, the Enlightenment, slowly replaced supernatural reasoning with one based upon an ordered nature, which God initially created but which, like an absent landlord, he had allowed to work according to his regular laws without any further direct interference. Some religious groups, especially the more radical Protestants, still believed in a God who continued to act directly on earth and therefore they still looked at illness as a punishment of God which he could remove at will. Catholics officially held to this view, but the combination of the reforms of the Council of Trent that led to the Counter-Reformation with the rationality of the Enlightenment meant that many took a more naturalistic approach to illness.

WITCHCRAFT, MAGIC AND MEDICINE

There was another way of explaining illness, one in which the patient did not have to blame him or herself for a bad life-style (as in Galenic medicine) or for having sinned (the religious view of illness). In the era of the witch craze, in which thousands of so-called 'witches' were burned in Europe, it was as natural to blame witches for illness as for other misfortunes. The patient did not need to reform either physically or morally, instead someone else could be blamed. Wise-women, white witches, were numerous in the countryside and they could be consulted to confirm a suspicion of bewitchment, to identify the witch and to take counter-measures. The law also could be used to try and punish witches (bystanders often looked to see if the symptoms of illness left the bewitched patient as the witch was being executed).

In continental Europe and in Scotland, witchcraft accusations in the sixteenth and seventeenth centuries were much more numerous than in England, where executions were only in their hundreds as opposed to over a thousand in Scotland and thousands in France and Germany. In England the accusation of witchcraft was generated from the village-level upwards, and reflected popular belief. Many of the continental and Scottish prosecutions were initiated by the State or the Church. Apart from formal accusations, it is difficult to know how often illness was thought to be caused by witchcraft. Many people, as Richard Napier, the early seventeenth-century minister turned healer discovered, suspected bewitchment but took it no further.

Similarly we know of the existence of white witches who might use magical charms or amulets or would recite parts of the Lord's Prayer as part of a magical healing ritual. In the Friuli in Italy, the *benandanti* who practised fertility rituals detected witchcraft and healed its effects, and also specialised in the cure of specific illnesses like the retention of urine. In Italy there were also 'signers' who marked the place where an illness seemed to lie (where there was pain or skin discoloration, etc.) with healing crosses. All across Europe white witches healed. Robert Burton in England wrote in 1621 ''Tis a common practice of some men to go first to a Witch, and then to a Physician; if one cannot, the other shall; if they cannot bend Heaven, they will try Hell'.

Both Catholic and Protestant preachers condemned white witches as being in reality black witches. Yet few were prosecuted as such, for in the popular mind although some might slide into the use of black magic and witchcraft, most were innocent of *maleficium*, of wishing ill – the defining characteristic of black witchcraft. Although we know that white witches were thick on the ground (one modern calculation is that in Essex, England, no village was more than 10 miles from a white witch), we know little about what they did except through the writings of the literate, who were nearly always hostile. Much of sixteenth- and seventeenth-century magical healing was part of oral culture and along with the rest of oral culture in general, it began to decline in the eighteenth century especially in urban areas. Magical healing also declined because of the Enlightenment's attack on 'superstition', which ironically also struck at magic's old enemy, religion.

It is difficult to know how the poor explained illness or what they thought about the medical provision that was available to them. Generally, they were illiterate and they remain silent to us. What we do know is what was done for the sick poor by the literate, their governors.

In the early sixteenth century a great change occurred in the perception of the poor by the well-to-do. In the Middle Ages the poor were seen in a positive light, as blessed by God and as objects for charity which would help the giver attain heaven. Although there were earlier prohibitions on strangers begging in a town, it was in the sixteenth century that beggars were generally seen as dangerous and in need of control and moral reformation, no longer viewed solely as representatives of Christ on earth. Economic necessity helped to shape new attitudes. The sixteenth century saw a rapid growth of population and, especially when famine struck, cities could not feed the crowds of starving peasants who came in from the countryside for food, let alone their own inhabitants. The old system of voluntary charity from individuals and from a variety of church and lay charitable organisations no longer appeared adequate. The answer for many contemporaries was to eliminate begging by the able-bodied and to provide for those too old or too sick to work.

Northern European towns (Mons, Ypres, Strassburg, Nuremberg, Bruges, and Lyons) from the 1510s and 1520s began to organise poor relief. They banned non-residents, often prohibited begging, and hoped to reform the manners of the able-bodied through the provision of public works (and thus also to avoid the expense of supporting them by making them self-financing). Tentative steps were taken to bring in all the monies from existing charitable institutions into an *Aumone-général* (a General Almony or Common Chest) out of which the poor could be supported. Luther's *Ordinance for a Common Chest* (1523) for the town of Leisnig in Saxony envisaged a compulsory rate levied on all parishioners as well as the appropriation of existing charitable funds. However, this is unusual and although later in the century, England and the Netherlands introduced poor rates, finance remained a problem for most poor-relief schemes.

The new initiatives in poor relief were published to the rest of Europe by the Spaniard Juan Luis Vives in his *De Subventione Pauperum* (*On the Relief of the Poor*; 1526) written to the councillors of the city of Bruges where he had settled (Bruges had already put its own scheme into practice). Vives saw vagabond beggars as sources of infection (they often presented a fearful sight when infected with syphilis) carrying plague and syphilis into a city. An English writer on poor relief, William Marshall, wrote in 1535 of the 'sundry and diverse diseases, contagions and infections' of the poor and of their 'heinous deeds, detestable sins, crimes and offenses'. The great fear of strangers bringing plague and other pestilences, as well as the fear of disorder and the economic burden of supporting a multitude of the poor helps to explain why wandering beggars were sent back to their places of birth on pain of savage penalties.

The new poor-relief schemes categorised the poor into undeserving rogues and vagabonds, wilfully refusing to work, and into the deserving, impotent poor, like the sick, young children, the very aged and widows. However, the institutional measures designed for the undeserving poor were at times applied to the deserving sick. They too were put sometimes into the large hospitals and work-houses which kept the dangerous poor off the streets, but which also provided medical care. Outdoor relief (in the street or in their houses), however, was also given to both types of poor, for there were never enough institutions to house all of them, and this would include provision for the care of the sick. Charity became increasingly organised and channelled by the civic or parish authorities, although voluntary charity was still seen as valuable. The result of the new poor law schemes was that the deserving sick poor also came under regulation and scrutiny, and became defined as marginal, special cases in relation to the rest of society.

This new approach appeared in Protestant and Catholic areas alike. Catholic cities like Venice initiated poor laws (the famine of 1528 was the spur for Venice). In Lyons a combination of Catholic humanist reformers and Protestants set up a Common Chest for the poor and imposed controls on begging. The Emperor, who was Catholic, also approved poor laws in the Netherlands and in Spain. The new attitude to the poor – more secular, more organised, and more negative about poverty – was not only the result of the famous Protestant sense of economic order and belief in the necessity of work so often referred to by historians. Both Catholic and Protestant governing classes felt the need to reform the management of the poor.

In England, the Reformation abolished all church institutions such as hospitals and hospices, and only St. Bartholomew's, St. Thomas', and Bethlem (or Bedlam, which took in mad people), all in London, survived from the medieval period. Even London did not, therefore, possess sufficient institutions to confine the incorrigible poor and the impotent and sick poor, as some reformers had envisaged. However, the regime at St. Bartholomew's was designed to deal with the new problems of the poor. Its beadles were ordered to search the streets of London for vagrants and to bring them to the hospital, whilst the sick who were also housed in the hospital were viewed as polluters of the city. The hospital claimed in 1552 to have cured 800 poor in the previous five years 'of the pox, fistulas, filthy blanes and sores... which might have....stunk in the eyes and noses of the city'. The financing of the hospitals relied largely on private charity with some contributions coming from the London parishes, but the latter were disinclined to continue their support, and an essentially parochial system of poor relief developed with the hospitals playing a minor role.

In 1601 the English Poor Law was established in its final shape. The poor were supported by the poor-rate levied on the houses in each parish, with additional charitable hand-outs in the form of money, fuel, or food funded by charitable bequests. To qualify they had to have been born in the parish and to be a child or aged or infirm or seriously ill. Above all, the parish gave long-term support to those who were of the respectable poor, perhaps fallen on hard times. In return for parish support, fit women pensioners of the parish might be required to act as 'searchers of the dead', or to help in the nursing and medical care of the sick pensioners of the parish. If need be, a parish supplemented this mutual support system with payments for the services of apothecaries or doctors. Many of the stages of life were taken care of. Abandoned pregnant women were supplied with a midwife and with gossips who were paid for by the parish. Babies were sent out to wet-nurses, their schooling, subsistence and clothes were paid for and when old enough they were apprenticed to a trade. If a pensioner of the parish was dying, a watcher might be appointed and paid to keep them company and a funeral would be paid for. In return the pensioner had to obey the parish authorities and carry out services required of them. If they were given money to pay for remedies or for the services of a medical practitioner, destitution was a necessary precondition.

Not all parishes could provide such a welfare service. The poorer

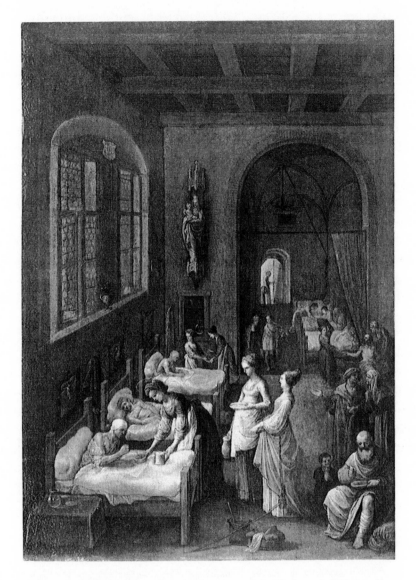

Fig. 32. St. Elizabeth visiting the sick. The statue of the Virgin and child as well as the pictures above the beds of the patients give a religious context to the hospital, and the slop bucket under the bed provides a practical one. Attributed to Adam Elsheimer *c*. 1598. (The Wellcome Institute Library, London. L12688.)

ones had few well-to-do households and many poor to support. In London especially, where parishes ranged from the rich to the very poor, the provision for the sick poor was very uneven. Other cities, like Norwich, contracted with lazar housekeepers (who no longer had any lepers) to house the sick, and with medical practitioners to cure them. The aim was to get those who could be cured back to work.

There was wide variation in the treatment of the sick poor. In rich Italian cities, like Florence, old systems of charity based on confraternities and on charitable hospitals often offered excellent care by the standards of the time. In Florence by 1500 some of the hospitals which had given hospitality to the healthy poor and to travellers (part of the medieval sense of a hospital) had become hospitals exclusively for the sick poor. The most famous, Sta Maria Nuova, founded in 1288 with 12 beds had expanded to 100 beds in the men's section and 70 beds in the women's part of the hospital by the beginning of the sixteenth century and provided lavish care by the standards of the time (p. 152). There is no doubt that some of the Italian hospitals were envied by the rest of Europe. Fynes Moryson (1566–1629), the English traveller, wrote of his stay in Florence in 1594, 'The Hospitall of Sta Maria Nova is said to passe all others in Italy, for all necessaries to cure and nourish the sicke, and for orderly attendance'. Luther had previously written of the hospitals in Rome in 1510–11, 'The best food and drinks are provided, the attendants are extremely diligent, the physicians learned, the beds and coverings very clean, and the bedspreads painted'.

However, incurables were often not admitted (many were sent to the hospitals for the *incurabili* or incurables established after the advent of syphilis). Conditions could be horrific, especially in times of plague. Cardinal Spada wrote of conditions in the pest houses of Bologna during the plague of 1630:

> Here you see people lament, others cry, others strip themselves to the skin, others die, others become black and deformed, others lose their minds. Here you are overwhelmed by intolerable smells. Here you cannot walk but among corpses. Here you feel naught but the constant horror of death. This is the faithful replica of hell since there is no order and only horror prevails.

Many hospitals continued to have traditional functions. For instance, the confraternity hospital of St. Spirito at Ferentino in central Italy gave hospitality to travellers and especially pilgrims going to Rome, and offered alms to priests and to the laity as well as feeding the sick and providing medical care. Many hospitals still took in abandoned children and women, the indigent poor. Rome in 1591 had 3666 people in hospitals out of a population of 116,695, Venice had around 4000 'perpetual poor' in hospitals and Florence in the mid-seventeenth century housed 2500 orphans and beggars (or four per cent of its population). Who the poor and who the sick poor were was unclear.

In France by the seventeenth century many of the civic secular schemes for the reform of the poor had failed. And from the 1620s a revitalised Catholicism took to reforming the charitable institutions of France. The Company of the Holy Sacrament composed of radical clergy and laity argued, from the 1630s until its suppression on the early 1660s, for the confinement of both the dissolute and of the deserving poor (the former would be reformed by punishment, the latter succoured and sheltered). The Company established the first institution for such confinement, the Hôpital-Général in Paris, in 1656–57. Over 100 hôpitaux-généraux were built by 1700. They were run on a mixture of religious discipline and forced labour. Their inmates numbered over a 100,000. Some were sick, and doctors visited the hôpitaux-généraux on a regular fortnightly or weekly basis. But the hôpitaux were not really medical institutions but rather workhouses and old-people's homes combining a brutal regime for those labelled work-shy with benevolence for the helpless, the aged, and the chronically sick.

The other charitable institutions, the large city and town hospitals, the hôtels-dieu, which had in medieval times provided hospitality, poor relief, and medical assistance gradually became more 'medicalised' by the end of the seventeenth century. Many employed surgeons and were visited daily by a doctor. Syphilitics and other infectious patients would be barred from entry into the hôtels-dieu by the surgeons, but otherwise the sick poor could use the hôtels-dieu for treatment.

Catholic reform also created nursing communities, usually female. Notable were the Daughters of Charity, founded by SS. Vincent de Paul and Louise de Marillac in Paris in 1633. The Daughters of Charity, often drawn from the poorer sections of society (in contrast to the wealthier cloistered nuns), supplied practical nursing skills and labour in French and foreign hospitals. Other confraternities of women provided medical care for the sick poor across the French countryside – just as Englishwomen provided informal charitable medical care for the poor in their area.

The care of the sick poor in sixteenth- and seventeenth-century Europe was not usually repressive, despite the reorganisation of charity in the early sixteenth century that brought about a change in the perception of the poor, which can still be seen in Western countries today. Although the sick poor enjoyed a more positive image than the incorrigible able-bodied poor, they were no longer part of the natural order established by God, but rather they were seen as victims of misfortune. Nevertheless, old attitudes to charity still persisted alongside new ones. And old institutions still continued at the same time as new ones were being created.

Learned medicine

Learned medicine, surgery, and medical botany based on the classical sources comprise the core of the Western literate medical tradition. In the sixteenth and seventeenth centuries it was renewed and then underwent change and challenge. The processes involved were intellectual as well as social.

THE RENAISSANCE

From the fourteenth century to the end of the sixteenth century there was a rebirth or renaissance of European social and cultural life. First in the rich commercial cities of northern Italy, then in Northern Europe, the arts and learning were, in the eyes of contemporaries, restored to the high levels achieved by the ancients.

Progress, it was believed, was achieved by emulating the ancients and by discarding the immediate medieval past. But outright innovation was also part of the renaissance. The feudal structure of society was in decline in Northern Europe by the sixteenth century (in the northern Italian cities it had never really taken hold) and new centralising forms of government were creating the nation states of France, Spain and England.

The geographical horizons of Europe expanded with the discovery of new routes around Africa to the Far East and of the New World of America. New inventions (in fact, they came from China) also changed the material world in which Europeans lived. Gunpowder, the compass and the printing-press all transformed the nature of wars, exploration and learning. The printing-press, invented in the mid-fifteenth century, meant that books became widely available and scholars did not have to travel large distances to consult a manuscript which might be the only copy of a particular work.

The Renaissance, although in reality it did not cut off all links with the Middle Ages, was thus a time of radical, often self-conscious, change.

THE REVIVAL OF GREEK MEDICINE

The early years of the sixteenth century witnessed the revival or rebirth of Galen and of Greek medicine, at least in the opinion of some contemporaries. But Galen had long been the great authority in medicine; the Arabs had translated his works and synthesised them. Western scholars in turn had translated the Arabic versions and a few had even gone to the original Greek texts. Their labours had formed the basis of the university medical curriculum in the Middle Ages, and this Greek-inspired medicine had been the subject of explanation, commentary, and disputation. On the face of it, to talk of a revival of Galenic medicine in the sixteenth century makes no sense, for long before this time it had formed the basis of learned medicine.

However, from around the mid-fifteenth century the love of all things Greek had grown apace and supplemented the earlier renaissance recreation of Roman literature and art that developed in the fourteenth century in the Italian city states. Greeks such as Theodore Gaza (*fl.* 1430–80) and his student Demetrius Chalcondylas (d. 1511) had come to Italy (even before the fall in 1453 of Constantinople, the repository of Greek culture) bringing with them from the city Greek manuscripts and the ability to read them. They quickly communicated their knowledge to Italian humanists (the students of classical literature who sought to re-establish and propagate the values of the classical world), some of whom came to believe that truth and knowledge were to be found in their purest form in Greek sources. Medicine was fertile ground for this later stage of the Renaissance, the hellenic (or Greek) Renaissance, for unlike much of classical literature, its major authorities were Greek rather than Latin.

There was a much wider dimension to this desire to go back to the original sources. In religion momentous changes were afoot in the first half of the sixteenth century. Luther and his fellow Protestants hoped to reform the Church by going back to the Bible as the sole fount of authority. Everything since the time of the New Testament, all institutional, Church-made, accretions such as Canon Law were to be rejected unless specifically authorised by the Bible. It was believed (also by reform-minded Catholics) that the study of Greek and of Greek (and Hebrew) manuscripts would lead to a better understanding of the Bible than using only the Vulgate Latin or medieval commentaries. The union of Reform and the Word was a powerful one, and what happened in religion found echoes in medicine.

Reference to the Reformation may help to explain a problem that faces the twentieth-century reader. For us, with our idea that progress always lies in the future, the often massive effort put into philological study, into the study of words, languages and texts, seems to have produced only a small return for medicine. But at that time words could be talismanic: if ancient enough, they might disclose eternal truths that had been lost in the intervening years. In the distant past lay progress, and philology was vital if the secrets of that past were to be reached. A necessary consequence was that the medical writings of the intervening years were disparaged.

A pressing concern to many humanists was the need for good new translations of the original Greek texts, since they felt that the Arabic and the medieval Latin translations were inaccurate and that the latter were often barbarously inelegant. Medical terminology it was felt was especially subject to corruption in translation. In 1492 Nicolaus Leoniceno (1428–1524) the long-lived doyen of Greek medical studies at Ferrara, focused attention on the issue in his *De Plinii ac Plurimum Aliorum in Medicina Erroribus* (*On the Errors of Pliny and of Many Others in Medicine*). He argued that Pliny the Elder in his Latin *Natural History* (which was important as a source of classical remedies) had erred when transmitting and translating Greek material, for instance, by confusing ivy and cistus (rock rose) because their Greek names (*Kissos* and *Kisthos*) were similar. Others, like Ermolao Barbaro (1454–93), came to Pliny's defence. Barbaro claimed in his *Castigationes Plinianae* (*Plinian Corrections*) (1492–93) that scribal error and not Pliny was to blame, and that a real Roman like Pliny who wrote correct Latin and was fluent in Greek could not have made the same type of errors in linguistic transmission of information as the barbarian scribes of the Middle Ages. The jurist Pandolfo Collenucio (1444–1504) also supported Pliny in his *Pliniana defensio* (*Plinian Defence*; 1493) by referring to his own and others' experience of plants.

 The controversy left some medical writers with the feeling that the Greeks were the supreme authority in medicine and that all intermediaries, including Romans, could and did err. In the years that followed, much work was done on terminology especially in medical botany; for instance in the 1530s there was debate on the true meaning and identity of *cinnamon* and in the 1550s of *akonitum* and *doronicum*. The precise meaning of texts was also a crucial issue in the blood-letting controversy initiated posthumously in 1525 by Pierre Brissot (d. 1522), who argued that the Greek texts of Hippocrates and Galen supported the view that blood-letting should be carried out on the same side as the source of illness rather than on the opposite side as Avicenna had stated.

In general, the polemical rhetoric of the medical humanists or hellenists was part of the wider renaissance condemnation of an entire epoch, the Middle Ages, the ages which separated them from the classical world. The picture they painted was one of darkness. In 1531 Johann Guinther von Andernach (1487–1574), a translator of Galen and teacher of the anatomist Andreas Vesalius (1514–1564), praised the times he lived in when 'medicine has been raised from the dead,' and Hippocrates and Galen who had been 'both almost utterly corrupt' are 'only now at last rescued from perpetual darkness and silent night'.

In 1525 the Aldine Press in Venice published the complete works of Galen in Greek. This marked a major step in the attempt to retrieve the pure and original medicine of the Greeks, the *prisca medicina* of the ancients. Yet for most medical men it had little direct relevance; for only a few could read Greek. What they used were the new Latin translations, which after 1525 tended to be based upon the Aldine Greek text rather than a variety of manuscript sources – a fact which some humanists deplored as too limiting because the possibility of finding good variant readings was lost. In anatomy, and in physiology especially, the new scholarship exerted a significant influence. Galen's physiological treatise *On the Natural Faculties* was published in 1523 in a new translation by Thomas Linacre and in 1531 Guinter von Andernach published his translation of the newly discovered, though still incomplete, text of Galen's *On Anatomical Procedures*, which produced a radical reappraisal of the order in which a dissection should be carried out. The printing press was the new and indispensable ally of those who wanted to propagate and promote the new Galen as widely and as accurately as possible (scribal error was now a thing of the past, to be replaced by printers' errors).

Between 1500 and 1600 there were published around 590 different editions of works of Galen. The main publishing centres were Paris, Lyons, Venice, and Basle in that order, with the most significant editing and translating being located first in Italy and then by the 1530s in Paris. There was also a corresponding retrieval of Hippocrates. The first humanist Latin edition of Hippocrates appeared in 1525, and the first Greek edition of Hippocrates, from the Aldine Press, was published in the next year. There were numerous Latin editions of his complete works, of individual treatises, as well as of commentaries on his treatises by Galen and by renaissance commentators. The work of Paul of Aegina was also published in an Aldine Greek edition (1528) which in turn resulted in a variety of Latin translations. In 1542 Janus Cornarius (1500–58) translated into Latin the works of Aëtius. Greek medicine had certainly been retrieved.

How did this enterprise affect medicine? It could certainly encourage a strong belief in the truth of ancient medicine. In Paris, Sylvius (1478–1555), the first of a long line of medical men who made the Paris faculty of medicine into a stronghold of Galenism, viewed Hippocrates and Galen with quasi-religious fervour, 'After Apollo and Aesculapius they were the greatest powers in medicine, most perfect in every respect, and they had never written anything in physiology or other parts of medicine that was not entirely true.' Sylvius was not alone in his veneration of Galen in the 1530s and 1540s. For instance Matteo Corti (1475–1544) and his friends established the informal *Nova Academia Galenica* (New Galenic Academy) in Florence in the 1530s, which was devoted to supplanting Avicenna and the Arabs in the practice of medicine.

Not everyone wanted to throw overboard the medical works of the Arabs and of the medieval writers, Avicenna was defended outright by Lorenz Fries (d. 1531) in his *Defensio Medicorum Principis Avicennae ad Germaniae Medicos* (*Defence of Avicenna, Prince of Physicians, to the Doctors of Germany*; 1530) who pointed out that much useful knowledge could be lost to medicine if one abandoned Avicenna. Avicenna's *Canon* and Rhazes continued to be taught in the Italian universities and in most of the other European universities. Also the tradition of medieval *practica* or *vade-mecums*, the handbooks which listed illnesses in a head-to-toe order with a description of diseases, symptoms, and a lengthier section on treatment continued to be printed despite humanist attempts to produce new teaching material on practical medicine (on which see below). The *practica* genre was too useful to be abandoned. For instance Marcus Gatinaria's (d. 1496) *Practica* was reprinted at least six times in the sixteenth century whilst the *Rosa Anglica Practicae Medicinae* (*The English Rose of the Practice of Medicine*) by John of Gaddesden (*c.* 1280 to *c.* 1349) was reprinted as late as 1595.

The humanist enterprise in medicine, although it led to the discovery of new texts, the production of new translations, and the sometimes uncritical worship of Galen, clearly did not obliterate the relevance of the immediate past to medical practice and education. But there was more to the enterprise. The huge effort expended upon the literary study of texts was not just to give medical writings a better, more classical, style. Nor was it confined to the business of elucidating the meaning of medical terms, useful though that was. In three areas, application of method or order in medicine, anatomy, and botany, the humanist enterprise exerted a significant influence. These topics reach beyond humanism and it will be useful to discuss them in their own right.

PRACTICAL MEDICINE AND THE GALENIC METHOD OF HEALING

The central core of medicine for most learned physicians was concerned with illnesses and their cure. The standard way that practical medicine was taught in the sixteenth century was by lecturing on the affections (the ill happenings) of the body in terms of signs, causes, and cures, usually in a head-to-toe order; in Padua, for instance, the professor of the practice of medicine lectured on Rhazes' ninth book *ad Almansorem* which followed such an order. The student or practitioner could also go and buy a *practica* to serve as a handy stand-by, in which he could look up what affections might occur in, say, the head (headache, vertigo, apoplexy, etc.), its associated symptoms, its causes, and its cures. Also included in the *practica* (as in the lectures of the practice of medicine) would be descriptions of the different types of fevers with their symptoms, causes, and cures.

The *practica* were very popular; they supplied what people wanted, a ready guide to diagnosis and a good list of cures. But they came close to failing the test that distinguished Galenic from empirical medicine, that is, that therapy must be rationally connected to, or justified by, reference to the cause of the disease. Either there was no discussion of causes or it was brief and cursory, and often no connection was made between the causes given and the cures listed.

The *practica*, however, totally failed to satisfy another demand of Galenic medicine. This was that therapy should consider not only the cause of the disease (the first 'indication of cure') but also the different characteristics of each patient: his or her constitution or temperament, strength, age, and the condition of the surrounding air. In other words, the *practica* did not take the individual into account – so, to the committed Galenic humanist they appeared to be empirical. Galen in his

Method of Healing, a work little known in the Middle Ages, had declared that there should be more than one curative indication, and that physicians had to consider not only the cause of the illness but all aspects of the patient and their environment. These injunctions gained renewed force from the new translation of the *Method of Healing* by Thomas Linacre, published in 1519 and often reprinted.

However, the *practica* survived largely unaltered not only because they were useful but also because, as Andrew Boorde (1490–1549), the English priest turned minister and medical writer, put it in his *Breviary of Health* (1547), 'Every man now a dayes is desirous to rede brefe and compediouse matters'. They appealed to a different renaissance fashion; the application of method to a variety of fields, including law and medicine which, in the sixteenth century was something of a craze and was given intellectual prominence in the logical tables of the French philosopher and geometer Peter Ramus (1515–72), although medical tables preceded Ramus' work. Discussions of method might involve complicated philosophical issues and their analysis, but often method simply meant brevity, compendiousness, reducing information to its bare bones.

METHOD IN MEDICINE

At a time when learned medicine was concerned with retrieving past knowledge rather than creating fundamentally new knowledge, it turned some of its intellectual energy to reducing Galenic medicine to method and hence to greater certainty. Complex medical information could be presented methodically in tabular or schematic form, either at the beginning of a book or in one of its major sections, or replacing ordinary text altogether. The tables summarised, in a methodical way, what was to come, moving from the general to the specific by the use of inclusive brackets as in a family tree, but horizontally left to right across the page, a process akin to that of the modern flow-chart. This was used to simplify and to schematise medical knowledge as in the example in Fig. 33. The same process of division was used to cope with a number of variables that generated a large number of possibilities or choices – which was what happened when Galen's method of healing was put into practice. A variety of indications (the cause of the illness, the state and characteristics of the patient, and of the air) had to be considered, and within Galenic medicine there were very large numbers of causes of disease and possible states of a patient. Method, it was hoped, would lead the physician to choose the correct indications.

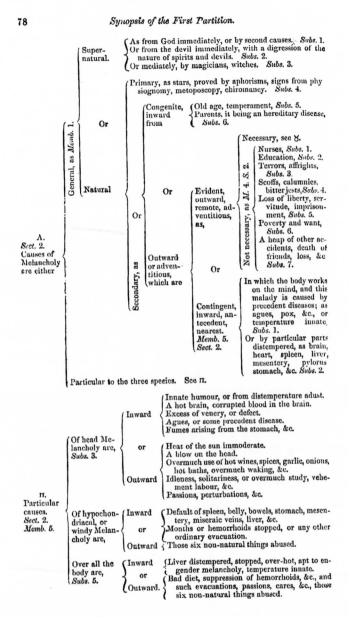

Fig. 33. An example of the methodical ordering of medical knowledge, moving from general categories on the left-hand side to more specific ones on the right. (From the 1881 edition of the *Anatomy of Melancholy*, London, Chatto and Windus, which follows the format of the first edition of 1621.)

The man most closely associated with the attempt to apply method to medicine was Giambatista da Monte (1498–1552), who became professor of the practice of medicine at Padua around 1540. From the start he was determined to reform teaching in the subject, not only to make medicine better, but to produce a more learned physician who worked according to the proper Galenic method, and so would be a cut above other practitioners. His students were clearly touched by his enthusiasm, for they continued to publish notes of his lectures after his death, some were later broken down to form the *Opuscula Varia* (*Various Little Works*; 1558) or reorganised into a huge compilation the *Medicina Universa* (*Universal Medicine*; 1587). Although nominally lecturing and commentating on Rhazes' ninth book *ad Almansorem*, he developed within the commentary format his 'universal method'. This involved moving by division from a general class of diseases to one of the specific diseases that comprised that group. What Da Monte held in his mind was the Galenic classification of diseases and signs, and with the hypothetical patient before him he would go through all the possibilities presented at each stage of the division until he arrived at a full account of the indications for cure. If the lecture was taking place within the hospital, the patient might well be in front of the class.

By beginning with universals, the most general categories of Galenic medicine, one ensured that its complete theory and practice were taken into account every time a patient was diagnosed and treated – because as the physician moved in his mind from general types of diseases and signs to the specific disease and its particular signs he would have gone through all the possibilities contained in Galenic medicine. This was a time-consuming process. Even more time consuming and far less clear was assessing the indications from the patient and deciding what weight to give to them and to the other indications, the cause of the disease, and the air. For this the physician would need to have at his finger tips every small detail of Galenic medicine and the ability to see how the indications related to them.

Da Monte is even more famous, however, for his clinical teaching. He took students to the bedside of patients in the Padua Hospital to show his method in practice. It is unlikely that this was the first time that bedside teaching had taken place at Padua, though daily clinical bedside teaching was formally required by the university only from 1578 onwards. It is significant that Da Monte went to the bedside, for the sort of knowledge he was trying to inculcate involved a habit of mind, a way of thinking about a patient which could be conveyed best by example at the bedside. It was more a form of knowledge which was 'tacit' and unwritten, gained by practice and apprenticeship rather than study. The paradox is that Da Monte believed that this almost intuitive process of taking minute particulars of the individual patient into account could be replicated by a mechanical method which would inevitably lead the student or the physician to the correct course of action.

Girolamo Capivaccio (d. 1589) and Alessandro Massaria (1510–98), who followed Da Monte as professors at Padua, discussed method at length. Both wrote *practica* which at times show the influences of Da Monte's teaching and especially his emphasis on the method of division from the general to the particular. As the quotation below from Massaria on the definition of vertigo indicates, this could be very tedious. It was no short cut, if carried out properly. Rather, as with present-day computers, all possibilities had to be considered in a step-by-step process:

> Now since vertigo is a thing contrary to nature, and the things contrary to nature are threefold, namely disease, cause of disease and symptom, the question is under which heading it is to be placed. First of all it is not a disease because it is not a dyscrasia, and not a lesion in the continuity of the body nor an abnormality in the composition of the body. Secondly, neither is it the cause of a disease since there is no disease produced by it and so it remains, as it should be, a symptom. Now since symptoms are of three kinds, injuries of the functions, change in the excrements, change in the qualities, and it is obvious that the excrement is not changed, nor the quality, therefore it will be an injury to the action. But once again since functions are threefold, the natural, the vital and the animal and since in the present case neither the vital nor the natural function are injured, it follows of necessity that it is an animal function which is injured. But since functions of this kind are threefold...

The Renaissance sometimes thought method a key to knowledge. But used in this way it was not a path to totally new knowledge. Both the universal and more specific categories were supplied already by Galenic medicine. Not only did Da Monte's method of division help to put Galen's *Method of Healing* into practice, but it was also a way of avoiding error and of creating a foolproof method of applying Galenic medicine to the individual patient. This was explicitly stated by Sanctorius Sanctorius (1561–1636), professor of the theory of medicine at Padua, who worked in a creative and innovatory fashion within the Galenic tradition. He wrote in his *Methodi Vitandorum Errorum* (*Methods for Avoiding All the Errors which Touch on the Art of Medicine*) of 1603 :

> I think that it is established that in the art of curative medicine infinite errors can be made, either in the recognition of disease, or of

cause, or in the contrivance of aids, or in prognosis or finally in the administration of remedies.

The method that Sanctorius favoured for achieving certainty in medicine was the running together or collection of signs or symptoms (*per syndromem signorum*), echoing Da Monte's method. Like Da Monte he stated that medicine did not begin with particulars, for no general conclusion could be derived from the particular patient *per se* or even from a number of them. Rather one had to begin with the most general forms and ideas which were then divided and divided again. These general ideas were Galenic and already pre-established, so what we have is a teaching device and not a method of discovery. It was a deeply conservative device appropriate for a learned medicine based on past knowledge. Its consequence was to preserve Galenic doctrine.

Seen in hindsight, the attempt by Da Monte and his followers to reform the teaching and practice of medicine by method was not very significant, but at the time it was perceived as exciting and progressive. But the truly methodical *practica* were too complicated, bulky, and time-wasting to use (Da Monte himself was notoriously long-winded in his lectures). Galen could be too perfectionist (though he himself did not always practice what he preached in the *Method of Healing*) for the majority of physicians, and it is significant that, except for the lectureships that Linacre endowed at Oxford and Cambridge, the *Method of Healing* was rarely included in university teaching and was not part of the formal curriculum in the Italian universities.

However, there is no doubt that at a more diffuse level Da Monte's methodical rebirth of Galen's method of healing as well as briefer 'methods of medicine' by others, helped to differentiate learned physicians from the crowd of competitors. They could advertise that they had a method, and that others did not.

INNOVATION IN GALENIC MEDICINE

Learned medicine was not totally conservative. Some of its practitioners were willing to go beyond Galen and put forward radical ideas about disease causation and the powers of remedies. In the orthodox account, disease was caused by an imbalance of the qualities and the humours; the inner temperament of the patient became unbalanced (there were eight main types of ill temperament: too hot, cold, dry or wet, or too hot and wet, hot and dry, cold and wet, cold and dry). An unbalanced temperament would be rectified by using a remedy with an opposing quality (too hot a temperament would be cured by a cold remedy of an equivalent degree to the heat). Both the nature of the illness and the power of the remedy could be felt by the touch of the physician, for he used touch to assess the degrees of heat, moisture, etc., involved. Knowledge of the different types of temperament of both the body and its individual parts and the ability to distinguish between them was a crucial part of the physician's learning and skill.

Some writers called attention to the fact that physicians were not certain in their judgement of a patient's temperament. Sanctorius believed that 'the medical art is conjectural in the calculation of the quantity of diseases, of the power of remedies, (and) in the understanding of their constitution,' and he tried to remedy the situation by devising the first thermometer and hydrometer. They measured degrees of heat and moisture respectively in an objective and more precise fashion. The thermometer, according to Sanctorius, would also allow the physician to judge if the patient was improving or getting worse, which might be impossible to do if the difference between the two states in the temperament of the patient was slight, 'for without the instrument physicians cannot perceive in any way [the differences in temperament] and so they are deluded in diagnosis, prognosis, and cure.' The instruments that Sanctorius invented, like his writings on method, were part of his campaign to make medicine more certain.

CAUSES OF DISEASE

As well as discussions about whether and how it was possible to have sure knowledge of temperaments, there were also debates as to whether temperament by itself could explain all types of disease. Diseases like syphilis and plague, which were new, devastating, and often appeared contagious, and for which cures did not easily come to hand, stimulated a search for causes other than the imbalance of temperament.

The source of the theory of disease as unbalanced temperament was the Aristotelian–Galenic synthesis of qualities, elements, and humours used in natural philosophy and medicine. But at this time there were other powers, other explanations available: God and Satan and their supernatural forces and followers might be seen as the cause of illness whilst God together with saints, icons, and prayers could also be appealed to for cures; then there were the influences of the stars, the powers of magicians and of witches, and in each person, the soul, immortal, life-giving, a powerful connection to the heavenly world, its presence serving as a constant reminder of the Christian repudiation of the materialism of the pagan philosophers.

Many of these powers and forces could not be felt by touch or any other sense, they were hidden to the senses, 'occult', and, by definition, therefore, they lay outside of Aristotelian–Galenic natural philosophy and medicine which was concerned with the sensory world. (According to Aristotle the four qualities of hot, cold, dry, and wet were the primary constituents of the world as they were perceived by touch, the primary sensory organ – but touch, of course, cannot sense the supernatural.)

Nevertheless, some were convinced that such powers could be the causes of diseases and of the efficacy of remedies. Occult, hidden, qualities, and sympathies might be at work. Similarly, the hidden qualities of the 'total substance' (*tota substantia*) of a disease agent or of a remedy could produce dramatic effects in the body. A poison or a remedy could act so quickly or powerfully to destroy or to heal that it was difficult to explain by its manifest qualities (of heat, moisture, etc.). There were similar phenomena in nature such as the power of the magnet and the electric discharge of the torpedo fish which appeared inexplicable using normal qualitative theory; and here also recourse was sometimes had to occult qualities or to the action of the whole substance.

Galen had referred to *tota substantia* in his *On the Powers of Simple Medicines* as an explanation for the actions of deadly poisons, amulets, purges, and many medicines which acted by attraction. But in the *Method of Healing* he stated that only those remedies which opposed a disease by their quality could be reduced to method; for those which acted by their total substance there was no method but they could be known by experience alone. Occult qualities and *tota substantia*, though referred to by Galen, had dangerous connotations for many sixteenth-century learned physicians, for, as the effects of occult qualities were known by sensory experience alone, they were associated with empiricism and empirics. And as their powers, although not their results, were unknown to the senses, they could be supernatural, originating in the stars or coming from God. In the Renaissance there was a close association between experience, the occult, the supernatural, and the unorthodox.

Jean Fernel (1497?–1558), one of the outstanding figures of the Paris medical faculty, believed that there were some things 'beyond the power of the elements.' He modified and developed Galenic medicine and physiology (a word he helped to popularise) in a creative way. For instance, he wrote that the spirits which governed many functions of the body (the nutritive, vital, and animal spirits) did not originate out of the humours as Galenic doctrine held, but came from the celestial regions. This was also the case, he believed, with some diseases and remedies whose occult qualities and powers from their total substance came from the heavens. The whole tenor of Fernel's medical philosophy was to emphasise that the body and its functions were enlivened and given particular characteristics by celestial heat and celestial spirits, some of which could be hostile and so produce disease. If in the process he downgraded the importance of temperament, he still remained a Galenist in his own eyes, if not always in those of his colleagues.

Evidence from plague (and 'new diseases' like syphilis) did force Galenic disease theory to become flexible. Johannes Argenterius (1512–72), who taught medicine at Pisa, was a sceptical Galenist who used the idea of a disease of the total substance to explain plague and syphilis. More significantly, the person to person contagiousness of plague seemed to be confirmed by bitter and widespread experience, but contagion did not form part of Galenic medicine. As is discussed above (pp. 196–8) the authorities responded to plague using a mixture of contagion and miasmatic theory. But the two were not totally at odds with each other. Da Monte, for instance, believed the putrid vapours of miasma could be communicated by people or goods and, then as putrefaction was a manifest quality, they would affect the temperament of the body that they had entered. So miasma could come close to contagion but still be a disease of the temperament. Similarly, Da Monte believed that syphilis was communicated by intercourse with an infected person from whom emanated a certain poison 'in which exists that evil and poisonous quality [putrefaction].'

Even ideas like those of Girolamo Fracastoro (c. 1478–1553) could become unremarkable in a short time. Fracastoro wrote a famous poem on syphilis (*Syphilis sive Morbus Gallicus* (*Syphilis or the French Disease*; 1530)) and a treatise on contagion (which has survived in several drafts) in which he argued that 'seeds of disease' capable of producing putrefaction were responsible for syphilis and other diseases, and, given a receptive medium, they gave birth to putrefaction. This, in fact, is very similar to what Da Monte thought, except that he argued that putrefaction acted directly through its own quality and required no seed to begin the process. Physicians, faced with strange and devastating mortality from diseases like syphilis and plague which appeared 'beyond the power of the elements', responded with flexibility in their thinking.

In the sixteenth century the theory and practice of Galenic medicine was consolidated by the linguistic endeavours of the medical humanists and by the attempt to reduce medicine into a methodical form. A few Galenic medical writers did become dissatisfied with the standard Galenic qualitative explanation of disease and advanced new causes of disease, but in its essentials Galenic medicine remained unchanged. Where change occurred was in anatomy, which at the beginning of the sixteenth century was a relatively unimportant part of medicine.

Anatomy

In the sixteenth century, anatomy underwent the same humanist renewal as the rest of medicine. Anatomy also seems progressive in a modern sense, going beyond the classical authorities and discovering new knowledge about the body. This impression is not confined to those nineteenth- and twentieth-century historians who were interested in tracing the accumulation of 'positive' knowledge (true factual knowledge) that led ever onward and upward to that of the present, and who saw renaissance anatomy as providing just such knowledge. Anatomists in the sixteenth century also believed that their subject was the most exciting and progressive part of medicine.

The following account of renaissance anatomy is in two parts. Firstly, a discussion of some of the formative factors that led to the growth of the subject together with an outline sketch of the work of the anatomists. Secondly, an analysis of how anatomy rose in status, how anatomists justified their subject, and what role they saw for it.

ARTISTS AND ANATOMY

The renaissance of anatomy owed much to artists. From the fifteenth century they begun to be interested in anatomical knowledge and brought with them a new representational, naturalistic, approach which shows itself in the illustrations of sixteenth-century anatomy texts. Leon Battista Alberti argued in his treatise *De Statua* (*On the Statue*; *c.* 1435) that a knowledge of the parts of the body was necessary for the sculptor just as a shipbuilder needed to know how the parts of a ship fit together. Behind Alberti's interest in the structure of the human body lay his belief that it could provide the artist with an insight into the nature of human proportion – an early intimation that to be representational was not unproblematic, for the cadaver on the dissecting table might well differ from an ideal representation of the body and its parts.

Lorenzo Ghiberti (d. 1455) in his *I Commentarii* (*Commentaries*; *c.* 1447–48) advised that the sculptor like the painter should be learned in 'these liberal arts' which included not only the traditional grammar, geometry, arithmetic, and astrology but also perspective, the theory of drawing and anatomy. Like Alberti he emphasised that knowledge of the bones of the body gives the artist an insight into how the body is formed and so allows him to create, or rather to imitate it, in a truly representational way. In order to aid the sculptor he gave a list of the bones, probably taken from Avicenna and Averroes.

By the end of the fifteenth century both art theory and artists' practice emphasised the importance of anatomical knowledge and experience of dissection. Underlying this view was a wish by artists to be more naturalistic, to imitate nature more closely, though with an eye to capturing idealised beauty as well. Their model for greater naturalism came from the ancient world, especially from the Roman statues that lay on or under the Italian countryside (as also in architecture where the remains of Roman buildings acted as examples of how to move away from medieval 'gothic'). In a sense, renaissance artists combined observation of nature with a reversion to classical styles and models that had similarities with the humanism of literary and medical writers, for artists felt that the ancients had observed and imitated nature best.

Artists began to learn the anatomy of the body as a matter of course. Andrea Verrocchio (1435–88; Leonardo da Vinci's teacher), Andrea Mantegna (d.1506) and Luca Signorelli (*c.* 1444–1524) all showed knowledge of the surface anatomy of muscles and perhaps of deeper anatomy (Verrocchio insisted his pupils study flayed bodies). However, it was Leonardo da Vinci (1452–1519), Raphael (1483–1521), Albrecht Dürer (1471–1528) and Michelangelo (1475–1564) who related most clearly to their art the knowledge they gained from anatomy.

The interest of artists in anatomical dissection put the subject into the public arena (literally so in some cases) and helped it gain popularity. The artists also influenced the content of anatomical texts. From the 1520s anatomical drawings became increasingly important in anatomy texts. Artists and anatomists alike aimed to give more representational and naturalistic descriptions of the body in pictures and words (though whether the observer's eye or classical authority provided this best was initially a matter for dispute). The end result was that the schematic illustrations of the Middle Ages were being supplemented if not entirely replaced by a new vision of the body.

Leonardo represents at the very highest level the involvement of artists with anatomy, even if he had little or no long-term influence on other artists or anatomists, since after 1570 his anatomical notebooks were locked and hidden from public view. That Leonardo dissected was known at the time, and significantly Giorgio Vasari in his *Lives of the Most Eminent Painters, Sculptors and Architects* (1550 and 1568) gives an academic context to Leonardo's activity: 'He then applied himself...to the anatomy of man assisted by and in turn assisting, in this research, Messer Marc Antonio della Torre, an excellent philosopher [he was to teach medicine at Padua], who was then lecturing at Pavia'. (della Torre and Leonardo planned an illustrated Galenic anatomy book.)

Leonardo's anatomical notebooks date from 1489 to around 1514. They show Leonardo comparing anatomy with architecture, and using anatomy to investigate the secrets of the microcosm (the little world of man) which he believed was created by God using the same harmonies of proportion as in the macrocosm (the universe). Leonardo put into his drawings what he had learnt by reading anatomy texts and what he saw from the body before him (the latter increasingly so over time). He drew imaginary structures which Galenic and medieval texts told him were there. For instance, he localised mental faculties such as imagination in the ventricles of the brain in much the same way as had medieval (and contemporary) anatomists. However, in overall conception his drawings were naturalistic rather than schematic, and he was also interested in how the anatomy of the dead body related to the living body – his figures, although usually taken from cadavers in the hospital of Sta Maria Nuova in Florence, are as if alive (a characteristic of the best anatomical illustrations such as those in the *De Humani Corporis Fabrica* (*On the Fabric of the Human Body*; 1543) of Andreas Vesalius (p. 277). He drew extremely detailed and naturalistic studies of very specialised parts of the body such as the hand, foot, shoulder and arms, larger parts like the head, and views of the internal organs in which the individuality of each part is emphasised. These illustrations show that the medieval representation of the body, idealised and simplified perhaps for mnemonic reasons, has been mainly left behind.

From 1489 Leonardo planned an anatomical atlas of the various stages of man from the foetus to the grave – it was to have dealt with

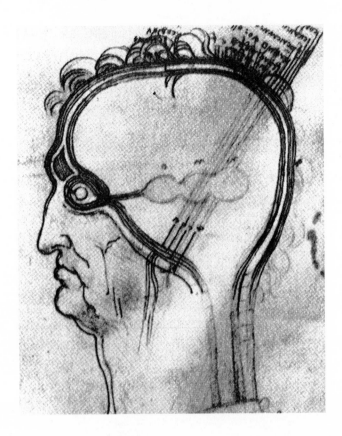

Fig. 34. Leonardo da Vinci's localisation of mental faculties in the ventricles of the brain following medieval examples. (Quaderni v, 6r, The Royal Library Leonardo Sketchbook, Windsor Castle.)

psychology (as seen in facial expressions) and physiology (around 1506 he read Galen's *On the Use of the Parts*) as well as anatomy, but it was never developed beyond some preliminary sketches. However, Leonardo's intense interest in drawing what he observed while dissecting, anticipates the new empirical approach to anatomy when realistic anatomical illustrations became a major part of sixteenth-century textbooks. Leonardo wrote that pictures could say more than words. (And such pictures, if traced on wooden blocks, could be accurately reproduced in their thousands by the newly invented printing press and so would not become corrupted through the errors of scribes in copying from one manuscript to another.) To conclude, both artists and anatomists wished as did Michelangelo, who collaborated for around

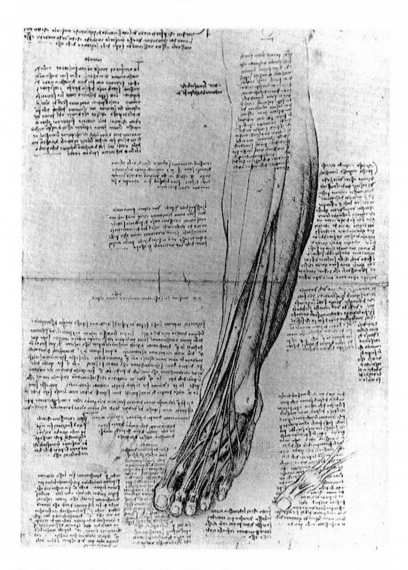

Fig. 35. Leonardo da Vinci's study of the surface anatomy of the foot and leg of 1510, based on dissection experience. (Windsor, Royal Library; 19017v.)

12 years from 1547 with the anatomist Realdo Colombo (d. 1559), to learn from 'nature herself', and it appears that this wish became commonplace first among the artists.

EARLY SIXTEENTH-CENTURY ANATOMY

Among the early sixteenth-century anatomists the wish to see for oneself arose from a variety of traditions. Berengario da Carpi (*c.* 1460 to *c.* 1530), who lectured on surgery and anatomy at Bologna, kept formally within the traditional bounds of academic medicine when he published in 1521 his *Commentary on the Anatomy of Mondino*. But the *Commentary* is many times longer than Mondino's text and one point that Berengario kept repeating in it, and in his short *Introduction to Anatomy* (1522), was his belief in *anatomia sensibilis* (the anatomy of observable things). Although ideally reason, observation, and the authority of Galen would be united together as his guides, in Berengario's view authority could not hold true in anatomy if it was against sense, nor did anatomy deal with insensible structures that might have been posited by reason. Early on, therefore, the sixteenth-century anatomists' credo that observation was the touchstone of truth was set out by Berengario. He also emphasised the visual by using a few woodcuts to illustrate his *Commentary* and *Introduction*, though the amount of detail in them is small (he also illustrated his surgical treatise on fractures of the skull, *De Fractura Calvae* of 1518).

Berengario's *Commentary* was not a typical product of the schools. Although he used Arabic sources like Avicenna and referred to medieval writers such as Guy de Chauliac, he discriminated in his choice of authorities and he castigated the practice of the 'aggregators' who piled authority upon authority. Here he had in mind works such as the *Liber Anathomie Corporis Humani* (*The Book of the Anatomy of the Human Body*; 1502) of the ill-fated Gabriele Zerbi (1444–1505) (who was sawn in half between two planks in Bosnia by the Turks), one of the last of the scholastic anatomies, which shared the humanist wish for good Latin terms together with a concern to list all the authorities on a particular topic. Berengario had a clear vision of anatomy being based upon a methodology that gave a high place to observation, and he realised that the pedagogically orientated public anatomies were not the occasions to undertake difficult investigations; instead he carried out private dissections when need arose. His major anatomical finding was to deny the existence of the *rete mirabile* or 'marvellous network' of blood vessels supposedly lying at the back of the neck (it is found in some animals but not in man) in which animal spirits were supposedly elaborated from arterial blood to convey sensation and motion in the brain and nerves.

The earliest 'hellenic' anatomy was that of Alessandro Benedetti (d. 1512). Benedetti, whose work was disliked by both Berengario and Zerbi, had lived for 16 years in Greece and Crete, and he corresponded with humanists like Giorgio Valla (whose list of Greek anatomical terms appeared posthumously in 1501). In 1490 Benedetti returned to Padua at the invitation of the Venetian Senate to take up the post of professor of practical anatomy. His little book on anatomy, the *Historia Corporis Humani; sive Anatomice* (*The Account of the Human Body: Or Anatomy*), was published in 1502 (earlier editions are possible but none has survived). The Greek word *Anatomice* in the title served notice of Benedetti's hellenicism. In the dedicatory letter to the Emperor Maximilian I, Benedetti condemned the moderns who had disgraced the Latin language with foreign, barbarous words, and he complained that things had come to such a sorry pass that the Arabs rather than the Greeks were being associated with medicine.

As a good hellenic humanist Benedetti, like Leoniceno, purified his text of Arabic terminology such as *siphac* (the anterior layer of the peritoneum) and *zirbus* (the great omentum) which had been used in the West from the twelfth century. Instead, like Valla, he self-consciously tried to use Greek words for his anatomical terms. Benedetti's book fits the pattern of the hellenic humanist revival in medicine described earlier – a return to the Greeks and a condemnation of the Arabs in order to clarify medical terminology. Its aim was philological rather than substantive. But it is worth noting his description of how to set up a temporary anatomy theatre. Anatomy was a spectacle with an audience and stage, the general public might not always be allowed in (Benedetti wrote that guards should be appointed to keep the public out), but as the century went on the university anatomies became more and more theatrical and members of the public increased in numbers. This open face of dissection reminds us that, as one would expect in a society where the private usually gave way to the public, anatomy was not something carried out in secret. It was sanctioned by the ecclesiastical and civilian authorities – and the highest in society allowed anatomy books to be dedicated to them. The subjects for dissection also came from the public domain – executed criminals killed in public – Benedetti recommended what type of hanged person to choose: neither thin nor fat, but tall so that the spectators had more material to look at.

The humanist revival of anatomy properly took off with the discovery of the first part of Galen's *On Anatomical Procedures*, which was translated into Latin by Guinther von Andernach in 1531 (although an earlier version by Demetrios Chalcondyles had been published in an edited volume by Berengario in 1529, it had far less impact than Guinther's). This was Galen's treatise on how to carry out a dissection, and it forced anatomists to re-order the stages in which they conducted a dissection. Mondino and the anatomists who followed him had begun with the internal organs in the body cavities because they were the parts of the body that putrefied first. Galen began in a more logical, if less practical, fashion with the bones of the skeleton for, he wrote, they were like the walls of houses, everything else in the body took shape from them. Galen then proceeded to the dissection of the muscles, nerves, veins, and arteries of the arms and legs, and the muscles of the hand. He then finally came to the internal organs of the cavities of the stomach and belly, the chest (the lungs and heart), and the brain. Not only was Galen's order of dissection more rational, but the quality of his descriptions was more detailed, clear, and sophisticated than that of the medieval anatomists. The humanist programme of going back to the pristine sources of medicine seemed to have paid off.

However, Galen's anatomy was animal rather than human. He made it clear that as human cadavers were not readily available, he had to use apes and other animals, though he advised that human material should be used whenever possible. And he had also enjoined his reader to look at the body for himself. The ground was prepared for anatomists to go beyond Galen in their investigation of the human body. The stress on personal and independent observation was reinforced in the *Liber Introductorius Anatomiae* (*Introductory Book of Anatomy*; 1536) of the Venetian physician Niccolo Massa (*c.* 1485–1569). Like Berengario, Massa stressed that anatomy depended on observation, on what was actually perceived (*anatomia sensata*), and he castigated those who wrote on anatomy without having seen or touched the things that they wrote about. However, he did not record any new anatomical findings. He did declare that the septum of the heart is in most cases solid and so by implication denied the existence of pores in the interventricular septum, but Massa still asserted the Galenic view that blood went across the septum from the right to the left ventricle of the heart. And, despite having read Galen's *On Anatomical Procedures*, Massa made it clear that he was going to follow the method of Mondino, 'a man most renowned for dissection', and begin with the stomach and belly. The Galenic programme in anatomy still had not been put into effect.

By the early 1540s an increasing number of anatomical texts were being published which produced significant developments in the subject. Johannes Dryander (1500–60), professor of medicine and mathematics at Marburg, carried out some of the first public anatomies in

Germany in 1534, 1536, and 1539 (others were being performed around the same time in Wittenberg, Leipzig, and in Vienna; in the latter they had been done for a century). He wrote up his earliest dissections in the *Anatomia Capitis Humani* (*The Anatomy of the Human Head*) published in 1536. His illustrations were detailed and showed the successive stages of the dissection of the head. This inserted a sense of systematic, if idealised, order into the relationship between the illustrations and the stages of the dissection as it was actually carried out – Vesalius was also to use such a series of illustrations. In the next year Dryander published the first part of his *Anatomia Hoc Est Corporis Humani Dissectio* (*Anatomy. That is the Dissection of the Human Body*), a misleading title for what was essentially the same as his anatomy of the head, but with additional woodcuts and textual material from Celsus and other authors.

Texts on particular parts or systems of the body were to be published throughout the century as well as anatomies of the whole body. A distinguished early example was Giovanni Battista Canano's (1515–79) study of the muscles of the arms in his *Musculorum Corporis Humani Picturata Dissectio* (*The Illustrated Dissection of the Muscles of the Human Body*; 1541). Canano's small treatise was the first to use copper engraved illustrations. In the treatise each individual muscle was depicted by the Ferrarese painter Girolamo da Carpi (1501–55/69) and related to the bones. Canano had studied the anatomy of muscles in his house at Ferrara (Italy) with his relative Antonio Maria Canano, while the brother of Andreas Vesalius, Francis, had looked in on the investigations. Here the importance of private dissections for anatomical research is apparent. In 1541 Canano was appointed professor of medicine at Ferrara, where he had studied, but he did not publish any further studies of muscles (six other books on muscles were projected).

By 1541 no one had carried out the full Galenic programme in anatomy. Galen himself had written that anatomy could be improved by observation so that a true Galenic anatomy could be critical and progressive. Galen's anatomical works were aimed at producing a single true description of the anatomy of the human body (allowing for the differences between the sexes). If one followed Galen's advice, his description should be checked by reference to the evidence of the dissected body laid out before the eyes of the anatomist and his spectators. In a sense, Galen's method of anatomy always had the potential to subvert his teaching on specific anatomical details. Furthermore, by giving observation a privileged epistemological status as a form of knowledge in its own right (discussed below), the anatomists made it difficult to preserve Galen's anatomical observations in the face of contrary evidence presented to their eyes (if other pairs of trustworthy eyes also witnessed the same contrary evidence, then the case against Galen was that much stronger – hence the anatomists' predilection for legitimating their discoveries in front of an audience who could act as virtuous witnesses).

Andreas Vesalius (1514–64)

In the event, Andreas Vesalius helped to restore Galenic anatomy, but only to correct it and go beyond it. Despite rearguard actions by some Galenists, anatomy after Vesalius moved beyond Galen's teaching in matters of observational descriptive anatomy.

Vesalius could be said to have been a true Galenic anatomist in the wider sense of following Galen's advice to see for himself (and he certainly kept to many of Galen's physiological theories and to their teleological conclusions), but Vesalius presented himself as a critic of Galen's and trumpeted aloud Galen's errors. He made an immense impact upon the discipline of anatomy. His fame was ensured by the publication of his massive *De Humani Corporis Fabrica* (*On the Fabric of the Human Body*; 1543) which, as well as being enormously detailed, was brilliantly and profusely illustrated. The rise of the Paduan school of anatomy that dominated the subject in the sixteenth century mainly stems from the time of Vesalius.

LIFE OF VESALIUS

He was initially trained in humanist medicine. Born in Brussels, he was the son of a pharmacist to the Emperor Charles V. After going in 1530 to study for the degree of master of arts at Louvain, where he learned Latin and Greek, he enrolled in 1533 in the Paris faculty of medicine. At this time Paris was at the forefront of medical studies and was enthusiastically promoting the humanist endeavour of reintroducing Galen's works into medicine. Vesalius was taught by Guinther von Andernach who, in his anatomical manual the *Institutiones Anatomicae* (*The Institutes of Anatomy*; 1536), praised Vesalius, his assistant, equally with Sylvius the die-hard Galenist. It was in Paris that Vesalius gained his skill in dissection, although in later years he castigated the uncritical teaching of the subject there which he believed led to the blind acceptance of Galenic texts. When in 1536 war between the Emperor and France forced Vesalius to leave Paris, he returned to Louvain where he helped to introduce dissection into the curriculum; in the same year he showed his enthusiasm for the subject by robbing a wayside gibbet of its victim, smuggling the bones back home and there reconstructing the skeleton (he had also robbed cemeteries in Paris).

In 1537 Vesalius left Louvain when he was invited to teach at Padua, one of the most lively and distinguished universities of sixteenth-century Europe, where he confirmed his reputation in anatomy. In the same year he received his doctorate in medicine from Padua and was immediately appointed lecturer in surgery and anatomy. Previously in Padua, anatomy had been demonstrated and carried out by surgeons and lectured on by one of the professors of the theory or of the practice of medicine. It had not been seen as essential for physicians. However, the rediscovery of Galen's *On Anatomical Procedures* and the better dissemination of his *On the Use of Parts* meant that humanist physicians took an interest in the subject, and the appointment of the young humanist physician Vesalius was one result. The holder of the Paduan lectureship in surgery and anatomy was now a scholarly physician (and enthusiastic anatomist) rather than a more lowly surgeon and this led to an increase in the status of the subject at Padua.

As a teacher Vesalius was popular (in 1539 the university added 30 florins to his annual salary of 40 florins because of the 'admiration' of his students), and he produced for them six anatomical charts of the body. The *Tabulae Anatomicae Sex* (*Six Anatomical Pictures*; 1538) were among the first anatomical illustrations specifically designed for students and were widely plagiarised. Single printed pages of anatomical figures of the whole body, 'fugitive sheets', began to appear just before the *Tabulae Sex* (the earliest known sheets are from 1536). The first three sheets in the *Tabulae Sex* were drawn by Vesalius and represented the liver and its blood vessels together with the male and female reproductive organs, the venous system centred on the vena cava and the arterial system. The other three drawings were by John Stephen of Kalkar (d. 1546), a pupil of Titian's, and depicted different aspects of the skeleton, posed as if alive. In his illustrations Vesalius was still seeing the body through Galenic eyes, he drew the *rete mirabile*, the liver was five-lobed in the medieval manner, and the heart was that of the ape.

Around 1539 Vesalius became more critical of Galenic anatomy. His increasing knowledge of human anatomy and of Galen's anatomical writings led him to his crucial realisation that Galen had dissected only animals and that animal anatomy could not substitute for human anatomy. Two trips to Bologna, in 1538 and 1540, gave him greater experience of dissection. On the second visit, when he gave anatomical demonstrations to accompany the lectures of the Galenist Matteo Corti (1475–1544) on the text of Mondino, Vesalius explicitly contradicted Galen and Corti on matters of anatomical detail. He asserted that anatomy could not be learned by reading Galen but only by the direct observation of the human body. In the *Fabrica* he wrote that the Bologna demonstrations prefigured the plan and approach of that work. In Padua, Vesalius' critical outlook increased when he took to performing the dissections regularly himself and also giving the lectures, and when in 1539 he was given a much larger number of cadavers of executed criminals by Marcantonio Contarini, a Paduan judge.

In the two years after his trip to Bologna, Vesalius worked on his great masterpiece, the *De Humani Corporis Fabrica*. He finished it in 1542 and took it across the Alps to Basle where the press of Joannes Oporinus published it in 1543 as one of the jewels of renaissance printing.

THE *FABRICA*

The book marks a turning point in the medical view of the structure of the body. Vesalius consistently tested the anatomical teaching of Galen by reference to the human body. Others had criticised isolated pieces of Galenic anatomical doctrine but Vesalius was the first to do this systematically, frequently using animal evidence to demonstrate how Galen had been mistaken. (The essential point about the *Fabrica* is its emphasis that it is the first proper account of *human* anatomy.) Additionally, the *Fabrica* gained immensely by the contribution of the artist (most probably John Stephen of Kalkar) who provided the text with a series of naturalistic yet technically precise drawings which showed the dissected body in life-like poses.

As well as correcting Galen, the *Fabrica* introduced novel methodological principles. It was the first in the long line of texts by the Paduan lecturers in anatomy to assert that anatomy was the basis of medicine. The *Fabrica* also emphasised that the anatomist-lecturer must perform the dissection himself (its frontispiece shows Vesalius dissecting) and that, in matters of structure, eyesight was preferable to the teachings of past

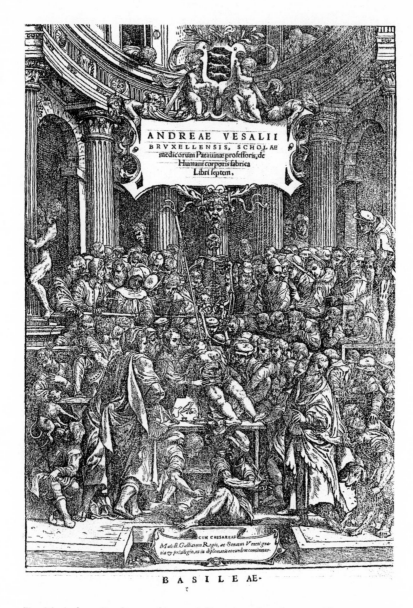

Fig. 36. Andreas Vesalius teaching and dissecting: the title page of his *De Humani Corporis Fabrica* (Basle, 1543). (The Wellcome Institute Library, London. M8925.)

authority and, indeed, served as a check upon them. Although Vesalius' empiricism was confined to bodily structures, rather than to function and use, for he was correcting Galen's descriptive anatomy and on the whole he kept to Galen's physiology, the *Fabrica* came to symbolise the

276

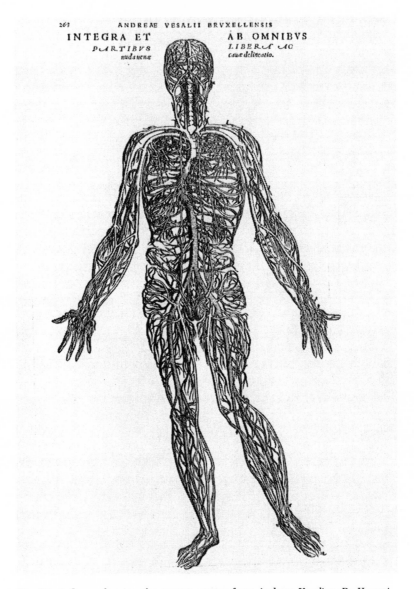

Fig. 37. A figure showing the venous system from Andreas Vesalius, *De Humani Corporis Fabrica* (Basle, 1543), p. 268. (The Wellcome Institute Library, London. M9545.)

power of personal observation, and the anatomists who followed Vesalius in the sixteenth and seventeenth centuries saw him as one of the major founders of the new anatomy. More generally, his book was one of the roots of the new view that developed in the seventeenth century that knowledge should be generated empirically.

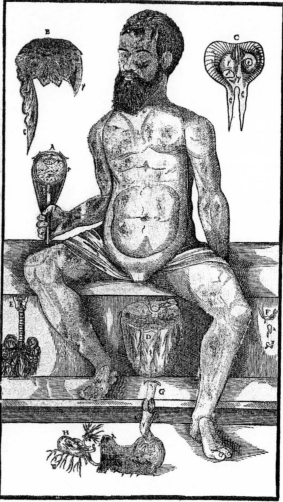

Fig. 38. An anatomical fugitive sheet. They were often bought by students to learn the basics of anatomy (Wittenberg, 1573). (The Wellcome Institute Library, London. L23188.)

STRUCTURE OF THE *FABRICA*

Book I of the *Fabrica* began in a Galenic fashion with the bones rather than with the internal organs as had been the medieval practice. Vesalius' osteology corrected various Galenic errors, for instance, the human sternum has three segments and not seven, and the mandible is not made of two bones. Book II dealt with the muscles and included the famous series of illustrations showing 'muscle-men' at different stages of dissection. Book III, on the vascular system, was less accurate than the previous Books because Vesalius was influenced by Galenic physiology and because he partly based his descriptions, despite his condemnation of the practice, on animal material. Book IV described the nervous system, in it Vesalius followed the Galenic classification of the cranial nerves into seven pairs despite tracing more. Book V described the abdominal organs and the organs of reproduction. Vesalius corrected Galen's belief in the five-lobed human liver, substituting an undifferentiated liver in humans and pointing out that it was only in lower animals that the liver had lobes. Vesalius accepted the fundamental tenet of Galenic physiology that the liver produced blood from chyle (the product of the stomach's digestion of food), but he denied that the vena cava originated in the liver. From this observation might have begun the destruction of the established Galenic view of two distinct vascular systems: the venous originating in the liver and the arterial stemming from the heart, but this was not the time. Book VI was devoted to the organs of the thorax. Vesalius followed Galen in describing the heart as muscular in structure but not in function, as it was not subject to voluntary control. However, Vesalius threw doubt on the permeability of the intraventricular septum. He wrote that he could not see any pores and expressed his wonder at the workmanship of God which produced invisible passages for the blood. In the second edition of the *Fabrica* (1555) the denial of the permeability of the septum was explicit. The impermeable septum was a crucial discovery of renaissance anatomy for it allowed anatomists like Realdo Colombo to conceive of the pulmonary transit of the blood, which in turn was used by William Harvey (1578–1657) as a stepping stone to the systemic circulation of the blood. Another crucial correction of Galenic anatomy came in Book VII which dealt with the brain. Vesalius, like Berengario da Carpi, denied the existence of the *rete mirabile*. Vesalius showed that the *rete mirabile* existed in some animals but not in humans. He expressed doubt as to how nerve conduction took place. He also denied that mental faculties such as memory and imagination were located in different parts of the ventricles of the brain, as his medieval predecessors had thought. In an elegant argument, Vesalius pointed out that the brains of animals showed little difference in structure from those of humans except in size, therefore, the functions of reason, which distinguished humans from animals, could not be materially located in the ventricles of the brain.

The *Fabrica* laid the ground work for a new anatomy of the body based on personal observation. The anatomists who followed corrected it as Vesalius had corrected Galen. In the process, a critical independence in observation became an established tradition among anatomists. They also became eager to establish priority in the discovery of new structures, achievement of such priority being increasingly important for gaining fame and reputation as an anatomist.

Anatomy after Vesalius

Anatomy took many different directions after the *Fabrica*. Anatomical accounts of the whole body continued to be published. Charles Estienne (1504–64) published in 1545 his *De Dissectione Partium Corporis Humani* (*On the Dissection of the Human Body*) that he wrote in the 1530s and which, if published earlier, might have lessened the impact of the *Fabrica*. Realdo Colombo, whose public criticisms of Vesalius whilst he was Vesalius' temporary replacement in his absence from Padua in 1543, provoked a bitter reaction from Vesalius, corrected some of the *Fabrica's* errors in his *De Re Anatomica* (*On Anatomical Matters*) published posthumously in 1559. It was much more succinct than the *Fabrica* and Colombo did not hesitate to boast of his achievements. His expertise in surgery and in dissection is shown especially in his vivisection experiments (see p. 328 for discussion). Another anatomy of the body was that of Colombo's former student, the Spaniard Juan de Valverde. His *Historia de la Composicion del Cuerpo Humano* (*The Account of the Composition of the Human Body*) of 1556 combined the teaching of Vesalius and Colombo, and excited the contempt of Vesalius who thought that Valverde had never dissected and had published only for profit. Less controversially, Gabriele Fallopia (1523–63), one of Vesalius's successors in Padua, wrote a detailed critique of the *Fabrica*, the *Observationes Anatomicae* (*Anatomical Observations*) of 1561. Later anatomists such as the Swiss Caspar Bauhin (1560–1624) still saw themselves as treading in Vesalius' footsteps when producing complete accounts of the body. In the *De Corporis Humani Fabrica* (*On the Fabric of the Human Body*; 1590) and in his best known work the *Theatrum Anatomicum* (*The Anatomical Theatre*; 1605) – which used Vesalius' illustrations – Bauhin emulated Vesalius in making it a matter of pride to be an independent observer, even though he was writing academic textbooks that mainly detailed the views of other anatomists.

One direction in which anatomists diverged from the *Fabrica* was the production of specialised studies of specific parts of the body, such as the treatises on the kidney, the ear, and the venous system published by Bartolomeo Eustachio (*c.* 1500–74) in his *Opuscula Anatomica* (*Anatomical Studies*; 1564). In them Eustachio criticised Vesalius for depicting the kidney of a dog instead of that of a man, and he described the suprarenal gland for the first time. He also produced detailed figures of the ear ossicles and the *tensor tympani* in man and in the dog, but priority in the discovery of the Eustachian tube should belong to Giovanni Ingrassia (1510–80) who discovered it in 1546. Eustachio, who taught in the medical faculty of Rome's university, the Sapienza, was a rather isolated figure in sixteenth-century anatomy; working away from the centre of anatomical studies, he referred with envy to Padua as 'that new Athens, source of all doctrines'. If his major work, the *De Dissentionibus ac Controversiis Anatomicis* (*On Anatomical Disagreements and Controversies*) with its 47 copper plates etched with the help of Pier Matteo Pini and the advice of Canano, had been published in his lifetime, it might have established Eustachio as a serious rival to Vesalius, as its illustrations, though not as elegant as those of Vesalius, were more accurate.

COMPARATIVE ANATOMY

The study of specific aspects of the human body came to be combined with the development of comparative anatomy in which different animals as well as humans were studied often in a self-consciously Aristotelian manner. Aristotle had been interested in comparing animal anatomy for the purposes of classification (using the anatomical similarities and differences between animals) and of discovering the essential structure and function of a particular part possessed in common by a variety of animals. Galen, on the other hand, had studied animal anatomy for the light it would throw on human anatomy.

It was Volcher Coiter (1534–1600?) who helped to initiate comparative anatomy. Coiter had been given a scholarship in 1555 to study abroad by the city council of his native Groningen (in the Netherlands). He studied with Fallopia at Padua, with Eustachio in Rome and with Guillaume Rondelet (1507–66) in Montpellier, so he was well versed in human anatomy, in the anatomy of specific parts of the body and in animal anatomy (Rondelet had produced in 1554–55 the *Libri de Piscibus Marinis* (*Books on Sea Fish*) – a good background for a comparative anatomist). In 1562 he went to lecture at Bologna on logic and then on surgery and anatomy. It was apparently a comment by the botanist and zoologist Ulisse Aldrovandi (1524?–1607) to Coiter while he was in Bologna that sparked Coiter's move into comparative anatomy. Aldrovandi said that the natural philosophers were ignorant and often mistaken in anatomy. As Coiter noted, anatomical knowledge of the human body alone was considered sufficient for physicians but philosophers (who studied all of nature) needed to dissect all animals. Aristotle was the major authority on comparative anatomy, and much of the work of Coiter and of the anatomists who followed in his footsteps was devoted to checking Aristotle's accuracy and, more importantly, repeating and developing his techniques in comparative anatomy (and they often focused on subjects such as embryology on which Aristotle had written). The anatomists were thus integrating Aristotle into their subject along with, and at times in opposition to, Galen and they were moving into an area which, unlike human anatomy after the *Fabrica*, was relatively unexplored.

Coiter systematically studied the skeletal structure of many different vertebrates, and, by vivisection, he gave accounts of the hearts of serpents, frogs, fishes, and cats and pointed out that excised hearts continue to beat. He also studied the anatomy and skeletons of birds. In embryology, Coiter repeated and expanded Aristotle's observations by describing the daily developments of the chick embryo in eggs (the human foetus had been studied by Julius Caesar Arantius (1530–89) his teacher at Bologna, who published in 1564 the *De Humano Foetu* (*On the Human Foetus*)). Coiter published his results in brief tabular form in his *Externarum et Internarum Principalium Humani Corporis Partium Tabulae* (*Tables of the Main External and Internal Parts of the Human Body*; 1572).

FABRICIUS AB AQUAPENDENTE

The greatest comparative anatomist of the age was another pupil of Fallopia, Hieronymus Fabricius ab Aquapendente (1533–1619), who succeeded to Fallopia's post at Padua in 1565 (it had been kept vacant after Fallopia's death in 1563). In anatomy he concentrated less on structure in the Vesalian manner instead he developed a comparative approach which stressed the utility of particular parts of the body, and one of his discoveries was to be crucial for the work of his student, William Harvey, on the circulation of the blood.

A long-term aim of Fabricius was to produce a large work to be called *Totius Animalis Fabricae Theatrum* (*The Theatre of all the Animal Fabric*), but only small sections of it emerged (and after a long gestation), and they did so in the form of specialised treatises which Fabricius hoped would be put together by his readers to form the *Theatrum*. In his first treatise, *De Visione, Voce, Auditu* (*On Vision, Speech, Hearing*; 1600), Fabricius set out some of his aims. He was concerned with three parts of anatomy: the description, action, and use of a part of a body (arguably Fabricius wanted to produce an account not, say, of a deer's or a man's eye but of *the* eye in general, something that is found in Harvey's account of the heart). He wrote that although Vesalius had surpassed the ancients in descriptive accuracy, yet he had written little on the action and usefulness of the parts (this was natural given Vesalius' emphasis on correcting Galen's description of the structure of the body). Fabricius hoped to remedy this defect. However, the emphasis on the action and usefulness of the parts was, as Fabricius himself wrote, nothing new. It was to be found both in Aristotle and Galen and it is clear that Fabricius was looking backward in order to progress. The result of his stress on action and utility was that the description of a part was merely a stage towards an understanding of its use. In this way Fabricius, more than other anatomists of the period, tried to integrate observation with theory. Another distinguishing characteristic was Fabricius' stress on comparative anatomy. His use of comparative anatomy, his emphasis on teleology – that each part of the body has a use and it is the ultimate aim of anatomy to discover it – and his choice of subject matter such as embryology point to an Aristotelian influence as does his very frequent citation of Aristotle's works. However, Fabricius himself did not seem aware of this change of emphasis and in his writings Galen often appears, and not in opposition but in support of Aristotle, when the general aims and methods of anatomical investigation were discussed.

In hindsight, one of the most significant of Fabricius' works was *De Venarum Ostiolis* (*On the Little Doors of the Veins*; 1603). The valves in the veins were to be crucial for William Harvey's demonstration of the circulation of the blood. Fabricius was not the first to discover the valves. In 1545 Canano told Vesalius of his discovery of valves in the opening of the azygos and renal veins but he did not publish his findings; other anatomists who have been associated with the discovery were Charles Estienne and Jacobus Sylvius. However, Fabricius was the first to discuss the valves at any length. In *De Venarum Ostiolis* Fabricius wrote that he first discovered the valves in 1574, and within four or five years he was demonstrating them to his students. The 29 year delay between Fabricius' discovery of the valves and his publication on the subject was typical of a man who often allowed a great deal of time to pass before publishing his treatises so that they could be subject to informal criticism and further revision. The delay can also be accounted for by the fact that in the sixteenth century a claim for priority for an anatomical discovery could be made during an actual dissection before witnesses as well as by means of publication.

Fabricius placed the function of the valves squarely within the traditional Galenic ideas of blood flow. He wrote that the valves had been constructed by Nature to prevent the extremities from being flooded with blood. This meant that the feet and hands would not be permanently swollen with blood, and that the other parts of the body would have a fair distribution of blood coming to them. This theory was integrated with the Galenic view that blood was attracted from the liver (the blood-making organ) by each part of the body as and when it needed nourishment. The valves thus helped the central and upper parts to attract blood by preventing the natural tendency of the blood to collect at the extremities.

Fabricius' embryological treatises also influenced Harvey. *De Formatione Ovi et Pulli* (*On the Formation of the Egg and the Chick*; 1621) and *De Formato Foetu* (*On the Formation of the Foetus*) published in 1604, but written after the former, are the two works upon which Fabricius' fame as an anatomist largely rested. The former deals with the development of the egg, and with the generation of the chick over time, whilst in *De Formato Foetu* Fabricius described how Nature provided the means for the foetus to grow, be nourished, be protected, have its 'residues' stored, and achieve a successful birth. He minutely described the development of the foetal structures, but his theoretical framework remained traditional. For instance, he agreed with Aristotle's view that the female contributed all the material and the male the form, so that the semen of the cock is the formative agent.

CONCLUSION

Renaissance anatomy changed and increased the observational knowledge of the structure of man and of other animals, but its debt to the ancients was two-fold. Firstly, the innovatory aspect of Vesalius' anatomy lay in its being a reaction against Galenic anatomy while following its precepts – in a trite yet true sense one can say that without Galen there would have been no *Fabrica*. Secondly, renaissance anatomy was profoundly conservative when it came to theory. No anatomist coherently opposed the traditional tripartite Galenic division of physiological function (venous centred on the liver, arterial on the heart, and sensory/motor in the brain), even when anatomical structures and vascular connections crucial to the scheme were being denied (for instance, the *rete mirabile* or an origin for the vena cava in the liver). Furthermore, at a fundamental epistemological level, although the anatomists elevated observation into a form of certain knowledge, they retained their belief in final causes, a belief they shared with Aristotle and Galen. The view that everything in nature including the parts of the body had a purpose, had been made purposefully, was to be denied and largely thrown out of the range of allowable explanations and causes by the new science of the seventeenth century. For the anatomists and natural philosophers of the sixteenth century such teleological reasoning was as acceptable as it had been to Aristotle who considered that a true explanation of something could only be given when its final cause had been discovered. In many senses, despite the anti-Galen rhetoric of writers like Vesalius, renaissance anatomy was a product of classical medicine and philosophy even while it was correcting their observational errors.

The anatomists' justification of anatomy

Renaissance anatomists had a high opinion of their subject. Yet this was not a view shared by other medical writers, nor, until late in the sixteenth century, did anatomy gain institutional equality with the other parts of medicine, even at Padua, its great centre.

The central problem for anatomy was that its place within medicine was a low one. It was not listed as being among the traditional major divisions of medicine – physiology, hygiene (the conservation of health), aetiology or pathology, therapeutics, and the three instruments of treatment – dietetics, pharmacology, and surgery. Writers like Leonhard Fuchs (1501–66) – who was favourable to anatomy – in compendia on the whole of medicine placed anatomy within physiology, and merely as a small part of it, after the temperaments, qualities, and humours of the body had been described – this followed the example of Avicenna in the *Canon*.

The response of anatomists such as Berengario at Bologna, Guinther von Andernach and Jean Riolan the Elder (1538?–1605) in Paris, Archangelo Piccolomini (1526–1605) in Rome and especially of the students and their anatomy lecturers at Padua to the low position of their subject was to assert that anatomy was the foundation of medicine (a claim which from the eighteenth century onwards was reflected in the medical curriculum.)

Together with the low status of anatomy within the divisions of medicine there was a corresponding disparity in the university status of the subject. Compared to the chairs of theoretical and practical medicine the lectureships or chairs in anatomy were low in dignity, power, and salary. The association of anatomy with surgery had helped to keep the status of anatomy low – often a surgeon was appointed to demonstrate and lecture on anatomy as well as on surgery.

But the appointment at Padua of the humanist physician, Andreas Vesalius, rather than a surgeon served notice that anatomy and surgery were to be incorporated into the overall humanist revival of medicine. And, indeed, Vesalius argued forcibly in the preface of the *Fabrica* for the unity of the different parts of medicine. He wrote that physicians should once again use their hands and become surgeons and apothecaries, something that they had come to despise 'after the devastation of the Goths.' In other words, the different parts of medicine should come to be unified in the person of the physician, something born out by Vesalius' background and career – his father was an apothecary (albeit to the Emperor), he himself was a physician who also later practised surgery. Vesalius felt that all the branches of medicine, and not physic alone, could be learned. Berengario, from the point of view of the surgeon-anatomist had earlier also deplored the physicians' disdain for the surgeons' manual labour in his *De Fractura Calvae* (1518). He pointed out that from the time of Guy de Chauliac back to that of Avicenna, physicians had also been surgeons and natural philosophers.

These were not pious sentiments. As is discussed further below, surgery came under the reforming gaze of the medical humanists. The surgical texts and the illustrations of the surgical instruments of antiquity were published, often in the vernacular, in order to raise standards and to make the subject more learned. As anatomy lay half-way between surgery and medicine, anything that raised the status of surgery indirectly affected anatomy.

After Vesalius, anatomy gradually became a *de facto* part of learned medicine (even in backward England in the 1550s John Caius (1510–73) the English Galenist physician who shared lodgings for a time with Vesalius in Padua was lecturing on anatomy to the College of Physicians of London and by 1584 the bequest of Lord Lumley and Richard Caldwell allowed the College to hold their own lectures on anatomy, in addition to those given at the Barber-Surgeon's Hall, though the numbers attending were initially very small). This was a spontaneous intellectual development among professors and students, which was recognised at the institutional level sometimes only after some time had elapsed.

THE DIGNITY OF ANATOMY

One reason why anatomy was held in low esteem was that its practice could provoke disgust. As Volcher Coiter admitted in 1572 anatomy appeared, 'unworthy of a free man' and 'they despise it and hold it in contempt as though useless. Those who do so, assert that it is disgraceful to touch the parts of a dead body polluted with blood and dirt.' Vesalius also had deplored the fastidiousness of men who were disgusted with dissection. And Valverde had explained the lack of anatomy in Spain as being due to the opinion of Spaniards that it was 'an ugly thing'. Coiter's reply to people's disgust was that it was not the disgrace of the body but of the spirit (the objectors' spirit) that was the issue. But this was a purist's reply. The business of anatomy could induce disgust even in experienced practitioners. Michelangelo, when collaborating with Realdo Colombo in carrying out a number of dissections, was reported to have had his stomach so affected that he could not eat or drink properly.

The anatomists tried to change people's mental perception of their subject by emphasising the worth of anatomy. Their prefaces and introductions were filled with encomia for their discipline. The gory spectacle of dissection was metaphorically transformed by constant references to the dignity and excellence of the body. Platonic and Hermetic references (the Hermetic writings were a collection of treatises purporting to disclose the ancient magical wisdom of the Egyptians, but shown to be forgeries in the seventeenth century) were made to man, the miracle of miracles, the microcosm of the world, the epitome of all things, the result of the divine handiwork. The body was also seen in Christian terms as the house of the immortal soul. Charles Estienne was not alone when he wrote in 1545, that of all things in the universe from

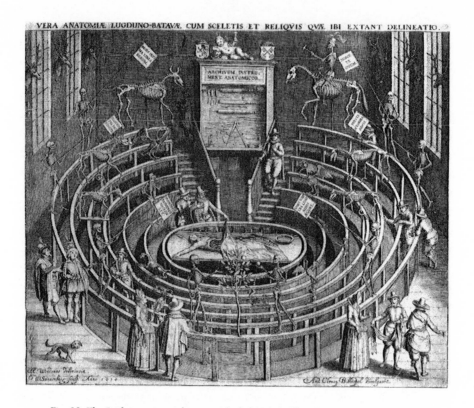

Fig. 39. The Leiden anatomy theatre with skeletons holding flags conveying moralistic sayings such as 'know thyself' ('*Nosce te ipsum*') which the image of the dissection reinforces. By William Swanenburgh after Jan Cornelisz wan't Woudt, 1610. (The Wellcome Institute Library, London. L9967.)

which the power and the workmanship of God could be contemplated, the human body was the best by far. And, he added, placing anatomy within the larger sphere of religion, we have been born with the duty of understanding God's creation and examining hidden things. Both Catholic and Protestant anatomists argued that contemplation of the body could lead to a knowledge of God's handiwork and hence of his nature and existence. Archangelo Piccolomini, who lectured on anatomy at Rome's Sapienza, made precisely this point in his *Anatomicae Praelectiones* (*Anatomical Lectures*; 1586), as did the Protestant Caspar Bauhin (in fact, Luther was reported to have said that anatomy was almost as important as religion in imparting morality, and John Calvin the leading Protestant Reformer after Luther, approvingly wrote of how Galen had shown the workmanship of God in the *Use of Parts*). The anatomists were placing their subject in the established and prestigious tradition of natural theology that was concerned with contemplating God's creation which had been the province of theologians and the natural philosophers, and in so doing they enhanced the status of their subject. At Wittenberg, the powerhouse of Lutheran theology, anatomy, in fact, became part of the religious curriculum. Philip Melanchthon (1497–1560), Luther's close associate who lectured on natural philosophy there, referred to anatomical knowledge to display God's handiwork and also in order to understand the soul. He wrote to Leonhard Fuchs in 1534 that the soul could not be properly understood without a knowledge of the workings of the body. The association of anatomy with religion undoubtedly helped it gain status and acceptance in the world at large.

The anatomists also gave their subject a history, both ancient and noble. Jean Riolan the Elder, one of the arch-conservative Galenists of the Paris faculty, but also a skilled anatomist, wrote that 'the sacred scriptures, the most certain indices of all things teach that the art of anatomy is clearly of great antiquity', and he cited Genesis 32.25 which referred to the patriarch Jacob's sinew or nerve in the 'hollow of the thigh.' Most writers began with the Egyptians or with Hippocrates and Plato as the founders of the subject, and so placed anatomy firmly in the tradition of the *prisca medicina* (the ancient, pure medicine). Piccolomini, for instance, stated in a marginal note to his text that 'anatomy was the first principle of medicine', citing Hippocrates' *Places in Man* and *On Diet* to the effect there was a need to know first of the composition of man before proceeding any further in medicine.

The nobility of the subject was asserted by the listing of emperors, kings and Roman consuls who had dissected or been interested in anatomy. Guinther von Andernach, in the *Dedication* to Francis I of France of his translation of Galen's *On Anatomical Procedures*, wrote that 'once anatomy was held in so much honour that not only the most distinguished philosophers or physicians but also patricians and men ... of the first quality were not ashamed to work on that subject.'

In typical humanist vein the anatomists wrote that anatomy's golden age had been and gone and that only in their own time was the subject being restored. They did not hesitate to boast of the achievements of the anatomists of their own day. Vesalius, despite the occasional criticism such as Colombo's comment to Lorenzo dei Medici that he was 'prolix' and made errors, was quickly set up as a hero-figure. Eustachio acidly commented how everyone in Padua believed that further efforts to improve upon or to contradict Vesalius' discoveries would be useless, and he noted, correctly, how Fallopia constantly referred to the 'divine Vesalius.' Vesalius, he also wrote, was universally considered 'the discoverer and almost the architect of the art of anatomy.' If historians have tended to concentrate on Vesalius, so clearly did his contemporaries, for whom he acted as a point of reference, personifying the success of anatomy.

However, Vesalius was not the only creator of 'modern' anatomy. Anatomists were quick to point out that their subject had developed through the efforts of a whole line of modern anatomists. Jean Riolan noted how 'many new things, unknown to the ancients' had been brought to light by 'Berengario, Zerbi, Massa, Sylvius, Vesalius, Fallopia, Colombo and a great cohort of young anatomists.' The articulation of a modern tradition in anatomy must have contributed to a sense of self-sufficiency and independence, for the creation of the modern heroes in anatomy not only enhanced the status of the subject but also allowed it to be favourably compared with classical anatomy.

Clearly the anatomists felt that their subject was in a progressive stage. They saw progress as the building up of more and more correct facts about the body. Piccolomini wondered why he was publishing his anatomical lectures if Hippocrates had invented anatomy, Aristotle enlarged it and Galen perfected it, and also if other anatomists like Fernel, Sylvius, Mundino, Corti, Vesalius, Fallopio, and Columbo had written on the subject. He answered that anatomy was not complete, there were quite a few additions yet to come. Jacques Guillemeau (1550–1613) wrote in his *La Chirurgie Françoise* (*French Surgery*; 1594) that Galen, the interpreter of Hippocrates, 'seems truly to have deprived posterity of all opportunity and means of having anything else to say', but added that the human body was infinite in its variations and 'Nature, as wondrous as she is infinite in her works, never stops producing every day something new.' The anatomists could stay in business.

ENHANCING THE STATUS OF SENSE OBSERVATION

The type of additional knowledge involved was sensory. It came not so much from books as from the eye and the hand (although, in the opinion of the philosophers, it was not knowledge in the fullest sense, for only knowledge of *causes* gave real knowledge). Piccolomini justified anatomical knowledge by stating that learning by the use of the hands and the senses was better than being taught anatomy by voice or by writing – it was more firm, more certain, and more stable. Piccolomini went as far as to argue that anatomical propositions were perceived immediately by the senses to be true (they did not need a logical proof by means of argument); they were like the premisses postulated by geometry: self-evident, commonly and universally agreed upon as most manifest and true. Hence, Piccolomini argued, anatomy could provide the basic propositions for medical demonstrations and it could provide the foundation for the rest of medicine.

Valverde wrote more simply that progress took place by downgrading the authority of books and relying on the senses. He opposed writing to sight: 'Andreas Vesalius started to open the eyes of many, showing that faith must not be given to everything which is found in writing' and books and authorities were also opposed to touch, 'the lazy should not try to defend their ignorance by means of the authority of this or that author and particularly in those things in which the contrary can be touched by hand.' There was agreement among anatomists that the way to get certain knowledge in their subject was through the senses, especially by 'autopsia,' seeing for oneself. Even Jean Riolan, conservative though he was, stated that in anatomy one should give more credence to the eyes than to the opinions of Hippocrates. This knowledge was validated if others saw the same thing, especially if they were skilled in anatomy in the first place. Eustachio doubted the usefulness of witnesses, for he wrote that the 'spectators at dissections .... usually have sharp ears but dim eyes for the most difficult things' and that they 'are easily persuaded into agreement with others,' but such doubts were few. The testimony of witnesses was often the conclusive demonstration of the truths of observation.

Elevating the status of observation was appropriate, given that anatomy concentrated on the structures of the body, their composition, site, size, shape, colour, and connections to the other parts of the body. All were matters for observation. It was only when the action and use of the parts of the body were being considered that the primacy of observation became debatable; this required discussion of causes, the traditional subject-matter of the philosophers, and, as such, involved both reason and the eyes.

CONCLUSION

When the Paduan Aristotelian philosopher Cesare Cremonini (1552–1631) denied in 1627 that anatomy could be the foundation of medicine, he declared that only causes, the subject matter of philosophy, and not observation could lead to true knowledge. The achievement of the anatomists was to counter the latter part of this claim, but it was a limited achievement, for they did not tackle the relationship between observational knowledge and that of final causes. If they had, the former might have cast doubt on the latter.

Despite Cremonini's worries, the anatomists remained part of the learned medicine of the time, developing the observational methods of Galen it is true, but they were not revolutionaries who would consciously destroy the theories of the ancients which provided the interpretive basis of medicine. As Helkiah Crooke (1576–1635) wrote in his Μικροκοσμογραφια (1631), which was an amalgam of two major anatomical textbooks, those of André Du Laurens and Caspar Bauhin, the ancients supplied the framework for the work of the anatomists: 'we must needes acknowledge, that the Groundworke of the building, and not onely so, but the whole frame was by the ancients reared up; and therefore now if any Ornaments be added, they must be fitted thereunto'.

Even if they were beholden in some ways to Galen, the anatomists were successful in upgrading their subject and giving it a higher profile. Anatomical dissections by the end of the sixteenth century could take on a carnival atmosphere; in fact at Bologna they were carried out during the carnival. They were popular, and an interest in the macabre and in the hidden nature of things, and a wish to be reminded of death by the *momento mori* of the body all contributed to their appeal to the public. Dissection also became more accepted in public and private life. Post-mortems were regularly carried out on popes and royalty and among private well-to-do families. Rembrandt's *The Anatomy Lesson of Dr. Tulp* gives us an icon of how the anatomists had succeeded in making their subject one of the accepted spectacles of early modern Europe.

Surgery

Surgery, one of the three branches of medicine along with physic and pharmacy, saw only a few significant changes in the sixteenth and seventeenth centuries. It was touched by the endeavour to recreate classical medicine and there were some innovations in surgical technique. But in its organisation and remit it remained unchanged from the Middle Ages. Surgery continued to be taught throughout most of Europe by apprenticeship and was organised around local guilds or colleges of surgeons and barber-surgeons. In Italy and Spain surgery was taught in the universities as well as by apprenticeship. There were also many operators who specialised in a single condition such as lithotomists and cataract experts, who travelled widely and often worked outside the guild structure.

THE SCOPE OF SURGERY

The separation between surgery and medicine which occurred in the Middle Ages also continued, but it was never a complete divorce. As in the Middle Ages surgery was largely but not exclusively operative and concerned with the surface of the body. Surgeons dealt with the many accidents that were part and parcel of life in pre-industrial Europe. For instance, they set the fractured bones that resulted from falls from horses, which were an important means of transport, or from working accidents in agriculture and in the fulling and tanning mills (legislation on safety at work or in the home was non-existent until the nineteenth century). Surgeons treated burns, which were most frequent among the old and among young children who often fell into unguarded fires at home. Contusions, knife, and increasingly, gunshot wounds, whether suffered in tavern brawls or in warfare, were another source of patients (in this case usually male).

Surgeons also dealt with the many disorders and blemishes that appeared on the skin such as tumours or swellings, ulcers, and the various spots, blotches and discolorations of skin diseases. The new disease of syphilis (see pp. 218 and 225), which often exhibited skin symptoms was viewed as a surgical condition and was often treated with mercury, guaiac, or sarsaparilla.

Topical remedies and lotions were used to treat skin disorders, but surgeons did not hesitate to employ the internal remedies and regimens of the physicians to strengthen the 'habit' or constitution of the patient before and after surgery. Literate surgeons, from whom our knowledge of surgery comes, were often close intellectually to the 'learned' physicians and shared with them a belief in the humoral basis of health and illness. Berengario de Carpi, who taught surgery at Bologna, advised on regimen and internal remedies as well as giving surgical instructions in

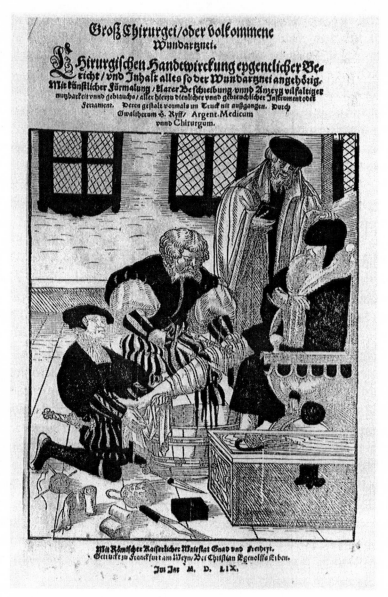

Fig. 40. Amputation of leg with clergyman in attendance from Walter Ryff, *Grosz Chirurgei* (Frankfurt, 1559–1562). (The Wellcome Institute Library, London. M17295.)

his treatise *On Fracture of the Skull* (1518). The most famous surgeon of the sixteenth century, the French royal surgeon Ambroise Paré (1510–90), had been trained by apprenticeship and wrote in French rather than in the Latin of the university educated physicians. But he similarly stressed the need for regimen based on the non-naturals, for instance, when treating gunshot wounds. The changing appearance over time of wounds, incisions, and other lesions was also often interpreted in humoral terms, for instance in the case of ulcers as movements of malign or corrosive humours into local areas of the body.

Surgeons also acted like physicians. Patients would frequently lodge in surgeons' houses or nearby inns or lodgings and look to the surgeon for their day-to-day care, not only for conditions such as syphilis which required extended treatments, but also for amputations and wound management, where the initial operative procedures often constituted only a small fraction of the time spent by the surgeon on the patient. Ships' surgeons, who were increasingly employed in navy and merchant ships on the long voyages that followed on the discovery of the sea routes to India, the East Indies, and America, had to act as surgeons, physicians, and apothecaries as they were the only medical experts on board ship. And in the English North American colonies, as in some parts of Europe, the three branches of medicine were also combined in one practitioner.

The wide scope of surgeons' practice should counter the view that is still commonly held today that in the days before anaesthesia and antisepsis the surgeons' business was bloody and all too often fatal. The case records of the apprentice-trained London surgeon Joseph Binns are typical and indicate the wide extent of the medical services provided by surgeons. Between 1633 and 1663 Binns recorded some 616 cases in detail. Of these 196 related to gonorrhoea or other sexual conditions with discharges and to syphilis (Binns seems to have made sexual diseases a speciality); 77 cases were of swellings and 61 were more properly medical including ague, stomach-ache, headache, insomnia, diarrhoea, and epilepsy. Fifteen suffered battle wounds, 14 were hurt at work, 19 suffered from falls from horses or coaches, and 41 were injured in fights. Of the 402 outcomes recorded, 265 were cured and 62 improved, while 22 showed no improvement and 53 died.

HUMANISM AND SURGERY

By contrast with physic and medical botany it is difficult to talk of a surgical renaissance. There were physicians and surgeons who hoped to create a learned surgery analogous to learned physic by using newly retrieved and translated classical surgical texts. But their endeavours had only a limited effect.

Many classical surgical texts remained obscure and uninfluential. Of the Hippocratic surgical treatises, only *On Wounds in the Head* attracted any commentaries, the first being by Fallopia in 1566. The surgical material in the works of Aëtius, Oribasius, and Celsus appears to have been little known, except for some sections from Oribasius' medical encyclopaedia which were included in the collections of surgical texts compiled by Vidus Vidius (d. 1569) and by Conrad Gesner (1516–65) in 1544 and in 1555, respectively.

The learned surgeons and physicians did recreate some parts of ancient surgery. Vidius, whose *Chirurgia (Surgery)* (1544) was a compilation of classical surgery drawn from a ninth- or tenth-century Greek manuscript, also printed in his *Chirurgia* illustrations of the surgical instruments described by Galen, Paul of Aegina, Celsus, and Oribasius. Vidius' volume was lavish and expensive, and out of the reach of impecunious apprentices of surgery, even if they had the Latin to understand the text and Vidius' commentary on it. Conrad Gesner hoped to influence German surgeons when he produced for them a collection of medieval and recent works in surgery which were distinguished by their good Latin style. But his *De Chirurgia* (1555) made little impression on the German market, where there were already a number of vernacular books on surgery by writers such as Hieronymus Brunschwig (1450–1512) and Paracelsus (1493–1541).

One solution was to bring the new learning to the surgeons in a language that they would understand. John Caius, the humanist English physician who searched the libraries of Europe for Galenic texts, gave anatomy lectures in English to the apprentices of the London Barber-Surgeons Company from 1546. In France a large number of classical surgical texts (including the surgical sections of Galen's *Method of Healing*) were translated into French by Jean Canappe (*fl.*1538–52), a Paris graduate physician and lecturer in surgery at Lyons and by Pierre Tolet (*c.* 1502–80), dean of the Lyons College of Physicians. In 1569 Jacques Daléchamps (1513–88), another physician who practised in Lyons, published his *Chirurgie Françoise (French Surgery)*, which condensed the ancient surgical writings and argued that ancient and modern surgery were in agreement and that the former was still useful. Daléchamps' volume was reprinted in 1570, 1573, and 1610, and with the translations of Canappe and Tolet brought ancient surgery within the view of the many surgeons without Greek or Latin.

INNOVATION IN SURGERY

Little changed in terms of surgical techniques in the sixteenth and seventeenth centuries. Most famously, Paré abandoned the standard use of boiling oil to cauterise gunshot wounds, substituting a salve instead. (Boiling oil was used to counteract the poisons which were commonly supposed to be produced by gunpowder.) Boiling oil or the use of a red hot iron ('actual cautery') fell into gradual disuse as patients increasingly objected to it, but it continued to be employed in cases of 'putrefaction' or gangrene until the early twentieth century. Paré also encouraged the revival of the use of ligatures in cases of amputation. Podalic version, where the child in the womb is turned so that it arrives head first, was another classical procedure popularised by Paré. In Italy Gaspar Tagliacozzi (1549–99) wrote up in his *De Curtorum Chirurgia per Insitionem* (*On the Surgery of the Mutilated by Grafting*; 1597) the procedure of rhinoplasty or reconstruction of the nose which had been a secret of the Sicilian Branca family of itinerant operators. Other family operators also kept their secrets. In London the Chamberlens hid from all eyes for a century the forceps that they had invented in the early seventeenth century. In France the Colot family of barber-surgeon lithotomists devised a procedure of lateral perineal lithotomy which they kept secret from the mid-sixteenth century until Francois Colot (d. 1706) made it public in his posthumous *Traité de l'Operation de la Taille* (*Treatise on the Operation of Cutting*; 1727). By the seventeenth century detailed written accounts of contemporary surgical procedures became increasingly common. Richard Wiseman (1621?–76), surgeon to Charles II, in his *Severall Chirurgiall Treatises* of 1676 interspersed detailed case histories, like Paré, often drawing on from his experience in war, with his descriptions of surgical procedures, and he depicted surgery as progressing through the accumulation of empirical knowledge.

Surgery, with its practical craft tradition and its lack of Latin was less influenced by the humanist revival of ancient medicine. The Dresden eye-doctor, Georg Bartisch (1537–1607?) in his famous book on ophthalmology, *Opthalmodouleia. Das ist Augendienst* (*Eye-Service. That is Eye-Work*; 1583) which for the first time recommended removal of the eye in cases of cancer, admitted that he employed a theology student to supply the appropriate classical quotes. The learned English surgeon William Clowes (1544–1604) acknowledged in 1585 that someone like

Paré, 'Who as it is thought hath small understanding in the Latine tongue, howsoever it is knowen, that he is not unskilfull in anie part of this arte of Chyrurgerie'. Paré and Wiseman were learned to the extent that they shared the Galenic physicians' humoral framework, but like the majority of their colleagues they were less scholars than craftsmen who relied on the traditional steady hand and a degree of insensitivity. As Paré wrote, following Celsus:

> A Chirurgion must have a strong, stable and intrepide hand, and a minde resolute and mercilesse, so that to heale him he taketh in hand, he be not moved to make more haste than the thing requires; or to cut lesse than is needfull; but which doth all things as if he were nothing affected with their cries; not giving heed to the judgement of the common people, who speake ill of Chirurgions because of their ignorance.

Botany and medicine

A large part of medical therapeutics was based on the products of the natural world, and pharmacy, which created medicines from them, was long established as a major division of medicine. The range of remedies available to pharmacy was extended in the sixteenth and seventeenth centuries as a result of the retrieval of classical drugs, the discovery of new medicinal products from America and the Indies, and by developments in medical theory that encouraged the use of chemical substances.

Herbs (which could include shrubs and trees) and their leaves, seeds, fruits, bark, and roots, were the most frequently used ingredients of medical prescriptions and were central to medicine throughout this period. When they were used individually medieval and renaissance physicians and apothecaries called them 'simples' or a number of herbs could be put together to make up a compound drug (animal and mineral ingredients might also be employed). Herbs were used as medicines throughout society, by university-trained physicians and by illiterate wise-women. The preparation of medical remedies was one of the skills expected of a housewife. Just as she had to be able to cook, so also she had to pick herbs and prepare them (by drying, pounding, boiling and, if rich enough, by distilling) for use as medicines. Many family manuscripts which have recipes for food also have recipes for medicines.

There was also a commercial side to herbal medicine. In their shops

CHAP. 32.   Of Dandelion.

¶ The Description.

1   THe herbe which is commonly called Dandelion doth send forth from the root long leaues deeply cut and gashed in the edges like those of wilde Succorie, but smoother: vpon euery stalke standeth a floure greater than that of Succorie, but double, and thicke set together, of colour yellow, and sweet in smell, which is turned into a round downie blowball, that is carried away with the winde. The root is long, slender, and full of milkie juice when any part of it is broken, as is the Endiue or Succorie, but bitterer in taste than Succorie.

‡   There are diuers varieties of this plant, consisting in the largenesse, smallnesse, deepenesse, or shallownesse of the diuisions of the leafe, as also in the smoothnesse and roughnesse thereof. ‡

1 *Dens Leonis.*
Dandelion.

‡ 3 *Dens Leonis bulbosus.*
Knottie rooted Dandelion.

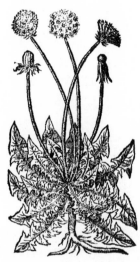

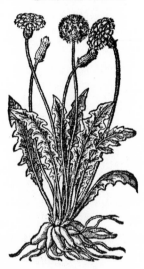

¶ The Names.

These plants belong to the Succory which *Theophrastus,* & *Pliny* call *Aphaca,* or *Aphace Leonardus: Fuchsius* thinketh that Dandelion is *Hedypnois Plinij,* of which he writeth in his 20. booke, and eighth chapter, affirming it to be a wilde kinde of broad leafed Succorie, and that Dandelion is *Taraxacon :* but *Taraxacon,* as *Auicen* teacheth in his 692. chapter, is garden Endiue, as *Serapio* mentioneth in his 143. chapter; who citing *Paulus* for a witnesse concerning the faculties, setteth down these words which *Paulus* writeth of Endiue and Succorie. Diuers of the later Physitions do also call it *Dens Leonis,* or Dandelion: it is called in high Dutch, **Bolkraut:** in low-Dutch, **Papencruit:** in French, *Pissenlit ou couronne de prestre,* or *Dent de lyon :* in English, Dandelion : and of diuers, Pisseabed. The first is also called of some, and in shops *Taraxacon, Caput monachi, Rostrum porcinum,* and *Vrinaria.* The other is *Dens Leonis Monspeliensium* of *Lobell,* and *Cichoreum Constantinopolitanum,* of *Matthiolus.*   ¶ The Temperature and Vertues.

Dandelion is like in temperature to Succorie, that is to say, to wilde Endiue. It is cold, but it drieth more, and doth withall clense, and open by reason of the bitternesse which it hath ioyned   A with it : and therefore it is good for those things for which Succory is. ‡ Boiled, it strengthens the weake stomacke, and eaten raw it stops the bellie, and helpes the Dysentery, especially being boyled with Lentiles ; The juice drunke is good against the vnuoluntary effusion of seed; boyled in vineger, it is good against the paine that troubles some in making of water ; A decoction made of the whole plant helpes the yellow jaundice. ‡

† The figure which was in this place was of the *Cich. Luteum,* where you may find it, but to what plant the description may be referred, I cannot yet determine.

Fig. 41. Description of the Dandelion, giving also its many names and its virtues, from John Gerald, *The Herball* (London, 1633) abbreviated from pp. 90–1. (The Wellcome Institute Library, London.)

the apothecaries did the same job as the housewife but on a much more extensive basis. They used not only local herbs but also plants and spices from the Middle East and Indies and from the 1520s and

1530s they began to employ the new American plants. The commercialisation of drug-making was not, however, as extensive as it was to become in the eighteenth century, when many household products came increasingly to be sold (so much so that historians talk of the 'commercial revolution of the eighteenth century'). However, in the elite part of the medical market-place, the physicians already relied on the apothecaries to make up their medicines.

THE RENAISSANCE OF MEDICAL BOTANY

In the first half of the sixteenth century, during the ascendancy of hellenism in medicine (p. 251), physicians were concerned that the remedies available to them were not as good as those of the ancient Greeks, and sought to retrieve the Greek *materia medica*. At the same time, the stock of West European plants known to medicine increased as botanists and medical men (often one and the same), especially those from north of the Alps where the Mediterranean plants of the Greeks could not be found or grown, noted down in their herbals plants that they had discovered on their field trips. In the herbals a plant would be identified by shape of leaf, given its names, and have its curative virtues described.

Botany in the modern sense did not exist in the sixteenth century. Classification of plants only began to be seriously considered in the next century. There was no uniform system of nomenclature, and this made the attempts to identify classical plants which had disappeared from the ken of Western Europe even more hazardous. However, there was a specialised interest in collecting and describing plants to which the term botany can be applied. By the 1540s the name *res herbaria* was being used for the study of plants, and physicians and their students were at the forefront of the field.

Botany went through the same process of humanism as did medicine. Medieval authors were denounced for their corruptions of ancient texts and their barbarian language. New 'purer' editions of major classical botanical works were published. Manuscripts of *The History of Plants* and *On the Causes of Plants* of Theophrastus, Aristotle's pupil, were brought anew from Constantinople in the early fifteenth century (the *History* had been unavailable to Western Europe during the Middle Ages) and translated into Latin around 1450 by Theodore Gaza. Pliny the Elder's *Natural History*, the classical encyclopaedia of nature, had many descriptions of plants, but it appeared to some late fifteenth-century writers that these were frequently wrong (p. 252) and not faithful to Pliny's Greek sources.

Galen wrote a treatise on the medicinal properties of plants, minerals, and animals, the *On the Powers of Simple Remedies*. This had been used in the medieval universities, but in 1530 a new Latin translation corrected by reference to 'old manuscripts' was published. The treatise in its new form was lectured on in universities such as Bologna (1534), Basle (1536), and Montpellier (1538), and the new Protestant university of Helmstedt (1576) for either its theoretical content or its description of *materia medica*.

More important, however, as a vehicle for medical botany was the *On Materia Medica* of Dioscorides (*fl.* AD 50–70) (discussed p. 57) which acted as the focus for the renaissance of botany and of medical botany. For the sixteenth century, Dioscorides' book served as a repository of ancient wisdom that had been used by the great Galen, and which could be retrieved if Dioscorides' plants were found again and securely identified. It also acted as an exemplar of how to discover by experience plants useful to medicine, something that those north of the Alps with less access to Dioscorides' plants took to heart. As Thomas Johnson, the editor of John Gerald's (1545–1612) *Herball*, wrote in 1633, Dioscorides was 'as it were the foundation and grounde-worke of all that hath been since delivered in this nature.'

On Materia Medica was known to the Middle Ages in a Latin version, but humanists collected new Greek manuscripts. The famous Venetian Aldine Press published a Greek edition in 1499, and in 1518 brought out a second edition improved by reference to manuscripts collected by Leoniceno. Barbaro's Latin translation and commentary on Dioscorides was published posthumously in 1516 as was the Latin translation of Jean Ruelle (1474–1537), which went through 25 editions. This was another example of the humanist enterprise of restoring an ancient classic to as pristine a state as possible.

HERBALS

Alongside the revival of Dioscorides, herbals underwent changes. The earliest printed ones were compiled from medieval sources, but in the first half of the sixteenth century, like the renaissance anatomy books, they became naturalistic and representational both pictorially and in their verbal descriptions. The first herbal which abandoned the stylised and difficult-to-identify pictures of medieval herbals was the *Herbarum*

Vivae Eicones (*Living Images of Plants*; 1530) of Otto Brunfels (d. 1534), a German theologian, botanist, and, at the end of his life, town physician of Bern. He wrote within the framework of antiquity and expected that the plants that he collected in the area around the Rhine at Strassburg would be the same as in his classical sources. Despite Dioscorides' own statement, he did not realise that different regions had different flora. His plants did not always tally with those in Dioscorides or in the *Herbal* of Apuleius (possibly written around the fifth century AD and well known in the Middle Ages), but he tried to force an identification. Where he could not succeed, he called the plants 'herbae nudae', destitute or poor plants, which had only German names.

The artist Hans Weiditz of the school of Dürer gave Brunfels' herbal its innovative dimension. As the title of the herbal indicates, Weiditz produced highly naturalistic depictions. He showed the individual plant in its actual state, with leaves torn or eaten by insects – at this time, the issue of depicting a type as opposed to an individual plant had not arisen. Weiditz, true to his belief in the reality or worth of every plant that he drew, insisted that Brunfels' *herbae nudae*, such as the pasque flower (*Pulsatilla vulgaris*), were put into the main body of the book despite Brunfels' wishes to the contrary. This new representational or naturalistic approach to plants flourished after Weiditz, and artists collaborated with the writers of herbals, as they did with anatomists.

Brunfels' herbal described 258 different plants; 93 years later Caspar Bauhin's *Pinax Theatri Botanici* (*A Catalogue of a Botanical Theatre*) included around 6000. This great increase was achieved through individual and collaborative efforts. The study of plants was seen as the pursuit of the scholar and the gentleman, one which gave aesthetic delight. The great humanist scholar Erasmus (1467–1536) praised the power of gardens to restore the soul, and Pier-Andrea Mattioli (1501–77), the focal point of much of Italian botany, wrote of the spiritual pleasure that looking at plants gave him. But it was its medical usefulness more than its association with sensual and spiritual pleasure that gave the subject a shape and an identity. As well as gaining a name, *res herbaria*, it begun to be taught in its own right in the universities. The first professorship in botany, essentially a lectureship on Dioscorides, was established in 1533 in Padua. University botanical gardens were created first in Pisa and Padua in 1544–45 (the decree of the Venetian Senate establishing the Paduan botanical garden stated that it should be created so as to avoid errors in pharmacy and to save lives by the rebirth of the *materia medica* of the ancients). Many other universities followed (Bologna, 1568; Leiden, 1577; Leipzig, 1580; Basle, 1588; Montpellier, 1597). Medical students were taken around the gardens and shown medicinal plants. This helped to meet the complaint of medical reformers like Leonhard Fuchs that physicians were ignorant of plants. In his *De Historia Stirpium* (*On the History of Plants*; 1542) Fuchs wrote that physicians so shrank from the study of plants that only one in a hundred knew anything accurately even about a few plants. 'Ocular demonstrations' of plants (echoing those of anatomy) were also given by university professors like Caspar Bauhin at Basle who took their students on field trips, *herbationes*, into the countryside to observe plants.

Plants, however, were not always available and they also altered with the seasons, and so the artificial garden, the dry garden or *hortus siccus* (our herbarium) was invented. Luca Ghini (1490?–1556), professor of botany at Bologna and director of the Pisan botanical garden, popularised the pressing and drying of plants, which were then gummed onto cards, and often collected into books. Such dried gardens allowed rare and exotic plants to be preserved, or to be sent by post, as well as acting as teaching material for students and as models for draughtsmen (who usually had to soak the plants to bring them back to something approximating their original state).

THE LOST DRUGS OF ANTIQUITY

There was large-scale international co-operation in sending and describing plant specimens. Physicians, pharmacists, scholar-botanists, travellers, diplomats, traders, and the Venetian State all became concerned with retrieving the lost drugs of antiquity. They co-operated informally with each other, sending plants and information. This is an early example of what in the seventeenth century became more usual; scientific networks changing science from an individual to a group activity – a change that is still taking place.

The great intelligence centre for botany was provided by Pier Andrea Mattioli, town physician of Gorizia, until he gave a copy of the 1554 edition of his *Commentaries on Dioscorides*, sumptuously illustrated in gold and silver, to the Archduke Ferdinand of the Tyrol, soon to be Emperor, who promptly made him his personal physician. Mattioli did no botanical work of his own but, bolstered by the Emperor's money, published the work of others who sent their results to his house in Prague and then later in Innsbruck.

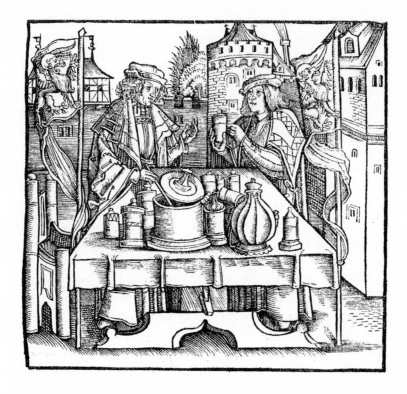

Fig. 42. The preparation of theriac in public, from H. Brunschwig, *Liber de Arte Distillandi de Compositis* (Strassburg, 1512), fol. 93r. (The Wellcome Institute Library, London. L751.)

In 1544 Mattioli translated into Italian Ruelle's Latin edition of Dioscorides. Ten years later he added a commentary and illustrations, which he published as *Commentarii in Libros Sex Pedacii Dioscoridis Anazarbei, de Materia Medica* (*Commentaries on the Six Books of Pedacius Dioscorides of Anazarbus on Materia Medica*). It was immensely popular; his Venetian publisher Valgrisi claimed that 32,000 copies of the early editions had been sold. It became the focus for much of Italian botany. Mattioli kept adding to the *Commentarii*, and in each new edition his notes on Dioscorides became larger, far outstripping the original text of Dioscorides. This reflected the information that Mattioli was eliciting from others such as Luca Ghini and Ulisse Aldrovandi (1524?–1607), who generously sent a large number of herbaria specimens and descriptions. The problem of identifying Dioscoridean plants necessitated con-

tact with the lands to the east of Italy, and Ghini, when asked to identify some of Dioscorides' plants which Mattioli had failed to do, had
plants sent to him from Greece, Crete, and the Levant by merchants
and by his brother who had lived in Crete. Mattioli noted how the
attempt to restore the *materia medica* of the ancients was progressing.
For instance, in his 1548 edition of Dioscorides he reported that true
Cretan dictamnus and true Dioscoridean rhubarb from the Bosphorus
had started to be imported into Venice.

Venice, the great commercial power and entrepôt of the
Mediterranean, the European city having the strongest links with the
Middle East, and the destination for the overland spice trade from the
Indies, was the natural centre for the enterprise of regaining the remedies of antiquity. Moreover, Venice controlled Crete and Cyprus, the
herb islands of the ancients. It ordered its diplomats, physicians, and
traders in the Middle East and in the Mediterranean to be on the look-
out for the plants that grew in Dioscorides' stamping ground. As Italy's
climate was not too different from that of the Eastern Mediterranean,
plants could be transplanted to gardens such as the one in Padua
(Padua was part of the Venetian territories).

The co-operative, informal, effort produced results. Drugs which were
unknown to Western Europe such as balsam, myrrh, and petroselinum
were rediscovered. Rhubarb roots, famous for their purging powers,
had entered Europe in the late Middle Ages through the overland trade
routes of the East. In the sixteenth century viable seeds or live plants
were eagerly sought. By the early seventeenth century seeds from
Bulgaria allowed one type of rhubarb (*Rhaponticum*, from the *Pontus* or
Black Sea) to be grown in Europe, but the search for the 'true' and
most efficacious rhubarb which Marco Polo had reported in 1295 as
coming from China continued into the nineteenth century. Theriac, the
fabulous panacea and antidote to poisons of the ancients, which had
been composed of at least 81 plant, animal, and mineral ingredients,
seemed in the 1540s impossible to make, many of its ingredients were
unknown and more than 20 substitutes had to be used. But by 1566
the Veronese botanist-pharmacist Francesco Calzolari was using only
three substitutes, and Mattioli could write in 1568 that the new theriac
was now as good as that mixed by Galen for the Emperors. By the end
of the sixteenth century physicians were confident that most of the
remedies of the ancients had been recovered.

DRUGS FROM THE VOYAGES OF DISCOVERY

There were other sources of drugs in the sixteenth century. The European vision of the world had been totally transformed by the Portuguese and Spanish voyages of discovery. The Portuguese sailed down the West Coast of Africa, rounded the Cape of Good Hope in 1487–88 and reached India in 1498. By 1512–13 they had found in the Pacific the legendary Spice Islands, the Moluccas, from where spices had traditionally reached Europe via India, the Middle East, and the Mediterranean (the 'overland' route). Africa, India and the Pacific coasts of China and Japan were no longer myths, but possible new regions for European commerce and empire. The Spaniards sailing to the West had discovered the Bahamas, Cuba, and Hispaniola in 1492–93 and then the Southern parts of America, which they quickly conquered. By 1522 Magellan's expedition had circumnavigated the globe.

Europeans looked for riches in the new-found worlds – gold and silver and also new remedies. The exotic was already present in the plant material from the Indies (cinnamon, cloves, nutmeg, etc.). More might come from India and the East, and from paradisical America much was hoped for. News of these far-off remedies reached the scholarly medical world and were integrated into it through the books of Nicolas Monardes (c. 1493–1588) and Garcia d'Orta (1501/1502–68).

The Spanish physician Nicolas Monardes popularised the new American drugs. Initially he doubted their value. In the *Dialogo Llamado Pharmacodilosis o Declarion Medicinal* (*Dialogue Called Pharmaceutical Account or Medical Declaration*; 1536) he wrote that the medicinal drugs of the New World were inferior to those of Spain. But Monardes changed his mind, and in his *Dos Libros. El Uno Que Trata de Todas las Cosas Que Traen de Nuestras Indias Occidentales* (*Two Books. One Which Deals With All The Things That Are Brought From Our Western Indies*) (in three parts, 1565, 1571, 1574) he enthusiastically publicised their therapeutic powers. Monardes did not travel outside Europe but learned about American plants from the material coming into Seville, where he practised, which was the centre for Spanish trade with the New World. He also had a botanical garden in which he grew and observed many of the new introductions (just as d'Orta observed plants in his gardens in Goa and Bombay).

In the *Dos Libros*, Monardes followed the standard format of botany books and gave for each plant its place of origin, its shape, colour, and general morphology. He then discussed its properties and uses. The plants from the New World posed problems for botanists, they were unfamiliar to Europeans and their powers were uncertain, though the public were eager to acclaim them as panaceas. This led Monardes not only to concentrate on the distinguishing marks of the new plants but also to describe how they were collected and processed. He frequently cited how American Indians used a plant, and he himself tested plants on animals to find out their properties. One of the best known of Monardes' plant descriptions was that of tobacco in the second part of *Dos Libros*. He praised it for binding wounds together, for dissolving obstructions of the stomach, and for curing pains in the head, 'toothaches, bad breath, chilblains, worms, pains in the joints, cold swellings, poisoned wounds, kidney stones, carbuncles, weariness, and so on'. Monardes used the classical theory of qualities as he did with other plants to explain that the marvellous powers of tobacco came from its hot and dry qualities. He also discussed the curative qualities of coca, sarsaparilla, and sassafras and, moving away from plants, the armadillo.

The *Dos Libros* was translated into Italian and English in Monardes' lifetime and after his death into French and German. The Flemish botanist Charles L'Ecluse also abridged and translated it into Latin in 1574. Europeans were eager to hear about new remedies, the English version of *Dos Libros* translated by John Frampton was entitled *Joyfull Newes out of the New Founde Worlde* (1577).

The Spanish in America were alert to the possibility of finding valuable remedies (both in the curative and monetary sense). In 1552 the Franciscan College in Santa Cruz, Mexico, which was interested in preserving Aztec culture, produced a manuscript account of Aztec medicine with drawings of hundreds of Aztec medicinal plants. It was written by an Aztec, Martin de la Cruz, then translated into Latin and sent to Europe. When in 1570 Francisco Hernández was appointed, by Philip II, *protomedico* to New Spain (the post involved the regulation of medical practice, see p. 231), Philip instructed Hernández before he sailed that he should gather information about the properties of all medicinal plants in New Spain.

Foreign remedies appeared to be godsends with the coming of syphilis into Europe in 1495 (see also p. 225). Mercury was soon established as the standard treatment but produced painful and dangerous side-effects (ulcerations, the loosening of bones, tremors, general paralysis). Patients hoped for easier remedies. In the Caribbean the Spaniards saw syphilis (or perhaps yaws which is very similar) being treated by decoctions made from guaiac wood (*Guaiacum Officinalis*) which grew there. Guaiac was being imported into Spain by 1508 and its use had become widespread by 1517, when Nicolaus Pol, personal physician to the Emperor Charles V, stated that 3000 Spaniards with syphilis had been cured by guaiac. In 1519 Ulrich von Hutten (1488–1523), (p. 218), described the distress and pain of the mercury treatment with its effusions of sweat and saliva, and the heat of the sweatroom in which patients suffocated, their throats so constricted that they could not vomit their own mucus. He then heard of guaiac and after repeated drinks of infusions of guaiac (taken in a warm room to sweat the body and so rid it of the disease, or the ill humours), he thought that he was cured (in fact, he later died from the disease). Hutten's treatise *De Guaiaci Medicina et Morbo Gallico* (*On the Guaiac Remedy and the French Disease*; 1519) was translated into German in the same year and into French in 1520 and helped to advertise guaiac. By the time Monardes wrote in 1565, guaiac was going out of fashion but he believed that it and the China root (*Smilax china*) and sarsaparilla (*Smilax aristolochiaefolia*) also from the New World, were effective against syphilis. The new drugs brought in large profits. The Fuggers, the most powerful bankers in Europe, acquired the monopoly of the guaiac trade from the Spanish Crown in return for a loan. The New World expanded the number of available remedies (cinchona bark, quinine, used by the Incas in Peru, was added to the list in the seventeenth century and was employed against intermittent fevers, which included malaria, endemic in many parts of Europe). Being plant remedies they were easily fitted into the Galenic qualitative model of therapeutics and their discovery did not challenge Galenic medicine. In fact, guaiac helped it, for the use of mercury had been mistrusted by Galen and was more associated with Arabic pharmacy.

India also supplied new remedies. In 1563 Garcia D'Orta published his *Coloquios dos Simples, e Drogas he cousas Mediçinais da India* (*Dialogues about Simples and Drugs and Medical Matters from India*). Printed in Goa, Golden Goa, the boom capital of Portuguese India, the book represents the experience that D'Orta had gained from his 29 years there. D'Orta brought the remedies of India and Asia further to the attention of Europe. He was a physician who had studied medicine in Spain at the universities of Salamanca and Alcalà de Henares and who also owned ships and traded in precious stones and *materia medica*. The book gives insights into Indian society and life in Goa as well as reporting his researches into Eastern drugs. In typical renaissance fashion, d'Orta began with the etymology of a plant's name and then he discussed its appearance, origin, preparation, and therapeutic uses. D'Orta used both classical and Arabic sources and had a good grasp of medical learning. He often favoured Arabic authors over classical ones and wrote that if he were in Spain he would not dare say anything against Galen and the Greeks. His support for the Arabs was understandable as they had written at great length on *materia medica* (see pp. 118–19) and also were more likely to have had a greater acquaintance with Eastern remedies. D'Orta repeated a common renaissance theme when he stated that because he had personally witnessed much of what he wrote about, he had the right to contradict the ancients who had often to rely on false, second hand, information. He described a number of Eastern products such as aloes, camphor, sandalwood, ginger, asafoetida, and betel. Like the Italian botanists, D'Orta was faced with problems of identification. For instance, he debated whether true cinnamon was 'canella', 'cinnamon', or 'cassia', and his solution drew on the experience of Chinese and Persian traders as well as on academic writers. Sometimes, as in the case of 'myrobalan', which had claims to be the balsam of the ancients, D'Orta could describe from his own observations several different species of 'myrobalan'. As well as creating greater clarity about Eastern drugs, he introduced new plants into European botany such as mangoes.

More descriptions of Indian and Asian plants were made by Christovao da Costa (1515?–80?) in his *Tractado de las Drogas y Medicinas de las Indias Orientales* (*Treatise of the Drugs and Medicines of the Eastern Indies*; 1578). Da Costa, a Portuguese physician and botanist who wrote in Spanish, based himself on D'Orta, but he had travelled further, reaching Malacca and China, and at times he corrected D'Orta. He produced good woodcuts of many of the plants that he described. L'Ecluse also translated Da Costa into Latin in 1582.

OPPOSITION TO THE EXOTIC

Exotic remedies were not always welcomed. As well as the danger that they might be counterfeited, they were often expensive and so out of the reach of the poor. It was widely believed that God of his mercy had put medicines on Earth for Man's use ('The Lord hath created medicines out of the earth', Ecclesiasticus 38.4) and more specifically that the diseases native to a country were best cured by the remedies to be found in that country. Such remedies were free, they could be picked from the fields, and so through God's mercy the poor as well as the rich might be cured. Most herbals mentioned how remedies were to be found growing all around, and a few physicians from the sixteenth to the end of the seventeenth century wrote specific books on medicines for the poor in which they stressed the use of common plants.

Medical reformers often expressed disgust with physicians and apothecaries for their prescribing and selling of expensive remedies. A powerful sense of Christian charity opposed the rapacity of learned medicine. Timothie Bright (1551?–1615) in his *A Treatise Wherein is Declared the Sufficiencie of English Medicines for Cure of All Diseases Cured by Medicines* (1580) stressed that Greek medicines were for the Greeks and English for the English; it was God's providence, his foresight, for the good of mankind that assured this. Just as animals were given by God the means to cure themselves when he gave them the knowledge of what curative plants to eat that grew near them, so God also provided healing plants for human beings. Paul Dubé in his often reprinted *Le Médecin des Pauvres* (*The Physician of the Poor*; 1669) lamented the cost and luxury of complex Arabic remedies. Dubé argued that God's providence had provided in one's own native countryside the remedies to cure native diseases, and that foreign remedies often lost their efficacy in France. Such treatises, stressing local remedies and written in the vernacular, challenged the hegemony of Galenic learned medicine which was often expressed in the universal language, Latin, and which claimed that its remedies (which now included those from America and India) applied universally right across Europe.

But within learned medicine, the retrieval of the *materia medica* of the ancients and the discovery of new remedies were matters for satisfaction. And, unlike anatomy, they provide an example of unity between ancient and renaissance medicine.

Paracelsianism

A new tradition, entering Western medicine with the work of Paracelsus (1493–1541) and his followers, gave shape and focus to the protests against establishment Galenic medicine. Only recently has the magisterial work of Walter Pagel and Charles Webster, among others, given the intellectual and reformist aspects of Paracelsianism the recognition that they deserve. Paracelsian medicine in the sixteenth and seventeenth centuries was praised by nineteenth- and twentieth-century German and English historians for its new and perhaps more effective therapeutic drugs, but its ideas were largely dismissed as an unfortunate episode, where a mystical, alchemical, magical, and astrological orientated system appeared on the scene and attempted to supplant Galenic medicine. Paracelsianism seemed superstitious while Galenic medicine was at least rational, even if it was not always 'scientific'.

However, in the sixteenth century, magic and witchcraft were believed in, both at government and legal levels as well as in villages. Religion could be the subject of intense belief, debates, and wars. What to us may appear non-rational was central to the consciousness of early modern Europe. It makes, therefore, no sense to emphasise and approve of only those pieces of Paracelsus' work which by hindsight seem to contribute to the formation of modern science and medicine.

LIFE OF PARACELSUS

Paracelsus, or Theophrastus Philippus Aureolus Bombastus von Hohenheim, was born in Switzerland, the son of a physician and probably of a bondswoman of the abbey of Einsiedeln in Switzerland where he was born. Around 1529, he adopted the name Paracelsus which probably meant 'surpassing Celsus', the Roman medical writer (incidentally, Bombastus was not a nickname, though it was appropriate, but the family name of Paracelsus' father). Paracelsus, according to his own account, was educated by his father in botany, medicine, mineralogy, mining, and natural philosophy. Four bishops and the abbot of Sponheim, Johannes Trithemius, also taught him. From Trithemius, who studied the occult and believed in the possibility of arriving at universal knowledge through magic and mysticism, he would have learned of the influence of celestial, spiritual, forces on earth and of the magical power of words and letters. Paracelsus went to the mining school of the Fuggers at Huttenberg close to Villach where he and his father had emigrated in 1502, and he also became an apprentice in the mines of Sigmund Fueger at Schwaz. This practical, religious and mystical education clearly shows itself in Paracelsus' work. He did not write in the elegant Latin of the humanists, but in a rough and ready variety, and he was happiest writing in German. Nor, like the humanists, did he venerate the wisdom of antiquity. Instead, he hoped to learn from peasants and miners and he immersed himself in magical and alchemical writings and in a popular spiritual Christianity inimical to organised religion. His education and his interests represent a break with the Western medical and scholarly tradition, based on ancient sources, amalgamated with mainstream Christianity and housed in the universities.

Paracelsus was nominally a Catholic, but he was reformist in religious sentiment and was probably influenced by the radical Protestantism of Sebastian Franck (1499–1543) and Caspar Schwenckfeldt (1490–1561). Although Paracelsus was called the 'the Luther of the physicians', like Franck and Schwenckfeldt he came to disapprove of Luther's insistence on an organised Church and of his creation of a new set of dogmatic beliefs to replace those of the Catholic Church. Spiritual knowledge was to be found in Nature, which was full of God's presence, and in oneself rather than, as Luther held, only in the literal words of the Bible and in a 'walled Church'. Together with religious independence went a social radicalism. Paracelsus, unlike Luther, sided with the German peasants in their wars against their feudal Princes.

Paracelsus, like many of his contemporaries, also had a sense of imminent change in the world. His *Prophecy for the Next Twenty-Four Years* (1536) presented a picture of a calamitous near-future ended by a vision of a utopia in which God's people were united to God after the defeat of Antichrist. Later radicals were attracted by Paracelsus' prophetic and reformist voice. When some English Protestants at the time of the Civil War looked for a medical model to replace that of Galen, they chose Paracelsus not only for his medical views but also for the context in which they were expressed – reformist in religion, prophetic of the coming of Christ, and charitable in its approach to the patient in contrast to what they saw as costly uncharitable orthodox medicine.

In his own lifetime Paracelsus expressed a contempt for the medicine of the universities (though he was clearly aware of its content). He may have studied at a university, perhaps at Ferrara (sometime between 1512–16), but he never accepted the authority of the Greek and Arabic medical writers. When he was appointed town physician in Basle in 1527 he also had the duty of lecturing to the medical faculty there. This he did in German rather than in Latin, and in his *Intimatio* or manifesto to the faculty he stated that he would not teach from

Hippocrates and Galen, but that his own experience would disclose the secrets of disease. He followed this up by burning Avicenna's *Canon*, the huge volume that encapsulated learned medicine, on a bonfire on St. John's day, 24th June, the student rag day. The hostility of the university authorities, combined with the alienation by Paracelsus of his natural allies, the Protestant town council, ensured that his stay in Basle, as elsewhere, was short-lived – his quarrelsome nature made him few friends.

THE IDEAS OF PARACELSUS

Paracelsus attacked learned natural philosophy and medicine on a variety of fronts. He created a new natural philosophy based on chemical principles. Salt, sulphur, and mercury were his new primary substances, which, although they did not completely replace the Aristotelian and Galenic system of qualities, elements, and humours, were considered by him as superior and more fundamental because they were 'male', active and more spirit-like rather than 'female' and passive, like the elements. The *tria prima* were principles of solidity (salt), inflammability (sulphur), and spirituousness (mercury) rather than material substances.

For Paracelsus the world was full of spiritual and vital forces. Some of them were the *archei*, the internal alchemists or principles which controlled processes like digestion, others were the *semina* or seeds coming from God, the great Magus or magician, who directed nature. The agents of disease might be poisonous emanations from the stars or minerals from the earth, especially salts.

Paracelsus has been praised by earlier historians for seeing the workings of the body in terms of chemistry, for his belief in chemical remedies, and for helping to create the subject of chemistry by moving alchemy from its secrecy and from its limited aims of making gold from base metals and of searching for the elixir of life into the broader field of iatrochemistry or medical chemistry. However, integrated with these views, and often condemned or ignored by earlier historians, was Paracelsus' belief in the spiritual nature of the universe and of human beings.

Again, Paracelsus' belief that every disease has a specific external cause and is an entity in its own right, what is sometimes called today the ontological theory of disease, sounds very modern until it is realised that his *essentia* or essence of the disease was a spiritual essence.

313

Andrew Wear

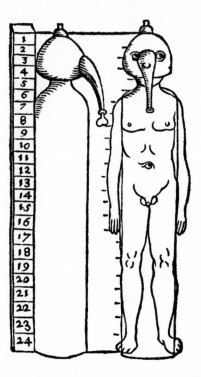

De fornace anatomica.
NOn abſimili ratione , noſtræ fornacis
proportio, correſpondeat præcedenti-
I s

Fig. 43. A Paracelsian 'anatomical furnace' for the distillation of urine and for discovering in the body the location of particular diseases. The cylinder corresponds in
size to the human body; where the different parts of the urine settle when distilled
indicates the presence of diseases. Anon, *Aurora Thesaurusque Philosophorum
Paracelsi... Preterea Anatomia Viva Paracelsi* (Basle, 1577). (The Wellcome Institute
Library, London.)

Behind such theories lay the belief in the correspondence and intercon-
nectedness of the macrocosm (the universe) and the microcosm (the little world of the body). An example of this correspondence is the
doctrine of signatures which was used to identify the curative powers of
plants. When a plant looks like a part of the body, then this signifies
that it can cure it (for example, the root of the orchid looks like a testicle and can heal its ills).

Paracelsus was consistently contemptuous of learned medicine. For instance, he called the anatomies of the universities 'dead anatomy' (which was literally true), for it did not disclose how the parts of the living body functioned and how they could be cured. A true anatomy would unravel the normal physiology of the body by discovering the particular nourishment that each part of the body needed. The influence of particular stars on particular parts of the body also had to be known. There was an anatomy of diseases and their remedies. Diseases could be known, not by the mere inspection of urine (uroscopy) but by a chemical 'dissection' of urine. Abnormal amounts of salt, sulphur, and mercury precipitated out of the urine could indicate particular disease. An early follower of Paracelsus described how to distill urine in a cylinder corresponding to the body and how, where, and in what order the different parts of the urine deposited themselves in different positions in the cylinder. In this way the types of disease and their location could be discovered; (see Fig. 43). On therapeutics Paracelsus stated, in direct opposition to Galenic medicine, that like cured like. A disease entity could be fought by knowledge of what was appropriate to the affected part rather than by giving something contrary. Moreover, if a poison or a star caused a disease, then it was to be countered by another poison or a star. (Paracelsus justified the use of drastic remedies like mercury, antimony, and arsenic along these lines, though their popularity may have owed more to their quick acting, visible effects upon patients, in contrast to the generally less dramatic Galenic simples.) By denying the significance of the humours and by stressing the importance in health and disease of the parts of the body and of the influences upon them Paracelsus was able to achieve a novel sense of specificity.

From where did Paracelsus get these ideas? Paracelsus poured scorn on the very act of learning through words, the basis of the medicine of the universities. The 'Book of Nature', he believed, held the key to knowledge. One had to learn and experience the 'Book of Nature' through one's feet, by travel, so that frequently 'one land is a page'. On the other hand, Paracelsus argued that logic, the foundation of university learning and disputation, darkened the light of Nature, and he termed Aristotle, the founder of logic and of much else in the university curriculum, 'the sharp illusionist'. Indeed, Paracelsus believed that 'the more learned, the more perverted'. In his view, the physician was born, not made. He knew the *arcana*, the secrets of Nature, and especially her cures, through the light of Nature. This knowledge could only be personally experienced; it was not to be taught by reading books in universities.

Religion and magic as well as observation held the key for Paracelsus to personal knowledge of Nature. A belief in personal religious experience was common in the fifteenth and sixteenth centuries. Widely acknowledged also was the existence of natural magic, the knowledge of how the celestial world interacted with the terrestrial and human worlds and how such knowledge could be used to achieve effects here on earth. Intellectuals like Marsilio Ficino (1433–99) and Agrippa von Nettesheim (1487–1535) found natural magic appealing, and many humanists were fascinated with the magical contents of the Hermetic writings. Witchcraft was held by both elite and popular culture to be another manifestation of the interaction between the supernatural and the natural. Similarly, astrology appeared to offer evidence of the influence of the heavens. Paracelsus disapproved of witchcraft and did not believe that the stars rigidly determined men's or women's lives (what was called 'judicial astrology'). But he did hold that the macrocosm and microcosm were connected by God, and that Nature largely consisted of the influences, emanations, and correspondences between the two.

There was little if any magic in Hippocratic and Galenic texts, and Greek medicine, despite its assimilation with Christianity, was essentially pagan and devoid of Christian context. Reformers of medicine claimed it especially lacked an ethos of Christian charity. In contrast, Paracelsus' medicine was explicitly Christian. For instance, he repeatedly stated that a remedy worked only when God willed that it should. This was also the position in Christianised Galenic medicine but only in a formal sense, for learned physicians rarely emphasised God's power and their own fallibility.

Paracelsus' writings thus represent a new medical tradition. In them not only were new medical theories and cures set out but their associated social and religious radicalism and the incorporation of contemporary medical and cosmological interests gave it a sense of relevance arguably lacking in a learned medicine based on ancient texts.

THE GROWTH OF PARACELSIANISM

In Paracelsus' own lifetime the existence of the new type of medicine was known only to a small number of people. Few of Paracelsus' medical writings were published before his death in 1541. During his life he was probably better known for his published prophecies and discussions of portents such as the comet of 1531 (Halley's Comet). Only after his death were the rest of Paracelsus' medical and chemical writings published. But starting in the 1550s and increasing in numbers from around 1570 Paracelsus' medical and chemical writings came to be disseminated in print around Europe. The lack of early publication partly accounts for the delayed impact of Paracelsus upon medicine.

By 1575 Paracelsianism had begun its rapid spread through Europe. This showed itself at two apparently opposite ends of the political spectrum: among court physicians and their royal patrons and among radical social reformers. The royal physicians often excluded the social radicalism in Paracelsianism, and if one looks for shared characteristics, it would be in religion, where both groups were usually Protestant, especially Calvinist.

Paracelsians looked for sympathetic royal patrons, partly because the universities, with the exception of Montpellier and some German ones, excluded them and partly because in terms of prestige, money and influence a position as a court physician in the sixteenth century could count for more than a university post. Royal or noble patronage helped to legitimate Paracelsianism, and to protect a practitioner against the attacks of a university faculty or a city College of Physicians with the power to regulate medicine in its locality. The financial backing of a ruler could also provide laboratory facilities. This personal patronage was as important for physicians and natural philosophers as for artists. (State support for science and medicine began in France in the later seventeenth century.)

Otto Heinrich, Duke of Neuburg and Elector of the Palatinate, was probably the first German noble to favour Paracelsianism. From the early 1540s he collected Paracelsian manuscripts which became the source for the later printed books. He supported a Paracelsian chemist, Hans Killian, and he employed the Paracelsian Adam van Bodenstein (1528–77), the son of the extreme Lutheran reformer Andreas Karlstadt von Bodenstein, as his personal physician. Adam von Bodenstein used the resources of the Duke's library to publish over 40 of Paracelsus' works. Another Protestant noble, the Landgrave Moritz of Hesse (1572–1632), was a prince-practitioner who carried out his own chemical experiments with the court physician Johannes Hartmann (1568–1631) and established a *Collegium chymicum* in 1609 at Marburg with Hartmann as the professor of 'Chymiatria' (medical chemistry).

At the Court of the Holy Roman Emperor, astronomers (such as

Tycho Brahe and Kepler) and alchemists and magicians were employed. Rudolf II supported Martin Ruland the Elder (1532–1602) and son, Martin Ruland the Younger (1569–1611), who were Paracelsian physicians. Oswald Croll (*c.*1560–1609), the personal physician of Prince Christian of Anhalt-Bernberg, also frequented the court in Prague. Croll's *Basilica Chymica* or *Royal Chemistry* (1609), which expounded Paracelsian philosophy and gave the ingredients of chemical remedies, became one of the major textbooks of Paracelsian chemistry. It emphasised the union of chemistry with medicine by stating that without the chemical philosophy all medicine was lifeless.

In 1604 Joseph Duchesne (*c.* 1544–1609), the personal physician to Henri IV of France, could write that, as well as the Emperor, the other German rulers who supported Paracelsian medicine were the King of Poland, the Duke of Saxony, the Elector of Cologne, the Margrave of Brandenburg, the Duke of Brunswick, the Landgrave of Hesse and the Duke of Bavaria.

Paracelsianism was many things to many people. Paracelsus' writings did not constitute a tightly knit philosophy. And two different types of Paracelsianism began to emerge: the full-blooded kind which incorporated the philosophical and cosmological elements together with a chemical *materia medica* (this was the version generally popular with the German princes), and a Paracelsianism denuded of its philosophical basis and consisting mainly of chemical remedies. The term iatrochemistry, or medical chemistry was used for both types. Compendia and textbooks set out Paracelsian philosophical medicine to the learned world in the linguistic respectability of Latin. As well as Croll's *Basilica Chymica*, there was the earlier *Idea Medicinae Philosophicae* (*The Idea of Philosophical Medicine*; 1571) of the Lutheran Dane Peter Severinus, who became physician to his king and helped to get Paracelsianism accepted in the medical faculty of Copenhagen University. Severinus attacked Galenic medicine for not curing new diseases (in other words, not being appropriate for the times). In Paracelsian fashion he exhorted his readers to burn their books, sell up their houses, travel, study the natures and differences of plants, animals and minerals, and not to be ashamed to learn from peasants about the stars and the earth. They were urged to buy coal and furnaces and to investigate by fire the properties of things (a favoured method of chemical analysis). Severinus coherently set out the major Paracelsian medical doctrines and the *Idea Medicinae Philosophicae* broadcast the Paracelsian message to Europe's intellectual classes.

However, a Paracelsianism which discarded the founder's philosophy or reconciled it with Galenic medicine became increasingly popular. Guinther von Andernach, the humanist physician, anatomist, and translator, towards the end of his life attempted the latter in his *De Medicina Veteri et Nova* (*Concerning the Ancient and the New Medicine*; 1571). As well as listing a large number of chemical remedies, Guinther equated the Paracelsian principles of salt, sulphur, and mercury with the Aristotelian elements. He stressed that the Greeks also had believed in the interrelationship between the macrocosm and microcosm.

In any case, the use of chemical remedies was not viewed as a purely Paracelsian innovation. Dioscorides had described mineral drugs as had medieval alchemists such as Ramon Lull (*c.* 1235–1315), Arnald of Villanova (1240?–1311) and John of Rupescissa (*fl.*1345–56) (though the medieval writers had also influenced Paracelsus). The practise of distilling herbs for their 'essences' had long existed in medieval Germany and increased in popularity with the publication of Hieronymus Brunschwig's (*c.* 1450–1512) books on the art of distilling simples and compound medicines: *The Book on the Art of Distilling Simples* (1500) and *The Book on the Art of Distilling Composite Remedies* (1512). Distillation acted as a bridge between herbal and chemical medicine by, as it were, chemicalising herbs. From the 1540s as the Catholic Counter Reformation gathered momentum Paracelsians went underground in Italy. The writings of Paracelsus were considered heretical, being tainted with Protestantism as well as magic. However, the distillation of oils and waters from animals and plants became very popular in Venice and helped to make the transition to chemical remedies. By 1642 the Collegio degli Speziali (the College of Apothecaries) was listing in its official price list hermetic and spagyrical (alchemical) medicines and those prepared by distillation.

Paracelsian and chemical remedies (the two were not always synonymous) had increasingly received formal recognition. Official pharmacopeias which set out acceptable remedies and listed their contents for apothecaries to follow had appeared in the German cities of Nuremberg (1546), Augsburg (1564), and Cologne (1565). The Augsburg pharmacopeia of 1564, the *Pharmacopeia Augustana*, listed distillations and a few chemical remedies for external use. In the 1613 edition a variety of chemical preparations were included, some of which had been described in 1582 by the Augsburg Senate as dangerous and poisonous (these included mercurial substances used to purge patients). In England, the London College of Physicians published its *Pharmacopeia Londinensis* in 1618. It included sections on 'salts, metals, minerals', 'chemical oils', and 'the more usual chemical preparations'; altogether 122 chemical remedies were set out in the enlarged second edition that appeared in the same year. In the 'Introduction' to the 'Reader', the College, which was still dominated by Galenists, wrote that the remedies of the chemists were placed at the end of the book so that they could act as subsidiary servants and helps to the medicine of the ancients.

From the end of the sixteenth century it was quite possible to conceive of chemical remedies without Paracelsian connotations. The German physician Andreas Libavius (1540–1616) published in 1597 his *Alchymia* (or *Chemistry* – this was a time when alchemy and chemistry were often indistinguishable), which has been seen as the first textbook in chemistry. Libavius argued for a chemistry which was devoid of Paracelsian cosmology. He did not believe in the theory of correspondences between the macrocosm and microcosm and, moreover, he attacked the Paracelsians for illicit magical practices in conjuring evil spirits. He believed that classical medicine could benefit from the use of chemical remedies, but saw no need for it to be overturned and replaced by a Paracelsian system of medicine.

PARACELSIANISM AND THE DECLINE OF GALENISM

Conciliation and assimilation were not enough to save Galenic medicine. By the later seventeenth century it had declined and lost its authority, helped in its downfall by iatrochemistry, although it too by then had lost authority especially in its Paracelsian guise. Socially, politically, and intellectually, iatrochemistry struck at the foundations of Galenic medicine. It took hold among empirics, apothecaries, and surgeons at the popular end of the medical market-place as well as in royal courts.

Galenic physicians fulminated against iatrochemists, placing them amongst disreputable mountebanks and charlatans peddling dangerous drugs, and at times accusing them like Paracelsus, of witchcraft and of consorting with the devil. The vilification betrays a deep anxiety at the threat posed by the iatrochemists to Galenic medicine, but it did not succeed in its purpose of marginalising and suppressing iatrochemistry.

In one sense this was because the learned physicians and their institutions, the university faculties of medicine and the city colleges of physicians, could not close down or effectively control the sixteenth- and seventeenth-century medical market-place. The iatrochemists were, as Galenist attacks indicate, merely one group among a highly diverse range of practitioners (which included patients and their families, neighbours, charitable gentlewomen or noblewomen, clergymen and their wives, wise-women, uroscopists, astrologers, herbalists, and empirics). The survival of the iatrochemists was connected with the failure of the monopolistic aspirations of learned medicine. The regulatory powers of the Galenic institutions were limited and liable to be circumscribed. In London, Queen Elizabeth and her ministers often supported unlicensed practitioners against the London College of Physicians, and in Paris successive French kings gave their protection to Paracelsian physicians, often from Montpellier, against the faculty of medicine in Paris, and they also helped establish the Jardin des Plantes, planned in 1626 and opened in 1640 which became a centre for chemical teaching, its chemistry professors being prolific writers of chemistry textbooks.

As the seventeenth century progressed, the picture drawn of the iatrochemists by the Galenists became evermore untenable for society at large. Not only was iatrochemistry practised on an increasing scale, but it gained increasing intellectual and social respectability, especially on account of its association with two potent symbols of the post-renaissance period: modernity and Christian charity.

Ethically, as well as intellectually, iatrochemistry acquired a wide appeal. In France an outstanding example of the conjunction of iatrochemistry and charity is found in the initiatives of the Montpellier-trained iatrochemist, royal physician and one-time Huguenot, Théophraste Renaudot (1584–1653), (the 'Gazetteer'), the founder of the *Gazette*, an early and significant news periodical. Around 1630 Renaudot established the Bureau d'Adresse, which acted as a clearing house in which the poor offered their services and employers registered their labour needs – an early labour exchange. It also offered free medical advice and treatment to the sick poor. As well as listing the addresses of physicians, surgeons, and apothecaries who would give free treatment to the poor, the Bureau from around 1632 began to offer free medical consultations and treatment. The Bureau's charitable physicians were iatrochemists and their remedies were chemical.

Renaudot hoped to extend the Bureau's services to the whole of

France. He therefore devised and published in 1642 *La Presence des Absens* (*The Presence of the Absent*), a booklet of 60 pages designed to allow the sick who could not visit the Bureau in Paris to have their illness diagnosed in their absence and a course of treatment set out by the Bureau's physicians. The pamphlet provided simple diagrams of the body for the patient to mark the position of the illness and lists of symptoms to choose from. Sufferers from syphilis, who might be ashamed of their condition, could use *La Presence des Absens* and benefit from the Bureau's chemical remedies (which were seen as especially effective for syphilis) without appearing there in person.

The Bureau became an all-round power-house for iatrochemistry. As well as providing free consultations and treatment for the poor, the Bureau was given royal permission to establish chemical laboratories and furnaces for investigating the medical properties of plants, animals, and minerals. In addition, at the Bureau weekly public 'conferences' took place and moral, literary, scientific, and medical topics were debated in public (unlike other seventeenth-century learned societies, whose meetings were held in private). Paracelsian and chemical medicine figured large in the discussions.

Although the Paris faculty of medicine, which until the 1660s was staunchly Galenist, fulminated against Renaudot, it remained powerless while he enjoyed the protection of Cardinal Richelieu. With the death of Louis XIII in 1643, Richelieu, Renaudot's patron, fell from power, and the faculty quickly moved to have Renaudot banned from practising medicine in Paris. But his free consultations had set a precedent, and the Paris parliament decreed that the faculty should provide free consultations for the poor. Paracelsianism, in this example as in others, was often part of the matrix of ideas associated with radical social and medical change.

By the 1660s Galenic medicine was buckling under a variety of pressures. Most of these were intellectual, but the social and ethical disrepute associated with learned medicine had probably the most corrosive effect. In France and in England, iatrochemistry occupied in the eyes of many the ethical high ground. As befitted its demotic Paracelsian roots, iatrochemistry appeared well suited to replace Galenism and to provide the theoretical and practical medical basis for a new type of state-organised medical service for the sick poor. The cost and avarice traditionally associated over the centuries with Galenic medicine finally counted against it, making it easy to portray it as mean and obscurantist.

MEDICAL REFORM IN ENGLAND

In England at a time of revolution, iatrochemistry was also associated with attempts to reform medicine. Puritans found iatrochemistry more Christian (the pagan roots of learned medicine were stressed) and more humane. The religious sentiments of Paracelsus appealed to Puritans in the 1640s; they empathised with his intense search for personal knowledge through the light of Nature and the experience of peasants and miners. They saw it as the counterpart to the intensity of their own personal relationship with God (no longer mediated through the Roman Catholic Church) and as echoing their belief that manual experimental knowledge would unlock the secrets of nature (either through the fire of the chemists' laboratories or by the labour of miners) which had lain hidden since the fall of Adam and Eve. Paracelsian medicine thus became the preferred medicine of the Puritan reformers. For instance, the minister and physician John Webster (1610–82) called for a reform of education in his *Academiarum Examen (The Examination of Academies;* 1654) whereby universities replaced disputations with manual experience in order to understand 'the centre of nature's hidden secrets, which can never come to pass unless they have Laboratories as well as Libraries and work in the fire, better than build Castles in the air'. Webster, in the same vein, argued that Galenic medicine and its foundation, Aristotelian philosophy, should be replaced by the medical philosophy of Paracelsus and his follower Johannes Baptista van Helmont (1579–1644).

A political revolutionary was often a medical revolutionary. Nicholas Culpeper (1616–45), 'Student in Astrology and Physick' and a prolific writer of popular astrological-chemical medical books (though he was eclectic enough to publish a Galenic treatise on practical medicine), fought in the Civil War on Parliament's side, and was a radical in medicine as well as in politics. He saw the ranks of the learned as part and parcel of the system of political tyranny, declaring that priests, physicians, and lawyers most infringe the liberty of the Commonwealth. In particular he castigated the pride, ignorance, fearfulness, uncharitableness, and greed of the physicians:

> Would it not pity a man to see whol estates wasted in Physick ('all a man hath spent upon Physicians') both body and soul consumed upon outlandish rubbish?... Is it hansom and wel beseeming a Common-wealth to see a doctor ride in State, in Plush with a footcloth, and not a grain of Wit, [knowledge] but what was in print

before he was born? Send for them into a Visited House [with plague], they will answer, they dare not come. How many honest poor souls have been so cast away, will be known when the Lord shall come to make Inquisition for Blood [will try felonies, crimes deserving execution]. Send for them to a poor mans house who is not able to give them their Fee, then they will not come, and the poor Creature for whom Christ died must forfeit his life for want of money.

The Bible, the ideological font for much of the political debate of the time, was used to justify or to denigrate medicine. The learned physicians appealed to the passage in Ecclesiasticus 38.1: 'Honour a physician with the honour due unto him... for the Lord hath created him.' Culpeper, instead, referred in a garbled form to Mark 5.25, which told of 'a certain woman' who 'had suffered many things of many physicians, and had spent all that she had, and was nothing bettered, but rather grew worse.'

The popularisation of medical knowledge in the mid-seventeenth century nearly always involved an attack on learned medicine for its cost and exclusivity together with a reference to the altruistic patriotism of the author in providing for the needs of the poor. Culpeper wrote that his motive for translating the College of Physicians' pharmacopeia was:

> Pure pitty to the Commonality of England (I assure you) was the motive, the prevailing argument that set my brain and pen a work upon this subject, many of whom to my knowledge have perished either for want of money to see a Physician, or want of knowledge of a remedy happily growing in the garden.

Latin was the language of the learned and its use in medicine was attacked by Culpeper and others as the language of monopoly and greed. Their rhetoric reflected changes in medical publishing, for the international and scholarly medicine of the universities was increasingly being replaced by a locally based medicine written in the vernacular and emphasising the cure of local diseases with local remedies if possible, which the poor could afford. As Charles Webster has shown, a large number of medical books were written in English rather than in Latin between 1640 and 1660 (207 out of a total of 238). The most pressing need for reformers was that medicine should be charitable and should be made freely available both in terms of knowledge and price. Gabriel Plattes in his utopian treatise, *Macaria* (1641), wrote that 'the parson of every parish is a good physician' and that clergymen could cure both the soul and the body.

As it was, such novel schemes did not come to fruition. But equally the College and Galenic medicine did not retrieve their authority with the Restoration of Charles II in 1660. Despite an establishment backlash against the 'enthusiasm' and intense zeal of the religious sectarians, which it was felt had created the turmoil of the Civil War, old modes of learning failed to make an effective come-back. Indeed, the Crown, which gave the Royal Society its charter in 1662 (the Society was founded in 1660), was associated with the modern, experimental natural philosophy.

There were other reasons for the decline of Galenic medicine. The discovery of the circulation of the blood from within learned medicine and then the creation of a completely new natural philosophy also helped to undermine learned medicine.

The circulation of the blood

The last achievement of renaissance anatomy was perhaps its greatest, the discovery of the circulation of the blood by William Harvey, a product of the Paduan school of anatomy. It also looks forward to the destruction of Galenic physiology and to the 'new science' which in the seventeenth century replaced Aristotelian natural philosophy and thus undermined the foundations of Galenic medicine. Before discussing Harvey's discovery and the vexed question of how to interpret it, the context to Harvey's work needs to be set out by considering Galen's views on the action of the heart and on the movement of the blood, and how they were modified by renaissance anatomists.

THE HEART AND BLOOD BEFORE HARVEY

In Galen's system of physiology there were two types of blood, the venous and the arterial. Their functions were radically different. From Plato, Galen had the idea that there were three centres in the body responsible for its vegetative, vital, and rational aspects (in a sense, the human body was seen as expressing the characteristics specific to plants, animals, and humans). The liver was responsible for nutrition and growth, the heart for vitality, and the brain for sensation and reason. The ability of the body to grow and to be nourished was ensured by the venous blood which originated in the liver, whilst life and motion were conveyed to the parts of the body by the arterial blood that had its source in the heart.

Arterial blood was a mixture of pneuma (spirituous elaborated air) and blood, and, like the venous blood, it was thought to travel to all the parts of the body and to be largely used up by them. The venous blood did not move regularly, whether in a circular or back-and-forth motion, but was attracted by the different parts of the body as and when they needed nourishment, while arterial life-giving blood, moved only outwards from the heart to be absorbed by the time it reached the extremities, it did not return back to the heart. Given the very different functions of venous and arterial blood, their two different points of origin and the belief that they were used up, the idea of the circulation of the blood, that is of the same blood being regularly moved around the body, was conceptually difficult.

The heart was not involved in moving blood through the arteries. For Galen the active phase of the heart's motion was diastole, when, like a bladder filling up, it sucked in blood. He explained the motion of blood through the arteries by a pulsative faculty or power of the arteries which moved the blood.

A crucial problem raised by Galen's cardiovascular system was to explain how the ingredients of arterial blood, originally venous blood and air, got into the left ventricle of the heart where they were changed into arterial blood. Venous blood had to move from the right side of the heart to the left. Galen argued that a little blood seeped from the right to the left side of the heart through invisible pores in the interventricular septum (the fleshy wall separating the ventricles of the heart). He did not believe in the pulmonary transit of the blood, that is that the blood passed from the right to the left side of the heart by making a loop across the lungs (through the pulmonary artery into the lungs, then into the pulmonary vein, and finally into the heart). Galen stated that only just enough blood to nourish the lungs left the right side of the heart, although occasionally a little blood would travel from the lungs down the pulmonary vein to the left side of the heart. Associated with this view was Galen's refusal to accept that what we now call the pulmonary artery was an artery not only in structure but also in function (he called it the artery-like vein, and the pulmonary vein the vein-like artery). The long-held teaching, originating even before Herophilus and Erasistratus, that veins were on the right and arteries on the left side of the body probably influenced Galen, as did the fact that out of the pulmonary artery there issued venous and not arterial blood.

On the question of how air entered the heart, Galen wrote that the function of the pulmonary vein was to convey air from the lungs to the left side of the heart. The air had been partly changed to pneuma in the lungs, but in the left ventricle of the heart it was completely altered by the heat of the heart, which at the same time made the venous blood that had come into the left ventricle through the pores in the interventricular septum finer. The end result of the mixture of pneuma and blood was arterial blood. This was thinner and brighter than the dull, dark-red venous blood. The concoction of arterial blood had as a by-product sooty vapours. These travelled back along the pulmonary vein to the lungs and were then breathed out (Galen argued that the mitral valve in the heart did not close completely: it prevented blood travelling back along the pulmonary vein, but allowed the exit of sooty vapours up the vein). Thus there was a two way flow in the pulmonary vein, of air down into the heart and sooty vapours up to the lungs. In hindsight, the lack of an observational basis to many of these details (the permeable septum, the denial of the pulmonary transit, no blood or very little in the pulmonary vein, the selective competence of the mitral valve, the two-way flow of air and sooty vapours in the pulmonary vein) appears an obvious weakness in Galen's cardiovascular system. But these details were embedded in a system that explained a great deal, and, most importantly, it did so in a rational and coherent fashion (which for learned medicine after Galen was probably more important than observational accuracy). Nutrition, growth, vitality, and also sensation and the faculties of reasoning such as memory and imagination were all subsumed into a theory whose parts seemed to fit logically one into the other. (On the third part of the system, Galen had argued that a small amount of the arterial blood was changed in the *rete mirabile*, the marvellous network of very fine blood vessels, and in the ventricles of the brain into animal spirits (very attenuated, fine, and spirituous arterial blood) which flowed through the nerves and the brain conveying sensation and motion.)

RENAISSANCE VIEWS ON THE HEART AND BLOOD

In the Renaissance, anatomists begun to contradict some of the observational details of Galen's account of the blood and the heart. Vesalius, as mentioned above, in the first edition of the *Fabrica* had written that the vena cava did not originate in the liver and in the second edition had explicitly denied the permeability of the interventricular septum. But he did not develop these findings and go on to doubt Galen's physiology.

It was Realdo Colombo, Vesalius' rival at Padua, who effectively publicised the discovery of the pulmonary transit of the blood and elucidated the action of the heart, and so provided Harvey with two important cornerstones for his discovery of the circulation of the blood. Colombo, perhaps because of his initial training in surgery, took up animal vivisection experiments, which he described in his posthumous *De Re Anatomica* (*On Anatomy*; 1559). He cut the pulmonary vein of a living dog as far away as possible from the heart and found that it always contained blood and not air (in the cadaver it was also always full of blood). Colombo observed that the blood in the pulmonary vein was like arterial blood, and concluded that it was in the lungs rather than in the heart that venous blood and air were mixed and altered into 'shining, thin, and beautiful' blood. He noted that when the lungs were injured, arterial blood came out, and that they, like every other part of the body, could not exist without vital arterial blood. He also observed that the pulmonary artery was so large that it probably had another function than merely to bring nourishment for the lungs, for it apparently contained more blood than the lungs needed.

His experiments led Colombo to the realisation that blood went from the right to the left side of the heart by means of the lungs, and his rejection of the permeability of the interventricular septum merely confirmed this. For Colombo this was a transit, or movement, of blood through the lungs, which was then used up and replaced by new blood produced by the liver from chyle (and ultimately from ingested food). It was not a circulation, or as it has sometimes been termed a 'lesser circulation', of the same blood through the lungs. Colombo, although he changed some important details, kept to Galen's view of venous blood being continually attracted and used up by the parts of the body. He could not, therefore, conceive of a 'lesser circulation', let alone a systemic or general circulation.

Colombo influenced Harvey not only on the pulmonary transit but also on the difficult question of the movement of the heart. As Harvey was to point out, this was very difficult to observe, since the different movements occurred very quickly. From vivisection Colombo concluded that the active phase of the heart was when it was raised up, swollen and constricted, and not when it dilated. He also wrote that while the heart was dilating the arteries were constricted and while the heart was constricted the arteries were dilated. The Galenic view had been that the arteries dilated when the heart also dilated in diastole. Colombo clearly perceived that the heart ejected blood out into the arteries when it constricted, and at the same time the arteries felt full and dilated. This was to be a crucial point for Harvey, as it led him to consider the amount of blood that left the heart every time the heart constricted. Unfortunately, at the end of his description of the action of the heart, Colombo used the word systole when he meant diastole, which confused later anatomists until Harvey grasped Colombo's real meaning.

Other anatomists wrote on the pulmonary transit at around the same time as Colombo. Juan Valverde, Colombo's student, described it in his *De la Composicion del Cuerpo Humano* (*On the Composition of the Human Body*; 1556), but clearly attributed its discovery to his teacher. Michael Servetus (b. 1511), anatomist, astrologer, theologian, and a heretic who contrived to offend both Catholics and Protestants and was burnt at the stake in Calvin's Geneva, also had the idea of the pulmonary transit. In 1553, the year of his execution, he published the heretical work *Christianismi Restitutio* (*The Restitution of Christianity*). In it he wondered how the divine spirit entered man. From the Bible, Servetus knew that the soul was contained in the blood and that the soul was breathed into man by God (Genesis 9.4). Servetus drew upon his anatomical training in Paris with Guinther von Andernach to argue that the optimum point of contact between the blood and the soul for their mixture was the lungs, which provided a larger area than the traditional left ventricle. He denied that blood could go through the interventricular septum (though a little might 'sweat' through it); instead it went to the lungs where it mixed with air (or soul) and became arterial blood. To support his view, he pointed to the large size of the pulmonary artery which, he stated, was too large merely to transmit blood for the nourishment of the lungs alone. Servetus' ideas had no influence on Harvey or on other anatomists for most of the copies of the *Restitutio* were burned with him, and it was only in 1694 that the English antiquary, William Wootton, published Servetus' discovery. But it is worth noting Servetus' work, for it exemplifies how in the Renaissance disciplinary boundaries were often permeable, and how anatomy could be joined with religion, the dominant ideology of the age.

WILLIAM HARVEY

In 1628, William Harvey, an Englishman who had studied anatomy at Padua, published a small book the *Exercitatio Anatomica de Motu Cordis et Sanguinis in Animalibus* (*An Anatomical Essay Concerning the Movement of the Heart and the Blood in Animals*, usually referred to by its Latin abbreviation, *De Motu Cordis*). In it he announced his anatomical discovery of the circulation of the blood. It was a discovery that others saw as having revolutionary implications with profound and destructive consequences for traditional medicine. The opponents of the Aristotelian-Galenic consensus which had dominated European learning for centuries eagerly took the circulation on board. For instance, René Descartes (1596–1650) included Harvey's discovery in his *Discourse on Method* (1637), which he wrote as a new and radical alternative to the philosophy of Aristotle. But, paradoxically, Harvey himself was unwilling to accept that it was revolutionary and far-reaching. What we have, on the face of it, is a typical ancients-versus-moderns debate. Was the discovery of the circulation of the blood one of the last achievements of the learned tradition of philosophy and medicine and more specifically of the anatomical tradition in medicine? Or was it an early product of the 'new science' of the seventeenth century?

Before directly discussing the question of interpretation it is necessary first to fill in the details of Harvey's life and then to look at the structure and content of the *De Motu Cordis*, while keeping the issue of interpretation in mind.

Harvey was educated at King's School, Canterbury and, from 1593 to 1599, at Gonville and Caius College, Cambridge. He took his Bachelor of Arts degree in 1597, and it is likely that after 1597 Harvey began to study medicine at Cambridge, but he did not take his medical degree there. In 1600 he went to Padua where he studied medicine and anatomy under Fabricius, from whom he developed an interest in the Aristotelian approach to the study of nature, especially comparative anatomy and embryology. Harvey, like Fabricius, was to dissect many different animals in order to build up a single picture of how a particular organ worked. In this way Vesalius' great stress on the difference between human and animal anatomy was blurred. Both Fabricius and Harvey also focused on function more than structure, which had been Vesalius' interest. Harvey's studies on the generation of animals (he wrote a book on the subject, *Exercitationes de Generatione*

Animalium (*Essays on the Generation of Animals*; 1651)) – often referred to as *De Generatione* – also drew upon the example of Aristotle and Fabricius.

In 1602, Harvey returned to England and began to practise medicine in London. In 1607 he was elected a Fellow of the College of Physicians of London (the centre for Galenic, learned medicine) and two years later he was appointed physician to St. Bartholomew's Hospital. Harvey quickly established himself in the upper reaches of the medical profession. In 1615 he was appointed Lumleian lecturer by the College of Physicians with the duty of lecturing on anatomy and on aspects of surgery, a post he held until 1656. From 1618 he was one of the royal physicians to James I and in 1630 he became Physician to Charles I. During the Civil War Harvey was frequently with the King.

Harvey's professional career indicates he was a conservative both in national and medical politics. In the College of Physicians he was appointed to some of its highest offices. He was frequently (1613, 1625, 1626, 1629) one of the four Censors who inquired into and prosecuted unlicensed practitioners and anyone accused of malpractice. That his colleagues chose Harvey for this post means they were convinced that he believed that the learned medicine of the College, the medicine of the ancients was best. (John Aubrey reported, in 1651, that Harvey advised him on what books to read and 'he bid me goe to the fountain head and read Aristotle, Cicero, Avicen[na] and did call the neoteriques [those who believed in the new philosophies] shitt-breeches'.) Harvey did not agree with the new mechanical and chemical views of nature. As Aubrey put it, 'He did not care for Chymistry, and was wont to speake against them with an undervalue.'

Intellectually, Harvey's experience in Padua placed him at the innovative end of learned medicine, where Aristotelian ideas were challenging Galenic ones and new approaches to anatomy were being developed. However, anatomy, even in its innovatory aspect under Fabricius, lay squarely within learned medicine. Professionally, Harvey worked within a conservative milieu and shared its values. Harvey's background of exposure to the cutting edge of new work in anatomy (Fabricius) and his very establishment career may explain some of the tensions and paradoxes in his work where the significance of novelty is often limited and put into an orthodox context. However, this was also an attitude that Harvey shared with many other anatomists, and is characteristic of renaissance anatomy.

As many of Harvey's papers were lost in 1642 when Parliamentary troops plundered his London lodgings, we have few records of Harvey's practice as a physician, and there is a lack of material with which to construct his intellectual biography. However, we do possess Harvey's notes for his Lumleian lectures for 1616 on the whole of anatomy, together with the additions of later years, and they allow us to see how he was thinking about the heart and the blood before the publication of *De Motu Cordis*.

The notes show Harvey as a typical academic anatomist, setting out the different opinions on particular controversies. His main source for material was the *Theatrum Anatomicum* (*The Anatomical Theatre*; 1605) of Caspar Bauhin (1560–1624) who had also studied at Padua. In addition Harvey referred to the *Historia Anatomica* (1600) of André du Laurens, which made a point of detailing the controversies between the physicians and the philosophers (the followers of Galen and Aristotle respectively) in matters of anatomy and physiology. As well as taking an academic, disputational, approach in his lectures, Harvey introduced his own observations and used his eyes to check upon previous anatomical findings, thus following the key injunction of Paduan anatomy (and also of academic textbook writers such as Bauhin – for the need for observation was embedded in the anatomical textbooks of the late sixteenth and early seventeenth centuries). Significantly, the lectures begin with the statement that 'anatomy is a discipline which '[deals with] the uses and actions of the parts [of the body] by eyesight inspection and by dissection'. Not only should the stress on observation be noted, but also Harvey's emphasis on the uses and actions of the parts, echoing Fabricius' view that after Vesalius this was what was left to anatomy to discover.

In the lecture notes, Harvey shows that he had taken some of the initial steps towards the discovery of the circulation. He had repeated and confirmed Colombo's work on the pulmonary transit of the blood (a finding now widely accepted by the younger anatomists), and in the notes it is clear that Harvey had concluded that the heart acted as a muscle with the ventricles contracting and forcibly ejecting blood outwards in systole rather than sucking it in during diastole. Essentially Harvey agreed with Colombo, and he sorted out the confusion in the *De Re Anatomica* between the terms systole and diastole. The circulation of the blood was very briefly mentioned in a late addition to the manuscript inserted, perhaps, around 1627.

DE MOTU CORDIS

De Motu Cordis itself is brief and to the point. The book divides naturally into two parts. In the first half of *De Motu Cordis*, Harvey began by pointing out the inconsistencies and contradictions of Galen's views of the movement of air and blood to the heart. He wondered how the mitral valve allows sooty vapours back along the pulmonary vein but not blood, and how the air and the sooty vapours are kept separate in the pulmonary vein, and he stresses that if the vein was opened, neither air nor vapours were to be found, but only blood. Harvey then proceeded, more positively, to demonstrate, in the anatomical sense of pointing out to the eye, the action of the auricles and the ventricles of the heart and the existence of the pulmonary transit of the blood. As his reader could not be at the dissecting table, Harvey described what it is that can be seen from the dissections and vivisections that he conducted. He wrote that he looked for himself to see the movements of the heart, but he found this very difficult: 'This was because of the rapidity of the movement, which in many animals remained visible but for the wink of an eye and the length of a lightning flash.'

He solved the problem by vivisecting frogs, small fishes, and other cold blooded organisms whose hearts were simpler and moved more slowly and distinctly than those in warm blooded animals. He also observed the hearts of dying dogs and pigs because then their hearts moved more languidly. In chapter six, Harvey forcibly argued that comparative anatomy should be used in order to produce a general picture of how the heart worked in all animals:

> those persons do wrong who while wishing, as all anatomists commonly do, to describe, demonstrate and study the parts of animals, content themselves with looking inside one animal only, namely man – and that one dead..... (like those who think they can construct a science of politics after exploration of a single form of government or have a knowledge of agriculture through investigation of a single field).

In chapters six and seven, Harvey demonstrated that the blood moves through the lungs, and he acknowledged Colombo's work on the subject. Up to this point Harvey had not written anything new, though he had been far more coherent, detailed, and exhaustive than Colombo, as one would expect in a specialised treatise.

It was in chapter eight of *De Motu Cordis* that Harvey came to novel matters, for in it he announced his discovery of the circulation of the blood. His fear of offending all men is more than conventional platitude, a conservative was being forced by his discovery to contradict ancient authority:

> The remaining matters, however .... are so novel and hitherto unmentioned that, in speaking of them, I not only fear that I may suffer from the ill-will of a few, but dread lest all men turn against me. To such an extent is it virtually second nature for all to follow accepted usage and teaching.... to such an extent are men swayed by a pardonable respect for the ancient authors.

Nevertheless, Harvey believed that someone with an eye trained in anatomy would agree with him – here the primacy that he and other anatomists gave to observation, especially by those trained in using their eyes was very clear, 'However, the die has now been cast, and my hope lies in the love of truth and the clear-sightedness of the trained mind'.

Harvey made quantitative experiments which indicated that far too much blood left the heart in a given time for it to have been absorbed by the body and replaced by blood made in the liver from the chyle pro-duced from the ingested food. The quantitative argument led to the conclusion that the blood must move continually in a circle, otherwise the arteries and the body would burst. The problem was to show the pathways of the circular movement. Harvey could not see the very minute connections, the capillaries, between the arteries and the veins (he was using a magnifying glass and not the newly discovered micro-scope). However, he showed that a connection must exist by means of a simple experiment which involved ligating, or tying a cord, around the arm. He ligated an arm very tightly so that no arterial blood could flow below the ligature down the arm. He then loosened the ligature so that arterial blood flowed down the arm, but the ligature remained tight enough to stop venous blood from moving up above the ligature. Whereas when the ligature had been very tight the veins in the arm below the ligature had appeared normal, now they became swollen, and this indicated that blood had moved down the arteries and then back up the arm inside the veins, so at the extremities there had to be connections for the blood to travel from the arteries to the veins. The last part of Harvey's anatomical demonstration of the circulation was to show that the valves in the veins always directed blood back to the heart and did not act, as Fabricius had believed, to prevent the lower parts of the body from flooding with blood.

334

After he had shown that there was a circulation and traced its pathways, Harvey was then able, in chapter 16, to point to previously puzzling phenomena, such as the rapid spread of poisons through the body, and to explain them by the circulation. At the same time, the existence of such phenomena was further support for the circulation. In the last chapter (17), Harvey, in a similar way, produced anatomical evidence, such as the greater thickness of the arteries near the heart, which, he argued, had been constructed in a purposeful way by nature to withstand the greater force exerted by the movement of the blood near the heart. This, he believed, supported his findings on the action of the heart (the forcible ejection of blood by the heart in systole) earlier in *De Motu Cordis*.

THE INTERPRETATION OF *DE MOTU CORDIS*

At first sight the work of Harvey looks very modern. He carried out experiments and he quantified. Both were to be constituents of the new science of the seventeenth century which replaced the qualitative Aristotelian view of nature by a mechanical and quantitative natural philosophy or science. The new science that men like Galileo, Descartes, Newton, and Boyle created conceived the world no longer in terms of qualities and elements but as consisting of particles of measurable sizes, and shapes and motions.

Harvey's methods appear to look forward to this new science for they seem to indicate a desire to quantify and a wish to act upon nature and discover her secrets. However, Harvey never deserted his Aristotelianism, and he was to reject the new science explicitly. Harvey did not see the body in a mechanical fashion – it was not a machine, but was enlivened and filled with vital forces. In chapters eight and 15 Harvey set out the reasons that impelled him to concentrate on the heart and to think of the circulation. He also considered the purpose of the circulation; for unlike the protagonists of the new science Harvey believed that teleology mattered. His language and ideas were vitalistic and heavily impregnated with Aristotelian concepts such as the belief that the heart was the most important organ of the body (Galen thought that it was the brain). The purpose of the circulation, wrote Harvey, using the traditional comparison between the macrocosm (the world) and the microcosm (the little world of man), was to transport life-giving blood to the periphery and then to bring it back to the heart where it could be enlivened again:

> So in all likelihood it comes to pass in the body, that all the parts
> are nourished, cherished, and quickned with blood, which is warm,
> perfect, vaporous, full of spirit, and, that I may so say, alimentative:
> in the parts the blood is refrigerated, coagulated, and made as it
> were barren, from thence it returns to the heart, as to the fountain
> or dwelling-house of the body, to recover its perfection, and there
> again by naturall heat, powerfull, and vehement, it is melted, and
> is dispens'd again through the body from thence, being fraught
> with spirits, as with balsam, and that all the things do depend upon
> the motional pulsation of the heart: So the heart is the beginning of
> life, the Sun of the Microcosm, as proportionably the Sun deserves
> to be call'd the heart of the world, by whose virtue, and pulsation,
> the blood is mov'd perfected, made vegetable, and is defended from
> corruption, and mattering; and this familiar household-god doth
> his duty to the whole body, by nourishing, cherishing, and vegetat-
> ing, being the foundation of life, and author of all'. (From the 1653
> translation.)

Given this type of language it is very difficult to place Harvey within
the new science of the seventeenth century. His basic ideas of how and
why the parts of the body worked as they did was Aristotelian. Harvey
not only shared with Aristotle (and Galen) a teleological view of the
body but also the belief that its uses were to be viewed as the powers or
faculties of the soul. This is why for Harvey the action of the heart was
kept going by a pulsative faculty, whilst Descartes, who rejected such
vitalistic explanations, believed that the heart acted mechanically,
rather like a combustion engine. (See p. 340.)

THE 'WAY OF THE ANATOMISTS'

It was not in the new philosophies that Harvey found his inspiration.
What gave him a sense of certainty about his work was the anatomists'
credo to see for oneself. Harvey was sure that he had *seen* the action of
the heart, the pulmonary transit and the circulation. In the *Second
Essay to Jean Riolan* (1649) he distinguished clearly between knowledge
of the existence of the fact of the circulation and knowledge of its purpose. He wrote that one had at times to talk of the causes of fevers, of
plague, or of drugs, yet he added, because we are ignorant of those
causes it does not mean that we deny their existence. So also with the
circulation:

> this is that I did endeavour to relate and lay open by my observa-
> tions and experiments and not to demonstrate by causes and

approvable principles, but to render it confirmed by senses and experience, as by the greater authority, according to the way of the Anatomists.

The way of the anatomist was based on observation, and this was more certain than the discussion of causes, which in chapters eight and 15 of *De Motu Cordis* he calls only 'probable.'

For Harvey anatomical experience had to be personal experience, seeing for oneself. Words were of no use. In *De Motu Cordis* Harvey wrote that 'I profess to learn and teach anatomy not from books but from dissections, not from the tenets of Philosophers but from the fabric of Nature'. The image of nature replacing books and their authority is a powerful and subversive one in this period. For Harvey nature was much more trustworthy than writers, and so personal knowledge of Nature had to replace public knowledge embodied in books. This belief in Nature as *the* authority is what leads Harvey to write that he teaches as well as learns anatomy from Nature. In order to teach, Harvey must take the reader to Nature herself: hence he must be given instructions how to see what Harvey had seen. Harvey constantly argued that books are no substitute for personally experienced knowledge.

> For whosoever they be that read the words of Authors and do not by this aid of their own senses abstract therefore true representations of the things themselves as they are described in the authors words, they do not conceive in their own minds aught but deceitful eidola and vein fancies and never true ideas. And so they frame certain shadows and chimaeras and all their theory and contemplation which, none the less they count knowledge, represents nothing but waking men's dreams and sick men's fancies. (*De Generatione.*)

Even theories and ideas, it seems, need to be checked by observation, if they are initially founded, or depend, upon observation.

Harvey believed that there were only two ways that the truth of an observation could be confirmed or grasped. He wrote in the Letter to Dr. Argent at the beginning of *De Motu Cordis* that the circulation had been confirmed by 'very many reliable witnesses'. Many eyes, especially if they were trained eyes, helped to ensure the truth of an observation. But, more importantly, Harvey believed that his reader had to see the observations and repeat the experiments that showed the circulation in order to have true knowledge of it.

In the end, it was Harvey's belief in the certainty of observational knowledge which gave him the confidence to defend his views. As he wrote in reply to Jean Riolan the Younger (1580–1657), the circulation of the blood was a fact of observation:

> it behoves him, whoever is desirous to learn, to see anything which is in question, if it be obvious to sense, and sight, whether it be so or no or else be bound to believe those that have made trial, for by no other clearer or more evident certainty can he learn or be taught. Who will persuade a man that has not tasted them, that sweet or new wine is better than water? With what arguments shall one persuade a blind man that the Sun is clear, and outshines all the Stars in the firmament? So concerning the Circulation...

Harvey's empiricism, his stress on observation and experimentation, might seem to lie within the new science. In fact its roots are to be found in Aristotle and Galen, for they also extolled the use of the senses, and in the renaissance anatomical tradition. Harvey was working within learned medicine and philosophy and they provided him with the intellectual means to create his empirical philosophy. Perhaps the question has been put wrongly by historians – it is not whether Harvey belonged to the new science (he would have repudiated the suggestion), but 'what did the new science gain from the renaissance anatomists and from Harvey?'

AFTERMATH

The major attack on Harvey's discovery came when Jean Riolan the Younger an anatomist with a European reputation and a leading Galenist in the conservative Paris Faculty of Medicine, tried to save Galenic medicine by limiting the effect of Harvey's circulation. Riolan realised that the circulation in its Harveian form had the potential to destroy Galenic physiology, for the liver could no longer be the blood-making organ of the body. Moreover, Galenic therapeutics was put in doubt because the rationale for bleeding, one of the major therapeutic procedures, had been damaged. For instance, the debate about the place where one bled and its relation to where the body was diseased, which had occupied physicians in the first half of the sixteenth century, was rendered meaningless now that the same blood went round the body. Riolan tried to produce a compromise. In his *Encheiridium Anatomicum et Pathologicum* (*An Anatomical and Pathological Handbook*; 1648) and in his *Opuscula Anatomica Nova* (*New Anatomical Studies*; 1649) Riolan conceded that there was a rather sluggish circulation in the aorta and vena cava, whilst in their offshoots, especially in the intestinal region, the blood did not circulate. In this way he tried to combine the circulation with a Galenic physiology where the liver still functioned to produce blood. Harvey replied to Riolan in 1649 in his two *Essays* published as *Exercitatio Anatomica de Circulatione Sanguinis* (*Anatomical Exercise on the Circulation of the Blood*). In the *First Essay*, Harvey showed that observationally Riolan's position was untenable, for the blood in *all* the arteries moved with force and in definite quantities, which clearly indicated the circulation. In the *Second Essay*, Harvey ranged more generally, giving new experiments in support of the circulation, and emphasising, as we have seen, how his philosophy of knowledge was based on observation and reflected Aristotle's own position.

Perhaps the most interesting reaction to Harvey's work came from René Descartes (1596–1650). Descartes saw the body as he saw the world, in mechanical terms. His new and influential philosophy was one which reduced biological processes to mechanical events. If the Aristotelian–Galenic consensus produced a common explanation for the macrocosm and the microcosm, so did Descartes' new philosophy. Instead of qualities, elements, and humours, matter in motion would now equally explain the world and the body.

In chapter five of the *Discourse on Method* (1637) Descartes discussed the circulation of the blood, which he believed could support his new philosophy. He carried out anatomical dissections which backed up Harvey's discovery of the systemic circulation of the blood. But he did not agree with Harvey on the action of the heart. Harvey's pulsative faculty, ultimately stemming from the soul, that kept the beat of the heart going was viewed with distaste by Descartes. In his philosophy the soul was no longer in the body and had no material existence; moreover, all the actions of the body had to have a mechanical explanation. Harvey's account of the heart was one based on vitalistic forces (for instance, his description of how the heart revivified the blood) which could not be explained mechanically, and so had to be rejected.

Descartes gave an alternative description of the action of the heart. He argued that the heart was active in diastole (rather than in systole), when its innate heat (like that of the heat inside a haystack) rarefied drops of blood in its chambers and made them expand and eject particles of blood out into the arteries. The smallest and fastest particles of blood went on to become the animal spirits that flowed through the brain, nerves, and muscles conveying sensation and motion. In this way

Descartes' heart was like a mechanical engine which gave motion to the rest of the body. It was started up by God, who put the initial heat into the heart, but God was acceptable to the mechanical philosophers.

By the 1660s the circulation of the blood was generally accepted. At this time the new mechanical philosophies were rapidly replacing the old order. But Harvey, even in his later work, never agreed with any of them. In his last book, *De Generatione* Harvey went beyond Aristotle, but only in the sense that he took Aristotle's vitalistic theories to their unmechanical extremes. He argued for a non-materialistic process of generation 'beyond the power of the elements' and in his old age confirmed that he remained unaffected by the new thinking:

> likewise in the Blood, there is a spirit of virtue, doth act above the power of the Elements (most conspicuous in the nutrition or preservation of each particular part) and also a nature, nay a soul in that spirit and the blood answerable in proportion to the elements of the Stars.

The new science

At a fundamental level the new mechanical philosophy replaced the Aristotelian cosmos of qualities and elements with a universe made from particles in motion, a universe which obeyed mathematical laws of motion. Just as Aristotelian natural philosophy had formed the basis for much of Galenic learned medicine, so the new philosophy which replaced it became the foundation of much of medicine. But it was not a complete take-over. A great deal of therapeutics remained untouched, and some of the more mechanical approaches to the body (comparing the body to a machine and implicitly questioning the role and existence of the soul) appeared too extreme to some.

Between 1660 and 1700, for reasons which still remain obscure (though historians have poured vials of vitriol over each other when debating them), European learned culture in large measure accepted the new philosophy, and its experimental and mathematical approaches to the study of nature. Possible factors encouraging this process include the practical work ethic of Protestantism, an increasing secularisation and demystification which, in England was given added impetus by the reaction that set in after the Restoration of Charles II in 1660 to the religious 'enthusiasm' of the Civil War period, and the growth of the absolutist state as in the France of Louis XIV. Such reasons may explain the popularity of a new view of nature, based on ideas of order, regularity, and of law-like behaviour with little scope allowed for any intervention by God on a day-to-day basis upon natural events, and also giving hope for practical technological results.

In England, which in the second half of the seventeenth century was *the* centre of the new science, an epistemology based on gaining knowledge from observation and experimentation became the norm and was contrasted with the wordy disputations of the 'rational' or learned physician. The institutional stronghold of Galenic medicine in England, the London College of Physicians, was in disarray. In 1665 a Society of Chemical Physicians was being planned in London and, although it was not in the end established, the project added to the sense of pressure felt by the College. By the late 1660s the College was weak and divided into factions, some members taking a Galenic approach, others a chemical one, whilst a few were sympathetic to the experimental philosophy of the Royal Society.

The Royal Society, the institutional flagship of the new science, was hostile to the old learning. Its members often attacked the Galenic physicians of the College in lively pamphlet wars. The Royal Society did not share the Galenists' contempt for empirical knowledge and empirics: indeed it came close to eliding the difference between the 'respectable' seeker after empirical knowledge whose motives were unsullied by commercial motives and the empirics of the medical market place. For instance, Robert Boyle (1627–91), who as the seventh son of the Earl of Cork inherited private means, was intensely interested in the chemical remedies of the empirics and the 'chemists' shops'. Such an interest helped to give respectability to the traditional enemies of Galenic medicine.

Moreover, the Society assiduously collected a hodge-podge of medical information about specific cures, the occurrence of monstrosities, and reports of diseases, all in the hope of putting together a natural history (a data-base of empirical information, sorted out into specific categories) which would provide the foundation for generalisations and universal laws in the inductive manner of the Society's source of philosophical inspiration, Francis Bacon (p. 343). Henry Oldenburg (1618?–77), the Secretary of the Royal Society, acted as an exchange centre for such empirical information. What before was disreputable and unacceptable to the old learning could be acceptable to the new learning. For instance, Boyle and Oldenburg were open-minded about the cures of the Irishman, Valentine Greatrakes (1629–83), 'the Stroaker' who healed by the laying on of hands in England in 1665.

Although Robert Boyle attempted to apply the mechanical philosophy to chemistry and to create a 'corpuscular philosophy' (in which chemical substances had particular arrangements of particles) that he hoped would replace both the Aristotelian four elements and the Paracelsian *tria prima*, iatrochemistry in its Paracelsian form remained buoyant until the last years of the seventeenth century. It influenced medicine throughout Europe and was often taken to be part of the new science. The work of Johannes Baptista van Helmont (1579–1644), the Flemish follower of Paracelsus, had gained wide currency and had revitalised Paracelsian chemistry by providing it with a down-to-earth approach (the use of chemical tests, quantification, the development of an idea of gas) whilst preserving a spiritual dimension to the chemical interpretation of matter as well as a strong Christian ethic. By the end of the seventeenth century the influence of Paracelsian medicine was on the wane, though chemistry in a corpuscular and mechanical guise was permeating the language of medicine.

In the Netherlands, the theoretical framework of the new science was generally accepted by the 1660s by many physicians but their energies went less into the making or extension of theories and more into observing and collecting information. In the 'Golden Age' of seventeenth-century Holland, the riches that came from trade paid for new anatomy theatres and herbal gardens like the one created by the Amsterdam city council in 1682. As the economic balance of power moved from Southern to Northern Europe the towns of Holland followed in the footsteps of the wealthy Italian cities of the previous century in encouraging the investigation of the body and the collection of nature's remedies.

In France the new philosophy of Descartes became dominant in the later seventeenth century. Although some universities continued to teach Aristotelian philosophy and Galenic medicine (as also in Italy) Descartes' physics were increasingly being taught in the two-year college courses (at the *collèges de plein exercise* which lay between schools and universities). The Académie Royale des Sciences, founded by Louis XIV in 1666 with salaried members and a well equipped anatomy theatre and chemical laboratories, contained France's scientific élite. Its members followed Descartes' version of the mechanical philosophy in physics, though in medicine the physician-academicians ranged from Galenists to iatrochemists and iatromechanists (the latter applied mechanics to medicine especially to anatomy and physiology). The Académie, unlike the Royal Society, was under government control and in 1686, for instance, when the king failed to respond to medication, it was ordered to discover new effective drugs, especially new herbal remedies. In the meantime the Académie had been chemically analysing remedies and carrying out a number of vivisection experiments. The picture that emerges is similar to that in England – largely haphazard empirical investigations usually in a chemical setting.

The effect of the new science on medicine was not uniform. This was partly because the nature of the new science was unclear and many different approaches came under its umbrella, and partly because medicine was a well established discipline with its own research interests, which, as in anatomy and medical botany, could be loosely integrated with the new science and share in its 'modern' label.

The relationship of medicine to the new science was complicated because the new science appeared in many guises. There were a number of different mechanical philosophies, for instance, Pierre Gassendi's (1592–1655), Descartes', Robert Boyle's and Isaac Newton's (1642–1727), and it was not until well into the eighteenth century that Newton's was invoked throughout Europe as the true mechanical philosophy, though Newtonianism was to mean many different things in different times and places.

There were also different styles of doing science. The English, following the philosophy of Francis Bacon (1561–1625), tended to favour an empirical and experimental approach. In the *Advancement of Learning* (1605) and in the *Novum Organum* (*New Organ*; 1620) Bacon had set out a programme for replacing Aristotelian learning. The sources of knowledge were to be observations, natural histories and experiments. By a process of logical induction the natural philosopher or scientist would progress from observations and arrive at generalisations and universal laws. Bacon's philosophy was one which encouraged a co-operative collective scientific effort (in *New Atlantis* (1627) Bacon set out a utopian vision of joint scientific endeavour) and in its early years the Royal Society saw Bacon as its exemplar.

In France, Descartes' followers began, not with observation, but with first principles created out of clear and distinct ideas in the mind. Descartes was by inclination a model builder. From general first principles he deduced how the world (and the body) might work mechanically. Experimentation and observation were usually to be employed at

343

the end of the deductive process to test the model against reality – though information from the outside world could also help to shape knowledge, as in Descartes' anatomical dissections.

Descartes' philosophy was an intensely personal one. Like Bacon he was sceptical of past authorities and of old learning. Moreover, like Bacon and later English experimentalists, he stressed the need for personal experience in order for knowledge to be valid (something that was to some extent also part of the earlier anatomical tradition). However, Descartes believed that what had to be personally experienced or perceived was not the outside world but the innate ideas which served as the foundation for reasoning out of the nature of the world. Such ideas were common to everyone and, as Descartes put it, they could be known to be true only if they had been personally perceived clearly and distinctly in one's own mind; it was not enough to rely on other people's opinions.

Pointing out such philosophical differences and similarities presents too tidy a picture of the new science in the seventeenth century. The development of the new science took decades and the old and the new learning could be mixed. Francis Glisson (1597–1677), who although a long-serving member of the College of Physicians of London was influenced by Bacon and Descartes and was an early member of the Royal Society, united scholastic disputation and terminology with experimentation, anatomy and chemistry. Rather than seeing the body as an inanimate machine, he ascribed the property of irritability to its parts in the *Tractatus de Ventriculo et Intestinis* (*Treatise on the Stomach and Intestines*; 1677), and earlier in 1672 in the *Tractatus de Natura Substantiae Energetica* (*Treatise on the Energetic Nature of Substance*) Glisson tried to show that all types of matter contained life. This deeply felt need to prevent the world from being reduced to complete lifelessness indicates the anxieties that might be aroused by too rigid an application of the mechanical philosophy which recurred throughout the seventeenth and eighteenth centuries.

Newton, the dominant figure in late seventeenth-century science, does not fit into neat categories. He could be an experimentalist in the Baconian manner (at least in his own mind), but he also went beyond Descartes in his use of mathematics in the *Philosophiae Naturalis Principia Mathematica* (*Mathematical Principles of Natural Philosophy*; 1687). Moreover, by his ascription of gravitational force to matter he appeared to some to be introducing the occult forms and powers of the

Aristotelian philosophy which many mechanical philosophers explicitly denied existed. Newton's life-long interest in alchemy is also at variance with an interpretation which sees the science of Kepler, Galileo, Descartes and Newton as the origin of our modern demystified science, from which God, let alone alchemy, has been largely banished. In fact, for the seventeenth-century mechanical philosophers God was still at the centre of their enterprise, for they were intent on revealing the laws and workmanship of God in order to praise Him and to confirm His existence.

The mechanical philosophy did have some profound implications for medicine. Most influential, even for those who did not agree with him, was Descartes' image of the body as a machine. He argued that it worked mechanically like the rest of the world, and was not kept alive and in motion by any activity of the soul. As he put it in the *Passions of the Soul* (1649), the body does not die because the soul leaves it, but rather because one of the body's principal parts has broken down, just as a 'watch or other automaton' stops when its parts are broken. This new materialistic and mechanistic view of the body as devoid of vital forces was based on Descartes' separation of the body from the mind. The former was material like the rest of the world, whilst the latter was immaterial. The source of the distinction was the famous statement 'cogito ergo sum' ('I think therefore I am'), which in the *Discourse on Method* Descartes took as the unshakable first principle upon which to base his new philosophy. He wrote that the truth of the statement did not depend upon the outside world or his body but upon the activity of thinking, for the world and his body could cease to exist, but as long as he was thinking he knew that he existed. Thought was immaterial, hence the mind was distinct from the material body.

Descartes' vision of life reduced to or equated with a mechanistic physics was fully developed in his *Treatise of Man*, written before 1637 but suppressed by him and not published until 1662, twelve years after his death, by which time his views were finding a favourable response. In the *Treatise* Descartes allowed human beings to have some degree of free will. He stated that the pineal gland at the base of the brain acted as a valve directing the flow of 'animal spirits' (Descartes was using the traditional terminology) composed of fine, quickly moving particles derived from the blood, which travelled through the nerves, muscles, and brain conveying sensation and motion. The mind could, by an effort of the will, control the action of the pineal gland on the animal spirits and consequently affect the body's movements. The pineal gland was thus the link between the mind and the body. But Descartes stressed that most actions were automatic, and that in the case of animals this was so for all their actions. In 1748 Julien de la Mettrie (1709–51) took the further step and declared that, man like animals, was a machine.

Not everyone agreed with Descartes. In the eyes of some he came close to eliminating the human soul, and his views might be considered as heretical, as happened at the Calvinist University of Utrecht in 1641, and in 1653 when the Pope declared Jansenism, a Catholic sect with a belief in predestination and in Cartesianism, heretical. Opposition to Cartesianism also came from England, where Newton (who, in fact, drew deeply on Descartes' work) set an example by attacking the mathematical and physical validity of Descartes' cosmos. There was a deep seated suspicion of Descartes' *a priori* method (i.e. beginning with first principles) and of his emphasis on the mind rather than the senses as the source of knowledge. This had implications for the theory of how we learn and understand (what later came to be called psychology). John Locke presented a radical alternative to Descartes in his *Essay Concerning Human Understanding* (1690), where he argued that ideas were not inborn but were formed out of everyday experience and sensations, especially when the latter constantly recurred in association with particular objects and events. Locke was a physician and philosopher who believed in experiment as the key to elucidating the details of the mechanical philosophy, and his theory of understanding was a justification of his empirical approach.

As this new learning, with a new interpretation of the world and new categories of what was acceptable for the investigator to study, was by-passing Galenic medicine, so developments within medicine also were pushing Galenic medicine to the sidelines. The potentially destructive significance of Harvey's discoveries for Galenic physiology became increasingly acceptable to the medical world. Moreover, new anatomical structures unknown to Galen were being discovered and they were given physiological interpretations antithetical to Galenic physiology. In 1622, Gaspare Aselli (1581–1625) saw the lacteal vessels. Their significance became apparent when Jean Pecquet (1622–74) described in 1651 the thoracic duct (the major vessel of the lymphatic system) and its connection with the venous system. Aselli had believed that the lacteals transmitted chyle to the liver to be made into blood, Pecquet's discovery that the chyle flowed into the vena cava and thence to the heart, put together with the Harveian circulation, was taken to have completely destroyed the food–chyle–blood system centred around a blood-making liver that was fundamental to Galenic physiology.

Galenic and renaissance anatomy of the brain was given a new direction by Thomas Willis (1621–75). Like Boyle, Willis believed in a chemical version of the mechanical philosophy and was a member of a group of Oxford experimentalists (p. 349), and placed his anatomical work into a chemical mechanical framework. In his *Cerebri Anatome* (*Anatomy of the Brain*; 1664), Willis traced and classified the cranial nerves more accurately (in modern eyes) and crucially he located the functions of the brain not in the ventricles as medieval anatomists had done, but in the different parts of the brain matter itself. He focused attention on the cerebrum and cerebellum – in the former movement and ideas were generated, whilst the latter controlled involuntary movements. His comparative studies on the anatomy of many different animals (he wrote that he had 'slain so many victims, whole Hecatombs almost of all Animals, in the Anatomical Court') indicated that the cerebellum was similar in all animals but that the cerebrum varied. Willis located traditional functions of the brain in different parts of its substance (imagination in the corpus callosum, the 'common senses' were in the corpora striata, memories were brought to mind by the animal spirits passing back along the convolutions of the cortex upon which previous sensations had left their marks). The animal spirits, Willis asserted, flowed through the different parts of the brain's flesh and evoked and transmitted ideas, sensation, memory, and imagination.

In the *Pathologiae Cerebri et Nervosi Generis Specimen* (*A Model of a Kind of Cerebral and Nervous Pathology*; 1667) Willis related psychological disorders to brain structures and also, using his favourite chemical explanations, described muscular contraction as a reaction that occurred when spirituo-saline particles from the animal spirits mixed with nitrosulfurous particles and exploded 'like the explosion of Gunpowder', thus inflating and contracting the muscle.

Willis' anatomy was congenial to his fellow English experimental philosophers. It was put into the right experimental mechanical framework, and it avoided theological controversy, for in *De Anima Brutorum* (*On the Soul of Animals*; 1672) Willis took care to give human beings a rational, immortal soul and a second physical or 'brutish' soul consisting of two parts: one located in the blood governing vitality, the other in the nerves and brain controlling sense and motion. His studies were centred on the 'brutish' soul. Willis' anatomy had less influence on continental Europe, where the Danish anatomist Niels Steno (1638–86) declared that both Descartes and Willis speculated too much, and that Willis' views were merely a modification of those of the ancients. In the wider sphere of medicine, Willis, who had a successful practice, was probably better known at the time for his writings on practical medicine such as his study of fevers and of the use of cinchona bark for fever than for his anatomical work.

The microscope also helped to move anatomy and physiology beyond the confines of Galenic knowledge. Invented between 1590 and 1609 in the Netherlands and then developed by Galileo, it became a serious aid for anatomists in the second half of the century. As Robert Hooke (1635–1703), Curator of Experiments and later Secretary to the Royal Society, put it in his *Micrographia* (1665), the remedies for the faults of human reason could come only 'from the real, the mechanical, the experimental Philosophy' whose 'groundwork' is 'sense'. The new science in English eyes had to be based on sensory knowledge, as Francis Bacon had taught. The microscope improved such knowledge, and Hooke wrote:

> The next care to be taken in respect of the Senses, is a supplying of their infirmities with instruments, and, as it were, the adding of artificial Organs to the natural; this in one of them has been of late years accomplisht with prodigious benefit to all sorts of useful knowledge, by the invention of Optical Glasses..... By this [the microscope] the Earth it self, which lyes so neer us, under our feet, shews quite a new thing to us, and in every little particle of its matter, we now behold almost as great a variety of Creatures, as we were able before to reckon up in the whole Universe it self.

Hooke's book was a celebration of what the microscope could discover in general (he showed how nettles and vipers stung, as well as depicting the magnified parts of spiders, ants, and other insects). But it soon became an instrument for the specialist researcher. The Italian comparative anatomist and embryologist Marcello Malpighi (1628–94) used a microscope to study the lungs of frogs. In his *De Pulmonibus* (*On the Lungs*; 1661) he provided the missing piece in the Harveian demonstration of the circulation. He described very thin vessels in the lungs of the frog which connected the veins with the arteries, something that

Harvey had to infer by the use of ligatures. Malpighi also used the microscope to see what we call the taste buds in the tongue with a nerve leading into each one of them and he also employed it in his investigation into how the liver and kidney functioned, in his dissections of the silkworm, and in his embryological studies. (The work of Malpighi and of Francesco Redi (1626–98), who showed experimentally that the popular belief in the spontaneous generation of maggots from decaying meat was impossible if flies were prevented from contact with the meat, indicates that medical-biological research continued to flourish in Italy despite the decline in Italian astronomy and physics in the later seventeenth century.)

Experimental investigations in physiology served further to make Galenic medicine appear irrelevant. The problem of respiration and the question of what it was in the blood that gave life to the body especially concerned a group of English researchers. Harvey had pointed out the contradictions in the Galenic theory of respiration, but he had not replaced it with a clearly developed alternative. From his later extant works it is clear that Harvey came to believe that life was located in the blood rather than in the heart as he had stated in *De Motu Cordis*. What was life-giving in the blood and how it got there became the focus of what we might call a post-Harveian research project located mainly at Oxford from the late 1640s to the mid-1660s, and involving a great deal of experimental vivisection, whose results were interpreted along mechanical or chemical lines or by using a combination of both. The role of air, or of something in the air, was quickly seen as crucial. Air began to acquire characteristics and properties. In 1643 the Italian mathematicians and followers of Galileo, Vincenzo Viviani (1621–1703) and Evangelista Torricelli (1608–47), showed that there was a pressure or weight associated with atmospheric air and that this determined how far a column of mercury could rise in a tube (the gap at the top of the tube was interpreted by some as a vacuum). Instruments too played an increasing role in the new discipline of pneumatics and in laboratory-based physiology. The force or 'spring' of the air was illustrated by the use of the air pump, originally derived from Otto von Guericke's (1602–86) well pump, which pumped out water from containers. In his 'Magdeburg experiment' of 1654 the force of a vacuum was demonstrated when teams of horses unsuccessfully tried to pull apart two metal hemispheres from which the air had been pumped out. In England when Robert Boyle read of Guericke's experiments, he got his assistant, Robert Hooke, to devise an air pump which was used to create vacua or partial vacua in containers. Animals were placed in the containers and their behaviour under different conditions noted. Their need for fresh air and their nearness to death, the greater the amount of 'exhausted air' (air breathed out), was observed, as was the effect of pumping out more and more air. It was clear that there were different types of air.

Experimentation on animals became common, and increasing skill enabled animals to be kept alive longer. In 1664 Hooke proposed an experiment in which a dog would be artificially ventilated 'by displaying his whole thorax, to see how long, by blowing into his lungs, life might be preserved, and whether anything could be discovered concerning the mixture of air with the blood in the lungs'.

There was soon general agreement that the air did unite with the blood in the lungs. Richard Lower (1631–91), one of the Oxford group, demonstrated that the blood leaving the lungs in the pulmonary vein had acquired the bright red colour of arterial blood before it reached the heart, so that Descartes' belief that blood was heated up in the heart became redundant (Lower felt the heart, and in his *Tractatus de Corde* (*Treatise On the Heart*; 1669) stated that it was not especially warm). Like Hooke, Lower blew into the lungs of a dog with bellows, with blood being forced into the lungs from the vena cava. As long as air was being blown into the lungs the blood in the pulmonary vein was bright, but when the bellows were stopped and the trachea blocked, the blood became dark and dull. Lower then performed an *in vitro* experiment to replicate what was taking place in the dog:

> That this red colour is entirely due to the penetration of particles of air into the blood is quite clear from the fact that, while the blood becomes red throughout its mass in the lungs (because the air diffuses in them through all the particles, and hence becomes thoroughly mixed with the blood), when venous blood is collected in a vessel its surface takes on this scarlet colour from exposure to air.

Lower also noted that when venous blood in a container was shaken and mixed with air it became bright red, the consequence, he believed, of a 'nitrous spirit' in the air entering into the blood and giving it its bright colour. His younger contemporary John Mayow (1645–79), who, like Lower, studied medicine at Oxford, used a mixture of the mechanical philosophy and chemistry to explain that the special part of the air, responsible for its elasticity, for its ability to support combustion

and for the colour of arterial blood, was composed of nitro-aerial particles. He stated that the heat of living organisms was the result of the
fermentation or combustion produced in the blood by the mixture of
nitro-aerial particles with saline-sulphurous particles.

Blood was increasingly seen by this group as a mechanical fluid conveying essential particles from food and air to all the parts of the body.
Blood was also viewed as a convenient experimental medium. In 1656
in Oxford, Boyle injected a dog with opium, and later in that year
Christopher Wren (1632–1723), another of the Oxford group also
injected 'Wine and Ale into the Mass of Blood by a Veine, in good
quantities, till I have made him extremely drunk, but soon after he
Pisseth it out'. Using such methods the effect of drugs could be demonstrated. The injection of colours into the blood was also used to help
trace and demonstrate the course and connections of different blood
vessels, such as the 'circle of Willis' – the connecting arteries at the
base of the brain described by Thomas Willis in his *Cerebri Anatome*.

In the mid-1660s, Boyle and Lower were transfusing blood from one
dog to another, often unsuccessfully, though Lower in 1666 managed
to keep one dog alive. The possibilities were exciting, for instance, an
old dog might be rejuvenated with a young dog's blood. The technique
was soon extended to humans. At a meeting of the Royal Society in
1667 Lower transfused blood from a sheep into a 'poor and debauched
man... crackd a little in his head'. He survived. But Jean Denis
(d. 1704) in Paris had carried out transfusions of animal blood into
humans earlier in the same year, and one of the subjects died, thus
halting blood transfusions in France and then in England.

Experimentation now routinely took place within an interpretative
framework that had nothing to do with Galenic medicine, except for
the age-old concern with the questions of the locus of life and the special properties that distinguish the living from the dead. When Thomas
Willis discussed the three philosophies available to a medical man, the
Aristotelian, the 'Epicurean' or mechanical, and the chemical, he was
contemptuous of the first. He wrote that it had 'no peculiar respect to
the more secret recesses of nature, it salves the appearance of things,
that 'tis almost the same thing, to say a thing consists of wood and
stones as a body of four elements'. The Aristotelian–Galenic synthesis
was seen as a tautology explaining nothing. Molière (1622–73) constantly satirised learned medicine and in his play *Le Malade Imaginaire*
(1671) made a now famous joke when, to the question why does

351

opium cause sleep, he gave the tautological answer of learned medicine: because it has a dormitive faculty. In fact, the mechanical and chemical approach was increasingly seen as 'real' science, and the Aristotelian–Galenic synthesis merely as ephemeral.

New observations and the new theories were combined together. The effective magnification of the compound microscope was only ×20 to ×50, though the self-taught Dutchman Antoni van Leeuwenhoek (1632–1732) using simple bi-convex lenses achieved ×400 magnifications and in his letters to the Royal Society, which encouraged his work, described what were later known as protozoa and red corpuscles, but no one followed his example. But when the microscope did discover something new, the interpretative framework or intellectual values of the new science often shaped the nature of the observations. Aristotle's (and Harvey's) theory of epigenesis, whereby the development of new parts in the embryo occurred by means of a formative virtue or by the actualising of what is potential, was condemned alongside other occult forces and virtues, for such a virtue could not be observed and did not work mechanically. Instead, the theory of preformation whereby the embryo was already perfectly formed in miniature and required no plastic or formative virtue of the Aristotelian sort to develop from unorganised matter, became the intellectual orthodoxy. Microscopists like the Dutchman Jan Swammerdam (1637–80), most of whose work was published long after his death in the *Bible of Nature* (1737), and Malpighi believed that in the egg was a preformed embryo. This 'ovist' view was opposed by 'animalculists' like Leeuwenhoek who described spermatozoa as perfectly formed humans. The ovist theory/observation was taken to its logical conclusion with the theory of emboîtement, which held that all the generations of men and women were contained in the eggs of Eve, like boxes within boxes, becoming infinitely small, until the last was reached, when the human race would end. No plastic virtue was needed beyond God's initial creative power; all the embryos had to do was to enlarge their preformed organs by the absorption of food. Explanations of living processes were no longer based on ancient, vitalistic, theories but on the mechanistic world view of the moderns.

It is clear that contemporaries increasingly associated Aristotelian–Galenic learning with empty speculation. In medicine chemical analysis gave a sense of realism to the new theories which from modern hindsight might also appear as speculation. For example, Nicholas Lémery

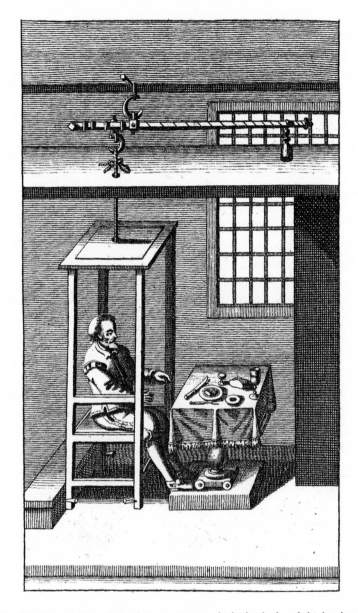

Fig. 44. The weighing chair of Sanctorius on which the food and drink taken is weighed as is the loss of weight due to insensible perspiration. Frontispiece of Sanctorius Sanctorius, *Medicina Statica* translated by John Quincy (London, 1718). (The Wellcome Institute Library, London. L17315.)

(1645–1715) in his popular *Cours de Chémie* (*Course of Chemistry*; 1675), which was influenced by atomistic and corpuscularian views as well as by iatrochemistry, explained how opium worked. A 'gummy and earthy matter' in opium produced sleep, and acted like other mucilaginous substances which, when mixed in the blood, gummed up the spirits flowing in the brain and moderated their speed. This slowing down of the spirits (which Lémery saw as composed of particles) produced sleep. At first sight there is little difference between this explanation and Molière's 'dormitive faculty' used by the Galenic physicians. Yet Lémery would have pointed to the empirical evidence he was presenting, for the gummy substance was the residue left after chemical analysis and, as he stated at the beginning of his book, he was not concerned with any opinion not founded on experience.

Quantification also served to give a sense of concrete reality to the new natural philosophy. For the eighteenth century, Newton's laws of motion and his optical experiments on colours seemed, through their mathematical language, to reflect nature herself (a point made by Galileo who had written that the *Book of Nature* was written in the language of geometry). Well before Newton, attempts were to make parts of medicine mathematical in the manner of the physicists; Sanctorius, who belonged to Galileo's circle, not only invented the thermometer to make medicine more certain (p. 261) but devised a weighing chair to calculate the amount of invisible perspiration lost after food, drink, and the evacuations of the body had been accounted for.

Sanctorius was working within a Galenic context but he clearly saw quantification as providing more secure knowledge. His work was taken up by iatromechanists who saw it as anticipating their own approach. John Quincy (d. 1722), a London apothecary physician who studied medicine in Edinburgh and was an avid follower of Newton, translated Sanctorius' *Ars... de Statica Medicina* (*Art... of Medical Statics*; 1614) in 1712 and wrote in the expanded edition of 1720 that 'those Rules and Laws of Motion, which we are furnished with from Mechanicks, are the only Guides we can have in discovering the Nature and Properties of all material substances whatsoever'. Quincy acknowledged that Sanctorius' theories were not mechanical but that his methods were in keeping with a mechanical approach: 'our Author, although he composed those Aphorisms, at a Time when this way of Reasoning was but very little made use of in Physick, and seems to have had very little Regard for it himself, yet the Means of Information

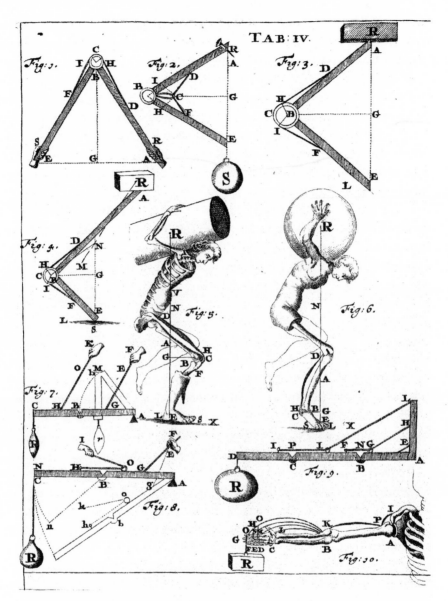

Fig. 45. Borelli's demonstration of forces exerted on the leg (fig. 5) and on the foot (fig. 6), and on the extended arm with weights at the end of the fingers (fig. 10). Figures 1, 2, 3, 4, 7, 8 and 9 demonstrate more generally the forces involved. Giovanni Borelli, *De Motu Animalum* (Leiden, 1685), plate facing p. 64. (The Wellcome Institute Library, London. L22127.)

he hath herein used, have so steadily guided him throughout the whole that there is but very little advanced but what is conformable and applicable thereunto' (i.e. to the mechanical philosophy).

Perhaps the most extensive attempt to give a quantitive description of the body was made by another disciple of Galileo, Giovanni Alfonso Borelli (1608–78). Borelli, who was also an astronomer and mathematician, in his *De Motu Animalium* (*On the Motion of Animals*; 1680–81) calculated the force exerted by the pull of different muscles, and analysed in geometrical terms how human muscles acted in walking and running. He also described geometrically the flight of birds and fish swimming.

In the first part of *De Motu Animalium* Borelli compared the body to a machine consisting of a series of levers. He wrote that God applied geometry when making animal organs, and that since the movements of animals are the proper subject of mathematics they can be understood in terms of levers, pulleys, winding-drums, and spirals, etc. Borelli ordered his book into 'propositions' as in geometry, first demonstrating, for instance, the forces involved in different types of lever with different weights attached and then applying his conclusions to the extended arm with weights attached to the ends of the fingers (Fig. 45, see 9 and 10). He also calculated the forces exerted in the lower muscles of the leg and in the muscles of the foot when a weight is carried on the back (Fig. 45, 5 and 6).

In the second part of *De Motu Animalium* Borelli discussed physiological processes such as respiration and the separation of urine from blood in the kidneys. Although he retained his mechanical approach Borelli was not able to quantify the mechanisms involved. As he wrote when discussing respiration, he hoped 'to investigate the properties of natural things... by using the knowledge of artificial things'. He argued that as in a clock the pendulum regulates its movement, so in animals and in humans, the particles of air entering the blood acted as 'small machines' whose oscillatory movement resembled that of a pendulum and imparted life (i.e. motion) and regularity to the animal. That Borelli was an iatromechanist rather than an iatrochemist is clearly shown by his denial that the separation of urine from blood occurred by a fermentive process (he pointed out that the spaces in the kidneys were too small for any chemical fermentation). Instead, the small vessels in the kidneys 'mechanically', like sieves, separated out water from blood.

Descartes' pervasive comparison of the body to an automaton, such as a clock, indicates how medicine (in the form of physiology) was now deriving its explanatory models from the physical sciences. For example, Daniel Tauvry (1669–1701) in his *Nouvelle Anatomie Raisonée* (*New Reasoned Anatomy*; 1690) set out the typical interpretative framework of the iatromechanist. He stated 'This treatise is only an application of physics and mechanics to the structures of the body'. And this led him to envisage the body as a 'static, hydraulic, and pneumatic machine' where 'the bones are the props and levers, the muscles are the ropes'.

A 'Newtonian medicine' also emerged in the last years of the seventeenth century. Taking their lead from the Scots Archibald Pitcairne (1652–1713), a physician who taught medicine at Edinburgh, Leiden, and Oxford, and David Gregory (1659–1708), the professor of mathematics at Edinburgh who had strong medical interests, a group of physicians, consisting of amongst others Richard Mead (1673–1754), George Cheyne (1671–1743), John Freind (1675–1728), James Keill (1673–1719) and his brother John (1671–1721), promoted a strongly mathematical Newtonian medicine. Pitcairne, who had been influenced by Borelli, saw in Newton's *Principia* a more precise model for iatromechanism. When in 1692 Newton showed him his essay 'De Natura Acidorum' ('On the Nature of Acids'), he took up some of Newton's ideas. In his lectures at Leiden, whilst professor of the theory of medicine (1692–93), he argued that fluids were not separated from the blood through differently configurated vessels (like sieves with different shaped holes); rather it was the size of the vessels' apertures and the forces exerted on the different fluids within the blood that was crucial. Part of this was derived from Newton's essay, but Pitcairne did not take up Newton's suggestion that secretion was affected by short-term attraction and affinity between the particular fluid and the receiving vessels. For Pitcairne the merit of Newton's physics for medicine was its precision and simplicity – attractive forces spoiled the simplicity, and in any case Pitcairne was probably concerned, like many iatromechanists and iatromathematicians (in Leiden he used the latter term of himself), to avoid re-introducing occult forms and powers, such as attraction.

The group around Pitcairne viewed Newton as their patron and popularised the idea of a Newtonian medicine. The Scot, George Cheyne, who had come to England to make good, in his *Essay Concerning the Improvements in the Theory of Medicine* (1702) called for a medical *Principia* ('Principia Medicinae Theoreticae Mathematica' – 'Mathematical Principles of Theoretical Medicine'). In the previous year Cheyne in his *New Theory of Continual Fevers* had presented a highly mathematical view of physiology, seeing the body as 'nothing but a congeries of canals'. He used the language of the new geometry to order his book and employed terms such as 'Postulata' and 'Lemma'. The book was a celebration of iatromathematics which, just as iatromechanics had identified the body with machines, equated the living body with geometry and hydraulics. Significantly, when Cheyne mathematised Pitcairne's ideas on secretion he did not take up Newton's suggestion of attractive forces to explain the phenomenon. But when in the 1706 Latin edition of his *Opticks* Newton in Query 23 discussed the possibility of attractive forces acting across short distances, John Keill in 1708 and Freind in the next year incorporated the idea in their explanation of animal secretion.

The starkly mathematical programme for a Newtonian medicine came to a gradual halt by the 1730s. Physicians began to draw on Newton's aether, 'a most subtle spirit' announced in the second edition of the *Principia* (1713) and then in the 1717 edition of the *Opticks*. The aether might explain gravity, and he thought it was the same or similar to the animal spirits in the nerves. Later Newton argued more subtly that the aether could be viewed as a vibration along the nerves. He wrote in Query 24 of the 1730 edition of the *Opticks* 'Is not Animal Motion perform'd by the Vibrations of this Medium, excited in the Brain by the power of the Will and propagated from thence through the solid, pellucid, and uniform Capillamenta of the Nerves into the Muscles, for contracting and dilating them?' Spirit had been brought back into physics and into physiology. The spell of iatromathematics was broken, and authors like Cheyne quickly followed their patron, the dominant figure of English science, and introduced spirit, and even the soul, back into the body.

Earlier Friedrich Hoffmann (1660–1742), who became professor of medicine at the new university of Halle which was founded in 1693 and was to be a centre for the German Enlightenment, had published in 1695 a short textbook on medicine, the *Fundamenta Medicinae ex Principiis Naturae Mechanicis* (*Foundations of Medicine from the Mechanical Principles of Nature*). In it Hoffman shows how a medical follower of Descartes found it necessary to water down Descartes' distinction between the mind and the body in order to capture the complexity of living processes. He did this by positing three types of soul: the immortal, one made from very fine material, and a gross material soul. The immortal soul influenced the second type of soul and that in turn influenced the third (only human beings had all three souls). There are analogies here with Plato's tripartite soul in the *Timaeus*, but what is significant is that the mechanical image of the body analogous to, or more often identical with, the crude machines of the time, was for some difficult to sustain given the complexity and apparent vitality of the body. It became clear to many eighteenth-century physicians and scientists that the body was indeed more than a machine, and that 'biological' concepts such as tissues and irritability might better express living processes.

THE END OF ANCIENT MEDICINE?

Despite what appears to be a revolution in medicine in which its philosophical basis was replaced, much of the heritage of the ancients continued to be influential. The great enemy of the iatrochemists and iatromechanists was Galen. Hippocrates, the father-figure of medicine, still appeared relevant. Paracelsus had praised him as someone whom God had chosen to bring medicine into the light of nature. Hippocrates was thus presented as being guided by experience, the new basis of knowledge for Paracelsians and mechanical philosophers, whilst Galen had introduced wordy and sterile sophistry into medicine. Thomas Sydenham (1624–89), the 'English Hippocrates' who became vastly influential in the eighteenth century, praised Hippocrates for his clinical medicine. The image of Hippocrates as the great observer at the bedside continued into the nineteenth century especially in the Paris school of medicine, which emphasised bedside teaching.

How and what Hippocrates observed are questions that would have elicited vastly different answers from a sixteenth-century Galenist and an eighteenth-century physician. The former read Hippocrates as observing the constitution of the patient, the latter as observing the symptoms that made up a disease. This transition owes much to the philosophy of Francis Bacon, who encouraged the making of natural histories of disease and their classification.

However, in the eighteenth century Thomas Sydenham was given much of the credit for the transformation in the medical perception of disease. Sydenham, a supporter of the Parliamentarian side in the Civil War practised largely amongst the poor in London after the Restoration of Charles II in 1660, and this together with his radical wish to improve medicine for the benefit of all, led him to study epidemic fevers rather than individual patients and their constitutions. As a follower of Bacon he was concerned to make general histories of diseases, collected from individual cases, which would allow diseases to be classified like plants. He wrote 'it is necessary that all diseases be reduced to definate and certain species, and that, with the same care which we see exhibited by botanists in their phytologies'. In his belief that diseases were real entities (or collections of symptoms) and could be classified into groups, Sydenham looks forward to the nosological systems of the eighteenth century.

Sydenham also was sceptical of hypotheses and of invisible causes, and was very doubtful that anatomy or the microscope would advance medicine. By stressing the value of eyesight observation and the uselessness of speculation, and by integrating his observations of diseases with their seasonality and relation to atmospheric conditions (which created 'epidemic constitutions') Sydenham became a hero-figure not only for eighteenth-century medicine but also for the 'bedside medicine' of the Paris medical school at the beginning of the nineteenth century which similarly suspected theory and valued clinical observation.

If concepts of disease were changing, this was less so with therapeutics. Although chemical remedies were well established, plant remedies continued to be used and procedures like bleeding, purging, vomiting, blistering, and cupping which had been developed on a humoral rationale were still being enthusiastically employed in the eighteenth century. Changes in physiological theories had little effect on medical practice, where the perceived need to evacuate the body of some malign substance, now often seen as chemical rather than humoral, still shaped therapeutic justifications. Uroscopy was the one diagnostic procedure that went into decline. In the Middle Ages it had been used to advertise the expertise of learned medicine, but in the sixteenth and early seventeenth century it was successfully condemned by learned physicians as part and parcel of quack medicine.

Other links with ancient medicine remained. Regimen, the way to lead a healthy life, continued to be structured well into the eighteenth century in terms of the traditional 'six non-naturals'. The environment and conditions of life especially were seen as determining general levels of health in populations, and this did not change until the 'bacteriological revolution' in the later nineteenth century. What was new was the way eighteenth-century medical men joined traditional ideas on health and the environment with a concern to reform the health of populations or groups in society; previously the emphasis was on reforming the health of the individual patient.

However, the theory of medicine, as opposed to Hippocratic experience and Galenic hygiene (preventive medicine) and therapeutics, had largely lost its links with classical medicine. The university of Leiden became the great centre of the new medicine, as Padua had been of the old. Franciscus Sylvius (or François de le Boë) (1614–72) taught at Leiden a chemical physiology founded on acid–alkali reactions which became immensely popular. By 1681 the lectures at Leiden were no longer based on specified medical authors (the medieval 'authorities') but were organised around medical subjects, and were given alongside bedside teaching and post-mortem dissections. The old authors were lost to view. Hermann Boerhaave (1668–1738), the greatest of the Leiden teachers of medicine and who trained the early professors of the Edinburgh school of medicine, praised the medical experience of the ancients, but condemned their theories as fallacious:

> The art of physic was anciently established (1) by a faithful collection of facts observed, whose effects were (2) afterwards explained, and their causes assigned by the assistance of reason; the first carries conviction along with it, and is indisputable; nothing being more certain than demonstration from experience, but the latter is more dubious and uncertain; since every sect may explain the causes of particular effects upon different hypotheses.

The results of applying the teachings of one sect, those of the mechanical philosophers, to medicine, can be seen in the history of eighteenth-century medicine: the constant rise and fall of different systems of medicine, and descriptions of diseases that emphasised experiential knowledge of symptoms rather than knowledge of the causes of disease. But, in the eyes of many contemporary writers around 1700, the new revolution in medicine, although incomplete, was not unsuccessful.

Chronological table for chapter 7

Year	Medical and scientific events	Year	Contemporary events
1700	Bernardino Ramazzini's *De morbis artificum*		
1704	Antonio Maria Valsalva's *De aure humana tractatus*	1704	Battle of Blenheim – English victory
1705	Raymond Vieussens describes left ventricle of heart and course of coronary blood vessels		
1707	Pulse watch introduced by John Floyer; Giovanni Maria Lancisi's *De subitaneis mortibus*; Georg Stahl's *Theoria medica vera*	1707	Union of England and Scotland
1708	Hermann Boerhaave's *Institutiones medicae*		
1709	Hermann Boerhaave's *Aphorismi de Morbis Cognoscendis et Curandis*		
1709	Great Plague in Russia		
		1711	Addison and Steele edit *The Spectator*
1714	Dominique Anel invents fine-point syringe Gabriel David Fahrenheit constructs mercury thermometer		
		1715	Jacobite rebellion in Britain
1717	Lady Mary Wortley Montagu brings to England Turkish practice of inoculation		
1718	Friedrich Hoffmann begins the nine volume *Medicina rationalis systematica*	1718	New Orleans founded by French

Year	Medical and scientific events	Year	Contemporary events
		1720	South Sea Bubble brings about crisis in British politics
1721	Smallpox inoculation introduced into America		
		1725	Death of Peter the Great; his wife Catherine I succeeds
1726	Stephen Hales measures blood pressure of the horse		
1728	Pierre Fauchard's *Le Chirurgien dentiste ou traité des dents* describes how to fill a tooth		
		1729	First performance of *St Matthew Passion* by J.S. Bach
1730	First tracheotomy for treatment of diphtheria performed by George Martine		
1731	John Arbuthnot's *An essay concerning the nature of aliments*		
1733	Stephen Hales's *Haemostaticks* describes his work on the measurement of blood pressure	1733	*Essay on Man* by Alexander Pope
1736	First successful appendicitis operation performed by Claudius Aymand American physician William Douglas describes scarlet fever		
1738	Death of Hermann Boerhaave		
		1740	Accession of Frederick II, the Great, of Prussia The War of Austrian Succession begins when Frederick II of Prussia invades Silesia
		1743	Excavations at Herculaneum begin

Year	Medical and scientific events	Year	Contemporary events
		1746	Victory of Culloden. Final defeat of Jacobites and escape of Charles Edward to France
1747	Bernhard Siegfried Albinus's *Tabula Sceleti et Musculorum Corporis Humani* Albrecht von Haller's *Primae Lineae Physiologiae* – first textbook on physiology James Lind discovers the curative effect of citrus fruits on scurvy		
1748	John Fothergill first describes diphtheria in his *Account of the putrid sore throat*		
1749	Count Buffon begins to publish *Histoire Naturelle; Traité des Systèmes* by Condillac		
1751	St. Luke's Hospital opened in London Robert Whytt demonstrates that pupil contraction in response to light is a reflex motion Death of French Physician Julien de Lamettrie	1751	First volume of *Encyclopédie* edited by Denis Diderot
1752	William Smellie's *Treatise on Midwifery* – first scientific approach to obstetrics Death of surgeon William Cheselden René-Antoine Ferchault de Réaumur discovers that digestion is a chemical action		
1753	*Treatise on Scurvy* by James Lind establishes curative effect of lemon juice		
1754	University of Halle graduates the first woman with a degree of medical doctor		
		1755	Earthquake at Lisbon (Nov)

Year	Medical and scientific events	Year	Contemporary events
1756	First description of casting models for false teeth in Philipp Pfaff's *Abhandlung von den Zähnen*	1756	Britain declares war on France Birth of Wolfgang Amadeus Mozart
1757	Albrecht von Haller's *Elementa physiologiae corporis humani* (1757–66) Death of psychologist David Hartley		
1759	Albrecht von Haller's *Experimenta physiologiae corporis humani* (1759–76); Kaspar Friedrich Wolff shows that specialised organs develop out of unspecialised tissue	1759	Capture of Quebec by Britain *Candide* by Voltaire
1761	Leopold Auenbrugger develops technique of percussion diagnosis of chest disorders Giovanni Morgagni's *De sedibus et causis morborum per anatomen indagatis*		
1763	First American medical society founded in New London	1763	Peace of Paris between Spain, France and Britain
1764	Robert Whytt's *Observations on Nervous Hypochondriacal or Hysteric Diseases* *Dictionnaire Philosophique* by Voltaire	1764	Expulsion of the Jesuits from France
1765	John Morgan founds first medical school in America at the College of Pennsylvania		
1766	Albrecht von Haller shows that nervous stimulation controls muscular action		
1768	Robert Whytt's *Observations on the Dropsy of the Brain* and first description of tuberculosis meningitis in children	1768–71	James Cook charts coasts of New Zealand and explores East coast of Australia. Confirms existence of Torres Strait

Year	Medical and scientific events	Year	Contemporary events
1771	John Hunter's *The Natural History of the Human Teeth* Death of anatomist Giovanni Battista Morgagni		
1772	Italian anatomist Antonio Scarpa discovers labyrinth of the ear	1772	First Partition of Poland James Cook makes a circuit of the Southern oceans and charts the New Hebrides
1773	Birth of Agostino Bassi Lazzaro Spallanzani discovers digestive action of saliva		
1774	William Hunter's *Anatomy of the Human Gravid Uterus* Franz Mesmer uses hypnotism to aid curing disease Karl Scheele discovers chlorine	1774	Louis XVI recalls the *Parlement; Werther* by Johann Wolfgang Goethe
1775	William Withering introduces digitalis to cure dropsy Percivall Pott suggests environmental factors can cause cancer (in chimney sweeps)	1775	American War of Independence begins
1776	John Fothergill gives first clinical description of trigeminal neuralgia		
1777	Death of physiologist Albrecht von Haller		
1778	John Hunter's *A Practical Treatise on the Diseases of the Teeth*		
1779	Lazzaro Spallanzani studies the development of eggs		
1780	Luigi Galvani experiments with muscles and electricity Death of physician John Fothergill		
1781	Henry Cavendish is first to determine the composition of water	1781	Joseph II of Austria issues the Toleration Edict: grants religious liberty to non-Catholic Christians

Year	Medical and scientific events	Year	Contemporary events
1784	German poet Johann Wolfgang Goethe discovers human intermaxillary bone		
1785	William Withering's *Account of the Foxglove*		
1786	Benjamin Rush's *Observations on the Cause and Cure of the Tetanus*	1786	Death of Frederick the Great; accession of Frederick William II Commercial treaty between France and Britain
1787	Death of physician Sir William Watson		
1787	Death of Scottish physician John Brown		
1788	Death of surgeon Percivall Pott		
		1789	the French Revolution
		1790	Death of Joseph II; succeeded by Leopold II
1791	Phillippe Pinel advocates a more human treatment of the insane in his *Traité medico-philosophique sur l'aliénation mentale*	1791	*The Magic Flute* by Mozart
		1792	The fall of the Monarchy in France. Republic declared
1793	Epidemic of yellow fever in Philadelphia	1793	Execution of Louis XVI Second Partition of Poland
1794	Death of German physiologist Kaspar Wolff Birth of Jean-Pierre-Marie Flourens Death of Scottish Physician James Lind		

Year	Medical and scientific events	Year	Contemporary events
1795	Matthew Baillie's *Morbid Anatomy of Some of the Most Important Parts of the Human Body* Sir Gilbert Blane makes the use of lime juice to prevent scurvy mandatory in the British navy Birth of surgeon James Braid Death of French surgeon Pierre-Joseph Desault		
1796	First vaccination against smallpox by Edward Jenner C. W. Hufeland's *Macrobiotics, or the Art to Prolong One's Life*	1796	Napoleon Bonaparte assumes the command in Italy
1797	Royal Society rejects Jenner's inoculation technique for smallpox Death of Richard Brocklesby		
1798	Death of Luigi Galvani	1798	Napoleon lands in Egypt Nelson wins battle of the Nile
1799	Death of Dutch physician and plant physiologist Jan Ingenhousz Death of physician William Withering		

7   The Eighteenth Century

ROY PORTER

The sixteenth and seventeenth centuries, as has just been shown, witnessed rapid growth in knowledge of anatomy, physiology, and pharmacology. Optimism about the advance of human knowledge deriving from the invention of printing and the discovery of the New World, coupled with the seventeenth-century scientific movement, created expectations of medical improvement. These, however, proved more impressive on paper than in practice. Greater knowledge led only rarely to more effective cures. And there was little sign that the war against ill health and disease was being won – throughout Europe the decades around 1700 saw epidemics rampant and mortality rates rising. The growth of giant ports and trading routes, increasing commercial contact with populations overseas and the mushrooming of the urban poor all created severe health hazards. There were, however, springs of hope. The spread of industry and affluence, the rise of literacy, the decline of religious wars and the containment of dynastic struggles, allied to the triumphs of the Scientific Revolution – all these elements spoke for healthier prospects. Better times, many believed, were at least within people's grasp – that was a theme destined to fuel the new faith in human potential characteristic of the Enlightenment. The last section of this book traces the growing confidence of, in, and for medicine in the eighteenth century, and assesses how far those aspirations and attitudes were translated into action.

The legacy of the Scientific Revolution in the age of Enlightenment

How did eighteenth-century physicians see their position in the long march of medicine? Most assumed eagerly the mantle of the Scientific Revolution, discussed in the previous chapter, and carried the torch of the Enlightenment, that drive for intellectual and cultural progress

371

(a)

(b)

(c)

(d)

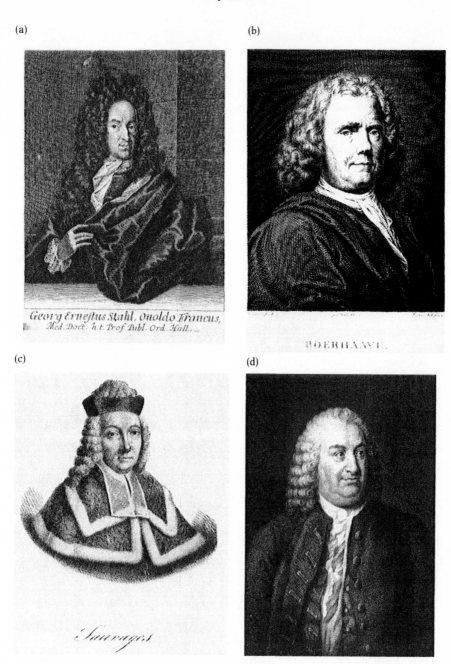

Fig. 46. (a) Georg Ernst Stahl; (b) Hermann Boerhaave; (c) F. Boissier de Sauvages;
(d) Albrecht von Haller. (The Wellcome Institute Library, London. V5595; V624;
M12032; V2526.)

(a)　　　　　　　　　　　　　　　(b)

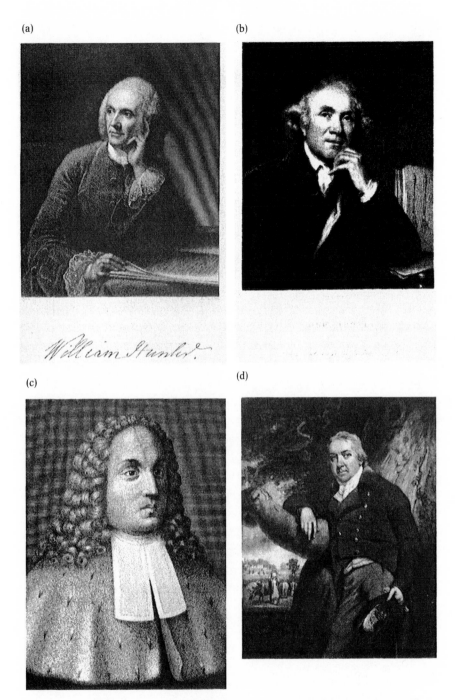

(c)　　　　　　　　　　　　　　　(d)

Fig. 47. (a) William Hunter; (b) John Hunter; (c) Giovanni Battista Morgagni; (d) Edward Jenner. (The Wellcome Institute Library, London. V2980; V2967; V4121; V3069.)

espoused by optimistic liberal thinkers in the Netherlands, Britain, France, and other parts of Europe. Enlightenment champions hoped to bring about a better world, marked by greater political, religious and personal freedom; they aimed to deploy science and technology to reinforce man's control over Nature, improve agriculture and industry, and enhance personal well-being. Medical progress loomed large in the agenda of such intellectuals.

Promoters of the Enlightenment like Voltaire (1694–1778) and Condorcet (1743–94) showed human history as a canvas on which good struggled against evil, reform against reaction, truth against error. In similar ways, eighteenth-century medical authors also dramatised the battles of reason against superstition, free inquiry against dogmatism, experience against bigotry and blinkered book-learning. William Harvey provided a superb model and mascot: his links with Padua and his impeccable experimentalism epitomised in Enlightenment eyes the alliance of medicine and science, enshrined in the image of the heart as a pump, proof of the happy marriage of medicine with the mechanical philosophy. By 1800, homage could also be paid to the surgeon John Hunter (1728–93) for demonstrating the Baconian union of hand and head, of manual and mental labour, thanks to which surgery was said to be ennobled into science. Medical propagandists thus reiterated key Enlightenment themes – the glories of Antiquity, rekindled by the Renaissance, the enduring importance of freedom, patronage, and public support – to conjure up a medical past that underwrote the present and foretold a glorious future.

A lofty mission was envisaged for medicine throughout the eighteenth century, contributing to what Bacon had called the 'relief of man's estate'. In North America, Benjamin Rush (1746–1813), physician and signatory to the Declaration of Independence, and in Britain, William Buchan (1729–1805), author of the best-selling *Domestic Medicine* (1769), portrayed health improvement as essential to human emancipation, ensuring freedom from suffering, want, and fear. The medical profession had all too often taken a leaf out of the Church's book, pursuing a closed shop and cynically keeping humanity in the dark; but this 'dark age' was coming to a close: physic, reformers claimed, would finally be laid open to the people, and health and humanity would advance in step.

To achieve such progress, medicine, it was argued, had to become scientific (in contemporary idiom, more 'philosophical'). For many, observation and experiment were the keywords: the bedside taught more than the bookshelf, and experience was superior to *a priori* rationalism – though what was valuable was 'philosophical' empiricism, not the 'vulgar' empiricism of so-called 'empirics' (alias quacks). Steering between the shoals of blind empiricism and the reefs of vain rationalism would require expert pilots.

Some physicians, like the Italian Giorgio Baglivi (1668–1707), believed medicine would become scientific by thinking arithmetically. In his *De Praxi Medica* (*On the Practice of Medicine*) (1699), Baglivi argued that 'the human body in its structure, and equally in the effects depending on this structure, operates by number, weight, and measure'. God, he explained, 'seems to have sketched the most ordered series of proportions in the human body by the pen of Mathematics alone'. For others, medicine's model would lie in mechanical physics. Baglivi's contemporary, the Leiden professor Hermann Boerhaave (1668–1738), saw health and sickness as questions of bodily structures and pressures, life depending upon the unobstructed motion of essential fluids. Boerhaave's hydraulic model of the body proved highly influential before 1750. It was eventually superseded, the accent shifting from the vascular to the nervous system, and new significance was set upon vital qualities like irritability, sensibility, and excitability through the work of Albrecht von Haller (1708–77) in Göttingen, William Cullen (1710–90) and his colleagues in Scotland, and Théophile de Bordeu (1722–76) and his fellow Montpellier 'material vitalists'. Despite such differences, throughout the century leading medical theorists agreed that elucidation of the 'animal economy' (physiology) depended upon systematic investigation of fibres and vessels. The development of morbid anatomy by Giovanni Battista Morgagni (1682–1771), with its conviction that post-mortem dissections would reveal disease lesions, eventually crowned the New Philosophy's confidence in structural/functional correlations and in the value of anatomical and physiological investigations.

Eighteenth-century medical thinking was heavily influenced by trends within science at large. But it was far from monolithic. Rival medical schools proliferated. Alongside those traditional centres of medical excellence, the Italian and French universities, new foci arose – Halle, Leiden, London, Edinburgh, and Philadelphia – each with its own ideas. In Halle, Georg Ernst Stahl (1659–1734) denounced the materialism he spied lurking in mechanistic theorisings, espousing instead an 'animism' that postulated the existence of a God-given, superadded non-mechanical soul ('anima') as the essential quality of living beings. Stahl viewed sickness less as structural/functional breakdowns than as the soul's attempt to counter threats to its well-being posed by morbific matter. He was not alone in underscoring the limits of mechanism; his doubts were echoed by Boissier de Sauvages (1706–67), who considered that life implied an inner organising principle. Likewise in their different ways Bordeu in Montpellier, Robert Whytt (1714–66) in Edinburgh, and John Hunter in London denied the sufficiency of mechanics for explaining animation and what was later called metabolic activity or homoeostasis, postulating instead some vital force or structured nervous organisation that transcended the merely mechanistic.

Only a very few radical physicians, notoriously the *philosophe* Julien Offray de La Mettrie (1709–51), truly sought, in the name of science, to reduce humans and every other living being to a machine. Even so, there is no disputing that theorists eagerly espoused the tenets of the new natural philosophy, especially the Newtonianism sweeping the Continent from the 1720s. To some degree this marks intellectual fashion, but weightier matters were also at stake, not least the nature and scope of medical explanations themselves. Confronted by sudden epidemics or strange symptoms – coma or convulsions – traditional thinkers had commonly looked beyond, seeking explanations in Divine will or Satanic possession, in astrological influences or the vagaries of human imagination. Enlightenment physicians, by contrast, maintained that such phenomena should be accounted for in terms of the internal organs and local operations of the body itself, viewed in its material environment. The mechanical model thus promised to consolidate medicine's unique authority to explain the body and its breakdowns.

QUANTIFICATION

In subjecting the organism to rational inquiry, Enlightenment medicine evolved certain characteristic strategies. Doctors participated in the enterprise of weighing and measuring Creation. William Petty (1623–87) had claimed that the real was what could be quantified; human understanding would be extended by the demystification of the marvellous and miraculous. This was to be achieved through fact-collection, through digestion of data into tables, equations, and ratios, and, finally, in the nineteenth century, through application of the

376

'law of large numbers'. What could be enumerated could be expressed as natural laws, even if they were only laws of probability. The empire of chance – so-called 'acts of God' – could be mastered by science.

Sickness had long been regarded as epitomising the hazards of this mortal world, or rather pointing to the essentially other-worldly meanings of things. When mortal affliction struck ('out of the blue'), pious eyes had looked Heavenwards for providential explanations. But, picking up cues from the New Science, Enlightenment physicians strove to plot biomedical regularities. From the balancing chair of Sanctorius (1561–1636), discussed above (p. 353), to the haemostatic experiments of Stephen Hales (1677–1761) a century later, the body's operations were increasingly tested and tabulated. The force of the blood's movement was measured and temperatures were recorded; this was the century when the Fahrenheit, Celsius, and Réaumur thermometric systems were devised. Collection of vital statistics stimulated compilation of life-tables and calculation of differential life expectations, essential for assurance, annuities, and other actuarial computations; life insurance now became big business. Originating in the seventeenth century, Bills of Mortality continued to be published, and morbidity profiles of city dwellers were built up and related to seasonal, environmental and climatic factors. Epidemic death rates and mortality crises became objects of investigation among army, navy, and civilian doctors, especially after 1750, in the expectation that demonstrating periodicities in outbreaks of disorders like smallpox, putrid and gaol fevers would aid prediction and containment. It is no accident that it was James Jurin (1684–1750), Secretary of the Royal Society of London as well as a prominent physician, who expressed the value of smallpox inoculation in numerical terms. By 1798, birth and death, so long the mysterious ministers of Providence, could be reduced to a mathematical formula in the ecological *Essay on ... Population* of the pioneer demographer, Thomas Malthus (1766–1834).

Arithmetical worldviews encouraged a secular mode of understanding, pointing to a human destiny whose key was not the decree of Divine Will but the balance of possibilities. Numerical laws also imply a certain determinism – trends seem to carry greater explanatory weight than personal free-will. Attention to the typical as well as the individual thus led medicine to gaze beyond the bedside to life-chances in the wider environment, thereby generating a new 'biopolitics', a state-led concern with the health of populations.

CLASSIFICATION

Science was also influential in the desire to create taxonomies. Naturalists like John Ray (1627–1705) in England, Joseph Pitton de Tournefort (1656–1708) in France, and notably Karl von Linné (Linnaeus: 1707–78) in Sweden, author of *Systema Naturae* (*System of Nature*) (1735) and inventor of the binomial system of taxonomy, sought to modernize natural history by taking the inventory of creation and classifying it. (Dispute raged whether such classifications were 'natural' or 'artificial'.) Medicine followed suit; Linnaeus (himself a physician, even if, so the tale went, he had studied medicine mainly to win the hand of a wealthy practitioner's daughter) produced a pioneering nosology (disease classification) in his *Genera Morborum* (*Types of Diseases*) (1763), with its groupings of common classes of disease. In France, François Boissier de Sauvages (1706–67) in his *Nouvelles classes des maladies* (*New classes of illnesses*) (1731) and *Nosologia methodica* (*Methodical Nosology*; 1768), and in Scotland, William Cullen, devised influential taxonomies. Sauvages endeavoured to classify diseases as if they were botanical specimens, subdividing them into 10 classes, 295 genera and no fewer than 2400 species. Seemingly endorsing Thomas Sydenham's (1624–89) proposal for a 'natural history of disease', such taxonomies bolstered the conviction (implied in the shift from traditional humoral fluidism to structural/functional solidism) that diseases truly were discrete entities, symptomatically distinct and stable. Even more ambitiously, in his *Zoonomia* (*Laws of Life*), Erasmus Darwin (1731–1802) advanced a disease taxonomy which he claimed was not merely heuristic but natural, being neuro-physiologically grounded. Diseases, Darwin argued, were to be identified as disorders of irritability, sensation, volition or association, according to the psycho-physiological level they affected.

There was no unanimity as to the truth or utility of such taxonomies. Cullen's elaborate nosology was vehemently challenged by his one-time pupil John Brown (1735–88), who insisted upon the unitary nature of sickness – there was only one disease, asserted Brown, though it assumed myriad forms and intensities. Yet Brunonian medicine depended no less, in its own way, upon contemporary scientific idiom. Brown envisaged a disease thermometer, calibrated upon a single arithmetic scale, running from zero ('asthenic' disorders, lethal bodily under-stimulus) up to 80 degrees (fatal over-excitement), the mid-point of which represented healthy equilibrium. The device of a single axis thus objectified illness into something quantifiable, and, in turn, dictated a therapeutics dependent upon dosage size – for Brown, treatment was essentially a business of larger or smaller measures of opiates and alcohol, sedatives and stimulants.

Rhetoric, reality, and historiography

Eighteenth-century medical authors thus attempted to set their discipline upon more 'scientific' footings; yet 'scientific medicine' was also a party badge – and the relations between medical reasoning, rhetoric and reality remained perplexing. Maybe such bold claims were being staked for medicine precisely because its actual state seemed just the reverse, an intellectual quagmire? To many it was scandalous that medicine never had caught up with chemistry or experimental physics. Towards 1800, Thomas Beddoes (1760–1808), a Bristol practitioner and pioneer of respirable gases for the treatment of lung disorders, reflected on medicine's situation. Like many another scientific doctor, Beddoes exulted in contemporary advances in physics and chemistry: the achievements of Henry Cavendish (1731–1810) and Joseph Priestley (1733–1804), Carl Wilhelm Scheele (1742–86) and Antoine Laurent Lavoisier (1743–94), Luigi Galvani (1737–98) and Alessandro Volta (1745–1827), Benjamin Franklin (1706–90) and James Watt (1736–1819). In 1793, Beddoes predicted that 'from chemistry, which is daily unfolding the profoundest secrets of nature, we can hope for a safe and efficacious remedy for one of the most frequent painful and hopeless of diseases', that is, tuberculosis. The physical sciences, he affirmed, would provide the paradigm for progressive medicine, for 'however remote medicine may at present be from such perfection', there was no

> reason to doubt that, by taking advantage of various and continual accessions as they accrue to science, the same power will be acquired over living, as is at present exercised over some inanimate bodies, and that not only the cure and prevention of diseases, but the art of protracting the fairest season of life and rendering health more vigorous will one day half realise half the dream of Alchemy.

The freeway of medical progress was clearly signposted. Medicine, in Beddoes's judgment, must become more experimental and collaborative; data-banks had to be founded and research laboratories established. Pondering the chemical revolution recently effected by

Lavoisier's discovery of oxygen, Beddoes announced in 1793 to his friend Erasmus Darwin,

> Many circumstances indeed seem to indicate that a great revolution in this art is at hand.... you will agree with me in entertaining hopes not only of a beneficial change in the practice of medicine, but in the constitution of human nature itself.

Yet Beddoes had to concede that medicine was still deplorably 'remote .... from such perfection'. Clinical practice – history-taking, diagnosis, prognosis, therapeutics – ought to be systematic and objective, but it was still, he lamented, the reverse, waylaid by know-all patients and mercenary physicians. And, for all his hopes, Beddoes's personal research programme came to nothing. Other promising medical movements, like hypnotism, did not bear much fruit.

STERILE RATIONALISM?

Indeed, it is these frustrations that have dominated conventional histories of eighteenth-century medicine. The influential historian, Fielding Garrison (1870–1935) judged that 'aside from the work of a few original spirits like Morgagni, Stephen Hales, the Hunters, Caspar Friedrich Wolff, and Edward Jenner, it was essentially an age of theorists and system-makers'. Garrison explained this wretched situation in terms of the spirit of the age: 'tedious and platitudinous philosophizing (upon *a priori* grounds) was the fashion', it being 'natural that the period preceding the outburst of political revolution should be as a lull before an approaching tempest'. In short, Garrison concluded, 'everything tended toward formalism, and every theory, however idealistic, soon hardened into a rational methodistic 'system''.

Later medical historians have often dismissed the Enlightenment as a wasteland of abstruse theorising ('the lost half-century in English medicine', is one verdict). There was no medical Newton or even Franklin, medical historians have insisted; no radical transformation was wrought in the understanding of the laws of life, of health and disease, until the nineteenth century with the investigations of Karl Ernst von Baer (1792–1876), Theodor Schwann (1810–82), Carl Friedrich Wilhelm Ludwig (1816–95), Claude Bernard (1813–78) and Louis Pasteur (1822–95), with their pathbreaking developments in patho-anatomy, histology, cell biology, and bacteriology. Charles Rosenberg has argued that there was no 'therapeutic revolution' till the nineteenth century (the date might be set even later). And, discussing the 'birth of the clinic', Michel Foucault (1925–84), contended that medicine did not achieve a 'scientific gaze' till the reform of the Paris Hospital during the French Revolution, whereafter the sick came to be seen, not as objects of charity but as specimens of disease. It has been claimed that medicine came of age only with the 'Pasteurization' of the laboratory from the 1870s.

TANGIBLE BENEFITS? MEDICINE AND THE SCIENCES OF MAN

Not all scholars take such a doleful view. Indeed, the Enlightenment historian, Peter Gay, has launched a counter-attack. Far from being trapped in arid system-building, medicine, Gay has contended, was integral to the *philosophes'* practical drive to transform the world. The plausibility of this view is enhanced by the fact that numerous Enlightenment luminaries were physicians. In England, the philosopher John Locke (1632–1704), leader of progressive thought in fields as diverse as epistemology, pedagogics, rational religion and liberal politics, was medically trained and active. A friend of Robert Boyle (1627–91) and Thomas Sydenham and a Fellow of the Royal Society, Locke provided in his *An Essay Concerning Humane Understanding* (1690) the philosophical basis for scientific empiricism, as well as offering an influential secular theory of insanity, in terms of the (false) association of ideas: mad people do not lack reason, but rather reason faultily. Many prominent Enlightenment spokesmen were physicians: Bernard Mandeville (c.1670–1733), satirist and controversialist; David Hartley (1705–57), promoter of a physiological psychology; Julien Offray de la Mettrie (1709–51), the most strident 'vital materialist' of the age; the Chevalier Jaucourt (1704–79), a prolific contributor to the Encyclopédie; François Quesnay (1694–1774), the physiocrat and economist; Erasmus Darwin, poet, inventor and evolutionary theorist; and Pierre Jean Georges Cabanis (1757–1808), leader of the Idéologues – to name but a few. Other key thinkers enjoyed close ties with medicine. Bishop George Berkeley (1685–1753), whose *Treatise Concerning the Principles of Human Knowledge* (1710) challenged Locke with a metaphysical Idealism (what is truly real is what is in the mind), and promoted Tar Water, a celebrated panacea. The Scot, David Hume (1711–76), based his own highly influential scepticism, his doubts about the knowability of the outside world set out in *An Enquiry Concerning Human Understanding* (1758), upon a theory of the passions and mental operations owing much to his acquaintance with medicine

– and to introspection into his own nervous breakdown. The controversy arising from Locke gave philosophy a new direction: traditional deductive logic and analysis of innate ideas supposedly implanted in the soul by God yielded to a quest for knowledge derived from the sense organs, informed by studies of the nervous system and experience of the learning process. The blossoming sciences of psychology, psychiatry, and sociology, and understanding of mental and social development were linked to medicine and physiological investigation.

Medicine furnished the intellectual foundations and idiom of the budding Enlightenment sciences of man. In his *L'Esprit des Lois* (*Spirit of the Laws*; 1748), the political thinker, Charles Louis de Secondat Montesquieu (1689–1755), clinched his theory of the climatic determination of national temperament with a physiological experiment – showing, by putting ice on an animal's tongue, how cold produced sluggishness and diminished mental sensations. Not least, the fierce debate in the 1790s regarding the guillotine as a mode of execution (was it humane, as was claimed, or might the severed head experience hideous sensations?), hinged upon the testimonies of rival doctors, including those of its inventor, Dr Joseph Ignace Guillotin (1738–1814). In short, numerous *médecins-philosophes* were convinced that a science of man – that grand Enlightenment design – required sound biomedical foundations. Such a claim was cardinal to the *Idéologues*, a group of radical medical thinkers. They averred that true knowledge of man necessitated a science of ideas, which must be grounded on a physiology of consciousness. Cabanis, himself in medical practice, demonstrated in his *Rapports du physique et du moral de l'homme* (*Relations between the Physical and the Moral Aspects of Man*; 1802) that mind was not a superadded religious principle but a function of higher nervous organisation. So objectionable were the materialist undertones of such teachings that Napoleon (1769–1821) retaliated in 1803 by abolishing the section of the French Institute devoted to the moral sciences.

In Britain, Cabanis's contemporary, Erasmus Darwin, advanced a rather similar biomedical theory of the material basis of human powers, expounded as part of a daring hypothesis of cosmic evolution. Drawing upon Haller and on the physiological psychology of Hartley, Darwin delineated the gradient of neurologically-based activities (irritability, sensation, volition, and association) that marked the ascent from micro-organisms up to mighty man. No absolute divide separated beings endowed with mere life from those also possessing volition and finally those blessed with consciousness. Nor was human nature immutable. Man, argued Darwin, possessed unlimited capacity to improve his faculties through learning, and acquired characteristics and ideas were heritable. Hence, as claimed in his evolutionary poem, *The Temple of Nature* (1803), medical materialism guaranteed human perfectibility, social, moral, intellectual, and scientific.

Moreover, biomedicine was to supply many radicals with blueprints for social action. This is nowhere so plain as in the writings of La Mettrie. In his *L'Homme Machine* (*Man a Machine*; 1747), this former student of Boerhaave proposed a reductionist vision of man as a pre-determined being, his activity a function of material-organic needs. La Mettrie levelled his writings against theologians and metaphysicians who postulated dualistic views of man and so privileged the soul as separate from, and superior to, the body. Such views, La Mettrie insisted, were unscientific, feeding the prejudices of priests and potentates.

Less easy to assess as a biomedical materialist is Denis Diderot (1713–84). In a stream of provocative works, including the *Lettres sur les Aveugles* (*Letters on the Blind*; 1749), the *Rêve de d'Alembert* (*D'Alembert's Dream*; written 1769) – which significantly uses the Montpellier vitalist physician, Bordeu, as a fictional character – and the *Élémens de physiologie* (*Elements of Physiology*; written around 1774: the last two were too hot to publish in the author's lifetime), Diderot explored the relationship between the material and the moral. If man is determined by his biomedical make-up, does this rule out free will? Can man be held responsible for his actions? Is there a soul? Is consciousness independent, or is it just a by-product, or even waste-product, of the brain, as bile is a secretion of the liver? Is there, finally, any true difference between *homo rationalis* healthy and sick, sane and crazy, between man and beast?

Diderot brilliantly restated the old conundrum, expounded long before by Michel de Montaigne (1533–92) and Sir Thomas Browne (1605–82), of the dual nature of man, a paradoxical mix of body and soul, animal and angel, corporeal and spiritual being. The *philosophe* put the questions once again, from the viewpoint of Enlightenment bio-medicine. How far he thought them soluble remains unclear.

These examples show that Gay was right to contend that medicine provided materials used by Enlightenment thinkers in building their views of man's place in nature and society. Gay goes further, arguing that the success of medicine created a crucial morale-booster for the Enlightenment, contributing to the 'recovery of nerve' so vital for the 'pursuit of modernity'. The progress of medicine in turn bolstered Enlightenment optimism. In particular, thanks to smallpox inoculation, 'the recovery of nerve was visible on men's very faces'; such developments helped to make medicine 'the most highly visible and the most heartening index of general improvement', and medical advances contributed to fitter populations. In sum, Gay concludes, 'for observant men in the eighteenth century, *philosophes* as well as others, the most tangible cause for confidence lay in medicine'.

Garrison was too gloomy about eighteenth-century medicine; Gay, by contrast, is too sanguine. Nevertheless, his is a valuable perspective, not least because it draws attention to medicine's self-image in the Enlightenment. Innovation was in the air, and medicine became linked with social reform and political change. As ancien-régime Church and Monarchy came under fire, science and medicine offered fresh theories of man and blueprints of social order.

Scientific medicine: anatomy and physiology

As demonstrated in Chapter 6, investigation of the fabric and workings of the human body developed rapidly in the sixteenth and seventeenth centuries, in association with the anatomy theatre, hands-on dissection, medical practice (especially surgery), and the triumphs of the New Science. From Vesalius and Falloppio to Malpighi and Borelli, investigators had increased anatomical knowledge, and, equally importantly, had conferred a new prestige upon the once-humble anatomy, making it the *pièce de resistance* of medical training and science. These anatomical traditions continued with undiminished energy and status. It is no accident that the best-attended lectures at the Edinburgh University medical school (founded in 1726), were those in anatomy; or that artistic renderings of skeletons and the anatomy class became potent icons of medicine.

Italy's golden age ended, and the cutting edge of anatomy moved north. France, the Netherlands, England, Scotland, and certain German-speaking principalities became vigorous centres, thanks, in part, to the rise of the northern universities (see p. 375). For over half a century, Leiden led the field in anatomy, thanks initially to the eminence of Franciscus Sylvius (François de le Boë) (1614–72), and then through

Hermann Boerhaave (1668–1738) and his pupil, Bernhard Siegfried Albinus (1697–1770), who became professor of anatomy and surgery in 1718, rising in 1745 to the chair of medicine. In a symbolic gesture, Boerhaave and Albinus edited and re-published Vesalius's works.

THE ANATOMICAL TRADITION

By 1700, knowledge of gross anatomy – bones, joints, muscles, etc. – was well advanced. 'In an age like the present, and upon a subject so much searched into as the human body', commented the Swiss physician, S.-A.-A.-D. Tissot (1728–97), 'we do not flatter ourselves with discovering essential properties; all that we can naturally hope for, is to push farther those discoveries already made, which require no more than dexterity and patience to bring them to perfection'. For this reason, the eighteenth century is mainly conspicuous for minute analysis of softer and more hidden fibres, the lacteal system, the lymphatics, and, of paramount long-term significance, the nervous system. Though Vesalius and his followers had traced the nerve pathways, they had not seriously explored brain and nerve function. Thomas Willis's (1621–75) *Cerebri Anatome* (*Anatomy of the Brain*; 1664) had developed the idea of brain localisation; but it was eighteenth-century studies – especially by Jacob Winslow (1669–1760) and the Prussian, Samuel Thomas von Soemmerring (1755–1830) who delineated the brain and classification of the cranial nerves (1778) – that set investigation of the nervous system upon a modern footing.

Valuable work was done on specific organs. In his *Icones Anatomicæ* (*Anatomical Images*; 1743), Albrecht von Haller produced a major study of the blood vessels and the viscera, while Soemmerring undertook meticulous explorations of the eye, ear, nose, and throat. Soemmerring's interests ranged widely, from hernia to racial anthropology and the evils of corsets. Like many of his peers, he was a superb draughtsman; his monumental treatise on anatomy (1791–96) was renowned for its illustrations.

Many first-rate anatomical atlases appeared, testimony to artistic skill and the transition from copper-plates to steel-plates. The finest specimens of anatomical illustration include folios like William Cheselden's (1688–1752) *Osteographia* (1733), Haller's *Icones Anatomicæ* (1743–56), and William Hunter's (1718–83) *Anatomia Uteri Humani Gravidi* (*Anatomy of the Human Gravid Uterus*; 1774), an astonishing depiction of the pregnant woman and foetus. Possibly the greatest

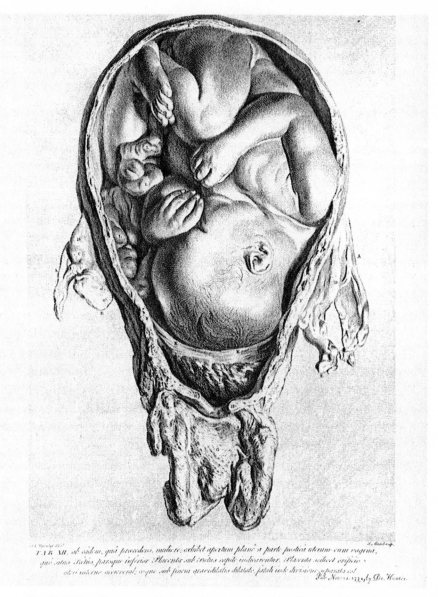

TAB XII. ab initio, qui præcedens, mulicre, exhibet apertum plane a parte postici uterum cum vagina, qui uteri fœtus, principio inferior Placenta sub cratus caput intercurratur. Placenta adest orificio; ubi a materno acceccit; aque sub finem graviditatis dilatata fætah iuste divisione expansus est.

Pub. Nov: 1 1774, by Dr. Hunter.

Fig. 48. William Hunter, *Anatomia Uteri Humani Gravidi* (1774). Hunter's work set new standards in the anatomy of the pregnant woman. (The Wellcome Institute Library, London. L4302.)

anatomical illustrator was the German-born Bernhard Siegfried Albinus (1697–1770), who studied under Govard Bidloo (1649–1713) and Boerhaave, holding the chairs of anatomy and surgery (1718) and then medicine (1745) at Leiden. Albinus edited the works of Vesalius,

Eustachius, Fabricius, and Harvey, and his publications on the bones, the muscles, intestinal veins and arteries, and the gravid uterus, were exquisitely illustrated. The finest general anatomy treatise was Soemmerring's *Vom Baue des menschlichen Körpers* (*On the Structure of the Human Body*; 1791–96). He was the first anatomist to juxtapose male and female skeletons. His depictions exaggerated the larger size of the male cranium and the greater breadth of the female pelvis, as if to make the point that anatomy was destiny, the female form being designed for child-bearing, and the male for rational thought.

FORM AND STRUCTURE

Anatomists inquired into form itself, starting a trend that led to the philosophical morphology of the nineteenth century. Some compared different vertebrates, judging them against an ideal of the plan of Creation or, occasionally, in the light of an evolutionary model. The most celebrated comparative anatomist was Felix Vicq d'Azyr (1748–94), permanent secretary of the Société Royale de Médecine, notable for his studies of bird and quadruped structures, the flexor and extensor muscles, and the morphology of the brain and vocal cords. Pursuit of anatomical systematics seemed promising, for form was thought to be the key to nature and function. For instance, on the basis of study of cranial angles pioneered by Pieter Camper, a new physical anthropology emerged, positing the differential characteristics of different racial types. Around 1800, German exponents of *Naturphilosophie* (philosophy of nature) were suggesting that Nature should be understood as a morphological unity, built upon a few elemental structural archetypes or anatomical building-blocks. Studies of cabbage buds, beans, and other plants led Caspar Friedrich Wolff (1734–94) to conclude that 'all parts of the plant except the stem are modified leaves', a view later endorsed by the poet and polymath Johann Wolfgang von Goethe (1749–1832) in investigations of plant metamorphosis (1790), in which he aimed to demonstrate the fundamental unity of leaf, flower, and fruit, and the 'descent' of all plants from an archetypal form (*Urpflänze*). Goethe interpreted insect jaws as modified limbs, and thought the skull was composed of modified vertebrae – a notion later developed by the illustrious philosophical morphologist, Laurenz Oken (1779–1851).

Early eighteenth-century dissectors pursued analysis of fine structures. Their work owed something to microscopy. Sustained scientific work had been carried out using microscopes late in the seventeenth

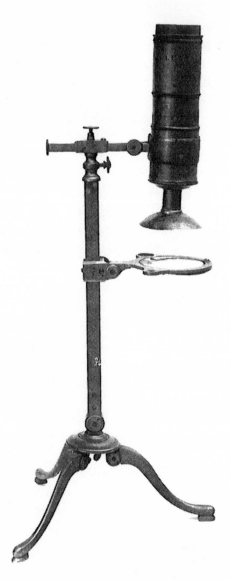

Fig. 49. Microscope by Dellebarre 1792. Eighteenth-century microscopes are remarkable mainly for their elegance as gentlemanly collectors' items. (The Wellcome Institute Library, London. M212.)

century; Robert Hooke (1635–1703) studied capillaries and Antoni van Leeuwenhoek (1632–1723) revealed micro-organisms and what would later be identified as red blood cells. Leeuwenhoek, however, was uniquely skilled in lens-grinding; his results therefore proved largely unrepeatable and he did not leave a thriving tradition behind him.

Partly by consequence, the eighteenth century saw only limited use of the microscope, though it became a favourite toy of gentlemanly science, popular books on miscroscopy being published and a market emerging in preparations for amateur use. Certain microscopical studies, however, bore fruit; Friedrich Hoffmann (1660–1742), for example, carried out new investigations of skin texture.

Fascination with individual parts followed from the New Science's concern with the elementary contrivances of nature. The fascination with bellows, syringes, pipes, valves, and so forth, found in Descartes, Thomas Bartholin, Malpighi, and others led many anatomists to explore the form/function relationship of small structures, in context of a model of the organism as a system of pipes, tubes, and fluids. The laws of mechanics thus underwrote anatomy. Boerhaave proposed that functional systems throughout the body comprised an integrated whole, maintaining a balance in which pressures and flows were equalised and everything found its own level. Spurning the earlier, crude 'clockwork' models of Borelli and others, Boerhaave treated the body as a network of vessels, which contained, channelled, controlled, divided, and released body fluids. The balance of health and sickness was primarily explained by movement, obstruction or stagnation of fluids in the vascular system.

Yet Boerhaave was no reductionist or materialist. The problems of life, volition and the soul were left rather nebulous in his writings. Their presence in living beings could be taken for granted, but inquiry into their ultimate nature was largely irrelevant to the real business of medical inquiry, which was to investigate discernible somatic processes. Consideration of the soul was best left to theologians and metaphysicians.

INVESTIGATING LIFE

Progress in physical science spurred investigation of the body machine. The mathematically-inclined Anglican clergyman, Stephen Hales, devised 'haemodynamic' experiments to measure blood circulation. As set out in gory detail in his *Statical Essays* (1731–33), Hales measured the force of the blood by inserting brass tubes into the jugular vein and carotid artery of a living horse, observing that the arterial pressure (calibrated in terms of columnar height) was far greater than the venous pressure. Through his quantitative estimates of blood pressure, heart capacity and blood-current velocity, Hales made the first advances

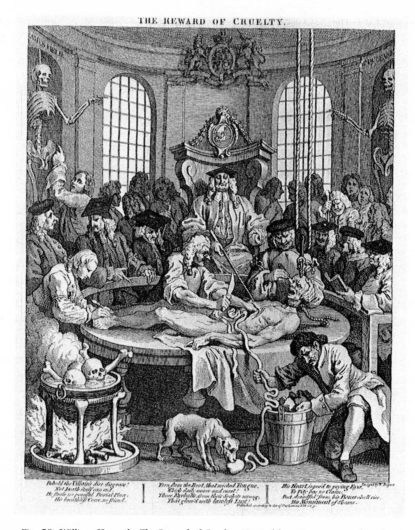

Fig. 50. William Hogarth, *The Reward of Cruelty*. Hogarth's satire suggests that the anatomists are as cruel as the criminal whose body is being dissected. (The Wellcome Institute Library, London. M10169.)

since Harvey in circulation physiology. Pursuing animal statics in the light of vegetable statics, he noted the constriction and dilation of the blood vessels under various conditions. A dauntless animal experimenter, Hales also followed up Descartes' interest in reflex action by decapitating frogs and then stimulating their reflexes by pricking the skin. Nervous responses continued, he found, until the spinal cord was obliterated.

Research on the nervous system using surgical extirpation led to protests against vivisection. Pigs, monkeys, and dogs had been experimentally sacrificed since the Greeks. But, from the chartering of the Royal Society (1662), there was a substantial increase in scientific experimentation upon animals for research and teaching purposes, and some experimenters assumed, with Descartes, that animals were automata that could feel no pain. Creatures were routinely employed for toxicological testing; Robert Hooke used animals to investigate hypotheses about gases, respiration and air pressure; and Hales performed the gruesome haemostatic experiments just described upon at least sixty experimental subjects, including horses. By 1758, the normally tough-minded Samuel Johnson (1709–84) was deploring the fact that animal experiments were being 'published every day with ostentation' by doctors aiming to 'extend the arts of torture'. Condemnation of animal experimentation formed part of a wider protest against cruel sports like bear-baiting and cock-fighting. William Hogarth's (1697–1764) 'Four Stages of Cruelty' print-sequence significantly opens with a boy tormenting pets, proceeds to show him turning into a murderer, and ends with his being hanged, and disembowelled at the hands of the Company of Surgeons. Murder, execution, and dissection were all of a piece: for Hogarth, the 'cruelty' of medical science was no less suspect than schoolboy viciousness.

Newtonian natural philosophy led investigators to transcend narrow scrutiny of the mechanics of solid structures, and to address wider questions of the properties of the living organism. This inevitably meant new debates over traditional doctrines of the soul and the divine order of being. Highly significant was the work of Stahl. The founding father of the distinguished Prussian medical school in Halle, Georg Ernst Stahl (1660–1734) adumbrated classic anti-mechanistic arguments. Co-ordinated and purposive human actions could not, he argued, be explained in terms of mechanical chain-reactions, like a stack of dominoes falling over. Wholes were greater than the sum of their parts. Human activity thus presupposed the presence of a soul, not as mere 'background music' (as postulated by the iatromechanists), but as a constantly intervening, guiding power, the very quintessence of the organism. More than a Cartesian 'ghost in the machine', Stahl's anima was the agent of consciousness and physiological regulation, and a bodyguard against sickness. For disease, according to Stahl, was a disturbance of vital functions provoked by misdirected activities of the soul. The body, strictly speaking, was passive and guided by an immortal spirit. As the

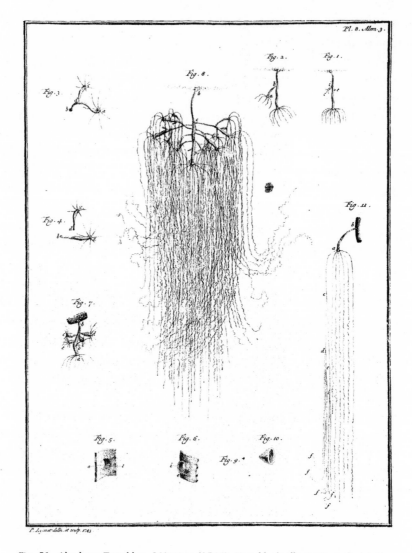

Fig. 51. Abraham Trembley, *Mémoires* (1744). Trembley's illustrations depict the remarkable regenerative powers of the polyp, thereby hinting that life was a phenomenon beyond explanation by mechanistic reductionism. (The Wellcome Institute Library, London. L21694.)

soul acted directly, independently of *archæi* (ferments) or other physical intermediaries, neither gross anatomy nor chemistry had, at bottom, much explanatory power: to fathom the operations of the body, he argued, required understanding the soul. Stahl's animism expressed an internally plausible biomedical logic, but it was also the product of a

Lutheran Pietism, an emotional variant of Protestantism common in eighteenth-century Germany.

Stahl's contemporary at Halle, Friedrich Hoffmann (1660–1742), looked rather more favourably upon new-style philosophical mechanism. 'Medicine', he announced in his *Fundamenta medicinae* (*Fundamentals of Medicine*; (1695), 'is the art of properly utilizing physico-mechanical principles, in order to conserve the health of man or to restore it if lost'. Hoffmann was an eclectic. While attracted by medical mechanism, he also postulated the presence of an ether-like fluid, whose function was to promote bodily motion and maintain tonic contraction of the muscles. Though regarding acute diseases as involving mechanically explicable spasmodic conditions (for instance, convulsions), Hoffmann also, more traditionally, judged humoral changes, faulty excretions, and fluid imbalances to be the sources of maladies, and relied heavily on time-honoured therapeutics like evacuants. Like many contemporaries, he kept a foot in each camp.

A perception of the limitations of mechanical approaches stemmed from renewed interest in the extraordinary powers of living things. Not least amongst these was a capacity to regenerate themselves, in a manner quite unlike clocks or looms. In 1712, René Réaumur (1683–1757) demonstrated the ability of the claws and scales of lobsters to grow again after being severed. In the 1740s, Abraham Trembley (1710–84) sliced polyps or hydras into several pieces, producing new individuals, and got a third generation by cutting up the latter. The Swiss naturalist Charles Bonnet (1720–93) similarly experimented on freshwater worms (1741–45), and in 1768 the Italian, Lazzaro Spallanzani (1729–99), succeeded in regenerating the heads, tails, and limbs of snails, salamanders, earthworms, and tadpoles. Clearly, there was more to life than mechanical philosophy had dreamt of; and such investigations compelled physicians to entertain subtler views of higher organisms.

THE MYSTERY OF VITALITY: ALBRECHT VON HALLER

Experimentation provoked new opinions regarding the character of vitality – and, by implication, the relations between body and mind, body and soul. The key figure in these debates was Albrecht von Haller (1708–77). An infant prodigy, born into the old upper bourgeoisie of Bern, Haller studied in Leiden under Boerhaave, Albinus, and Jacques Benignus Winslow, and taught for 17 years at the newly-founded

University of Göttingen, setting up the botanical garden, before returning to his native Switzerland in 1753. A linguist and polymath who
wrote poetry and novels and made contributions to botany, Haller's
forte was physiological experimentation, and he produced an essential
text, the *Elementa Physiologiae Corporis Humani* (*Elements of the
Physiology of the Human Body*; 1759–66). Building on Boerhaave's concern with the fibres, his finest contribution to the study of animal economy was his laboratory demonstration of Francis Glisson's (1598–1677)
hypothesis that irritability or contractility was a property inherent in all
muscular fibres, whereas sensibility was the exclusive attribute of nervous fibres. Haller thus established the fundamental division of fibres
according to their reactive properties, a division into 'irritable' and 'sensible' components. The sensibility of nervous fibres was their responsive-
ness to painful stimuli; the irritability of muscle fibres was their property
of contractility in reaction to stimuli. Haller thereby had a theory of why
the heart pulsated: it was the most 'irritable' organ in the body.
Composed of layers of muscular fibres, it was stimulated by the inflow-
ing of blood, responding with systolic contractions. On the basis of
experimental procedures employed on animals and humans, Haller's
theories thus distinguished organ structures according to their fibre
composition, ascribing to them inherent sensitivities independent of any
superadded soul or non-material force. As with gravity, Haller believed
the causes of such living forces were beyond knowing, or at least
unknown. It was sufficient, in Newtonian fashion, to study the effects.

Haller's stance possessed many strengths. It rejected the unspoken
dualistic mechanism of Boerhaave and his 'hydraulic' school as too
simplistic for solving the puzzles of life; it equally repudiated Stahlian
'animism' for smuggling certain theological notions back into physiology, and the atheistic reductionism of La Mettrie. The concepts of irritability and sensibility achieved widespread approval. Like their mentor,
Haller's successors chose to treat vitality as a property of the material
ensemble of living bodies themselves. Continuing his work in
Göttingen, Johann Blumenbach (1752–1840), best known nowadays
for his pioneering anthropological writings, delineated several additional vital properties, including the *Bildungstrieb*, an inherent life-force
or a 'moulding' quality responsible for regeneration. Blumenbach's
notion paved the way for *Naturphilosophie*, with its commitment to
viewing Nature as holistic, integrative, and purposive.

THE SCOTTISH POSITION

A Scottish school of animal economy also arose. Like Haller, Robert Whytt (1714–66), a pupil of Alexander Monro primus (1697–1767) and Professor of Medicine at Edinburgh University, explored nervous activity but contested Haller's doctrine of the inherent irritability of the fibres. In *On the Vital and Other Involuntary Motions of Animals* (1751), Whytt argued that the reflex involved 'an unconscious sentient principle ... residing in the brain and spinal cord', though he denied that this entailed any under-cover reintroduction of the Stahlian soul. Building upon Haller's concept of irritability as a property of fibres, William Cullen (1710–90), Professor of Medicine and the Institutes of Medicine at Edinburgh University and the most influential teacher in the English-speaking world, interpreted life itself as a function of nervous power, and, by extension, construed all disease as ultimately 'nervous'. Cullen's one-time pupil, John Brown, was to out-Haller Haller by reducing questions of health and disease to variations around the mean of irritability. In place of Haller's concept of irritability, however, Brown substituted the notion that fibres were 'excitable'. Life was hence to be understood as the product of the action of external stimuli upon an organised body – life, pronounced the Brunonians, was a 'forced condition'. Sickness was disturbance of the proper functioning of excitement, and diseases were to be treated as 'sthenic' or 'asthenic' accordingly, as the vital condition or 'excitement' increased or diminished. Though winning only a modicum of support in France and England, Brunonian medicine had the virtue of simplicity and was enthusiastically taken up in America by Benjamin Rush, and in Italy by Giovanni Rasori (1766–1837); Christoph Girtanner (1760–1800), and Johann Peter Frank (1745–1821) popularised it in German-speaking Europe.

MONTPELLIER MEDICINE

In France, Montpellier graduates led the vitality debate. Boissier de Sauvages denied that Boerhaavian mechanism could explain the source of motion in the body, and, like Haller, thought that *anatomia* needed to be undertaken as *anatomia animata*, study of the structure of a living (not a deceased) body, divinely endowed with soul. Later Montpellier teachers assumed a more materialist stance, stressing the inherent vitality of living bodies rather than an external soul. Théophile de Bordeu (1722–76) demonstrated that Boerhaave's reductive and mechanistic explanation for gland secretions was physically impossible, but he also denounced recourse to metaphysical explanations for bodily functions. Bordeu maintained that each organ was naturally endowed with an inherent capacity to respond to stimuli – vital function was native to the organs themselves. The Montpellier school culminated in Xavier Bichat (1771–1802), whose dissections led him to postulate the presence of 21 different sorts of tissues or membranes as the elemental biological units. Though he doubted the value of the microscope, Bichat's tissue studies of the 1790s must be seen as foundational for nineteenth-century medicine, especially pathological anatomy. Parallel researches were pursued in London. John Hunter (1728–93), Scottish-born but London-based, proposed a 'life-principle' to account for properties distinguishing living organisms from inanimate matter – the repository of that life-force was the blood. (Hunter is further discussed on p. 439.)

Post-1750 investigators thus accentuated the qualitative distinctions they discerned between living and non-living bodies, but treated the superior properties of living entities as deriving not from any divinely-added soul but from their innate organisation. Echoing the old notion of the Great Chain of Being, many posited a hierarchy of levels of complexity. Living things in general enjoyed powers of nutrition and reproduction; unlike mere vegetables, animals also had capacities for mobility and sensitivity, associated with the workings of a nervous system; 'higher' animals (vertebrates, quadrupeds, mammals), endowed with more intricate nervous systems, additionally had forms of 'will', thereby establishing the potential for self-directed action. Endowed with consciousness, man was typically seen as the apex of this pyramid of organised vital powers. The hierarchy of faculties was sometimes described in the idiom of 'development' (higher forms were more 'evolved'). But for most investigators, 'development' did not carry any implication of species transmutation over time, that is, organic evolution in the modern post-Darwin sense, but merely a pre-ordained plan of Creation, unfolding conceptually and possibly temporally, by divine law or special fiat. At the close of the century, however, Jean Baptiste Lamarck (1744–1829) in France and Erasmus Darwin in Britain were turning the 'stages' model of the hierarchy of organised powers into authentic transformationist terms, showing how lower forms transmuted into higher, thanks to inherent progressive drives and environmental challenge. Erasmus Darwin explained this capacity of life to evolve by postulating an inherent Hallerian motility, lodged in the fibres of organised, animated creatures. Living beings, in other words, did not merely react mechanically to outside interference, they possessed an animation of their own, sustained through nutrition and discharged through action, the ultimate ebbing of which spelt death. Living bodies, in short, responded purposively to their external environment.

Thus earlier philosophies of the 'machine of life' gave way to accounts of 'vital properties'. It is no accident that the very term 'biology' was coined around 1800, amongst others by Gottfried Reinhold Treviranus (1776-1837), Professor of Mathematics and Medicine at Bremen. The influential French historian, Michel Foucault claimed, in a phrase more arresting than accurate, that pre-1800 approaches to the study of the animal kingdom had no concept of 'life'; 'life' was invented with biology, Foucault maintained, at the dawn of the new century. Against Foucault, it may be argued that Haller's work on fibre responses and nervous organisation created from the mid-eighteenth century's recognisably 'modern' notions of life.

EXPERIMENTS INTO LIFE

It would be wrong, of course, to imply that all researchers were bent on revealing the secret of life. Most investigations were more circumscribed. The processes of digestion, for example, came under vigorous scrutiny. Were digestion and absorption effected by some internal vital force, by the chemical action of gastric acids, or by the mechanical operation of churning, mincing, and pulverizing? The digestion debate had rumbled on since the Greeks. Eighteenth-century inquiries were characterised by a new experimental ingenuity, initiated by the French naturalist, René Réaumur (1683–1757). Having trained a pet kite to swallow and regurgitate small porous food-filled tubes, Réaumur demonstrated the powers of gastric juices, and showed that meat was more fully digested in the stomach than starchy foods. By using pieces of sponge, Réaumur was able to obtain specimens of gastric fluids. Lazzaro Spallanzani followed up these investigations, experimenting upon himself by gulping down and regurgitating linen bags. Attempting to gauge whether digestion was essentially a chemical process, Spallanzani proved the solvent powers of saliva.

As is suggested by digestion studies, medicine and chemistry fruitfully interacted. Following up lines of inquiry developed by iatrochemists like J. B. van Helmont and Sylvius, chemists explored fermentation and the parallel between respiration and combustion. Joseph Black (1728–99), who formulated the idea of latent heat and in his *Dissertatio de Humore Acido a Cibis Orto et Magnesia Alba* (*Dissertation on the Acid Humour Arising from Food and on White Magnesia*; 1754), identified fixed air or what came to be known, after Lavoisier's revolution in chemical nomenclature, as carbon dioxide. Thanks to Black, gas chemistry advanced rapidly, and with it recognition that the atmosphere was not homogeneous but rather a mixture of distinct gases. In 1766, Henry Cavendish produced hydrogen, and Daniel Rutherford (1749–1819) discovered nitrogen in 1772. Soon after, both Joseph Priestley and Karl Wilhelm Scheele separately isolated the gas that Antoine-Laurent Lavoisier (1743–94) would style oxygen (1775). Major advances followed in the understanding of respiration. Black had noted that the 'fixed air', given off by quicklime and alkalis, was also present in expired air; while non-toxic, it was physiologically irrespirable. Priestley grasped that vegetating plants renewed vitiated air (which, as a devotee of the phlogiston theory, he called 'phlogisticated dephlogisticated air'). It was Lavoisier who best explained the interchange of gases in the lungs. He showed that the air inhaled was converted into Black's 'fixed air', whereas the nitrogen ('azote') remained unchanged. Respiration was, Lavoisier believed, the analogue within living bodies of combustion in the wider world; both needed oxygen, both produced carbon dioxide and water. He perceived that oxygen was indispensable for the human body, showing that, when engrossed in physical processes like digestion, the body consumed greater quantities of oxygen than when at rest. A little later, Spallanzani revealed that oxidation occurred in the blood and throughout the entire physical system. By 1800, it had been recognized that oxygen combined with the carbon contained in food to generate animal heat and discharge the carbon dioxide exhaled in breath.

GAS CHEMISTRY

Breakthroughs in chemistry seemed full of promise for medicine. Hopes rose that gases would furnish specific cures. The rationale of Thomas Beddoes's Pneumatic Institute, opened in Clifton (Bristol) in 1799, was to experiment with gases and launch new therapies. Beddoes (1760–1808) developed a partnership with James Watt (1736–1819), publishing with him *Considerations on the Medicinal Use of Factitious Airs* (1794) which adumbrated the project's rationale. Beddoes then discovered the Cornish apothecary's apprentice, Humphry Davy

(1778–1829), who, as his assistant, in turn discovered the anaesthetic properties of nitrous oxide (laughing gas). Beddoes envisioned that nitrous oxide would cure tubercular patients. In the event, Beddoes's aërotherapy or pneumotherapy achieved scant success – and the authentic anaesthetic properties of nitrous oxide curiously lay neglected for a further four decades.

There was also intense interest after 1760 in attempts to measure the salubrity of the atmosphere. Medicine had long been concerned with the 'bad air' (*mal aria*) supposedly given off by marshes and fens, and with the much-touted bracing qualities of coastal resorts and mountains. Now, advances in gas chemistry opened prospects of scientifically analysing the compositions of different kinds of atmospheres and gauging their healthiness. Pneumatic chemistry apparently held the clue to the progress of environmental medicine – though, once again, aspiration outstripped achievement.

ELECTRICITY

Advances in other sciences also promised medical pay-offs. Electricity made great strides and became a fashionable subject of experimental display, guinea-pigs being routinely 'electrified' out of curiosity and amusement. Haller's observations on sensitivity and irritability pointed to parallels between physiological and electrical events. What animated the nerves? The force in muscular activity might be mechanical (as with a bell-pull, or a wire under tension); or chemical (perhaps akin to a gunpowder trail, setting off a chain of minor explosions); but many thought it must be electrical. Animal electricity was observed in the torpedo fish by John Walsh (1725–95), and John Hunter was soon to undertake studies of other electric fishes. But experimental electrophysiology – the application of currents to nerve and muscle preparations – was pioneered by Luigi Galvani (1737–98). In *De Viribus Electricitatis in Motu Musculari* (*On Electrical Powers in the Movement of Muscles*; 1792) the Italian naturalist described animal experiments in which he suspended the legs of dead frogs by copper wire from an iron balcony. As the feet touched the iron uprights, the legs twitched, because of an electrical potential difference between iron and copper. Subsequently, Galvani systematically explored the electrical properties of excised fibres. His experiments were followed up by Alessandro Volta (1745–1827), professor at Pavia, whose *Letters on Animal Electricity* appeared in 1792. Volta showed that a muscle could be thrown into

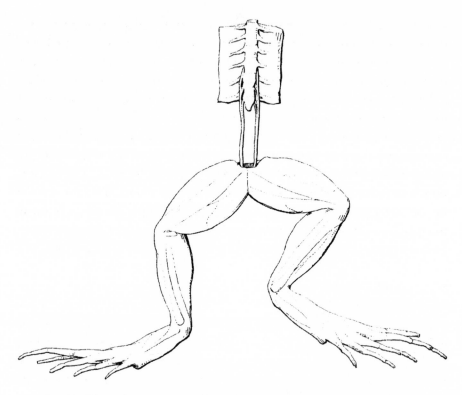

Fig. 52. Galvani, frog preparation. Galvani's experiments demonstrated the relations between electricity and nervous response, and so furthered debate about the nature of the life force. (The Wellcome Institute Library, London. L2011.)

continuous contraction by successive electrical stimulations. The connexions between life and electricity implied by such writings proved immensely suggestive for later neurophysiology, to say nothing of providing the inspiration for science fiction fantasies like Mary Shelley's (1795–1851) *Frankenstein* (1818), whose theme was the artificial creation of life.

EMBRYOLOGY

Embryology also developed. Aided in part by microscopical studies, so-called animalculist or *emboîtement* theories had risen to prominence after 1650. These typically claimed that a homunculus, a minuscule though fully-formed creature, was already present in the male seminal fluid. Reproduction was thus essentially a matter of implanting a ready-to-grow seed capsule into the female seedbed. William Harvey, on the other hand, had lent his authority to a different theory, ovism, arguing

– as a female version of preformationism – the indispensable role of the female egg in generation. The 'preformationist' dispute bubbled well into the eighteenth century, buoyed up by wider questions of theology (*emboîtement* could be seen as predestinarian) and gender politics (ovism dignified women). The most distinguished study of reproductive processes came from Caspar Friedrich Wolff (1733–94) of Berlin. His *Theoria Generationis* (*Theory of Generation*; 1759) supported Harveian epigenetic notions by offering experimental evidence of the gradual evolution of the foetal parts: organs appeared and became differentiated step-by-step, rather than being preformed and merely swelling in bulk in the fertilised egg. Wolff's work marks contemporary recognition of the inherent complexity of living processes.

Clinical medicine and disease theory

Anatomy and physiology thus advanced, both piecemeal and as part of a debate about the nature of life. The surge of science encouraged attempts to understand the laws of living beings. But the relations between biological knowledge and medical practice were complex and opaque, and few scientific breakthroughs had direct application to the mastery of disease. Renowned clinicians were not necessarily prominent in scientific advance, or vice versa. Some physicians shone by being figures of fashion, wits, literary lions, or through sheer force of personality. John Radcliffe (1652–1714) rose in London circles thanks to his bluntness with patients, Richard Mead (1673–1754) by virtue of his suavity. Like Sir Hans Sloane (1660–1753), Mead dabbled in science and built up a fabulous collection of antiquities, books, and *objets d'art*; bequeathed to the nation, Sloane's collection became the nucleus of the British Museum. Samuel Garth (1661–1719), Richard Blackmore (d. 1729), Mark Akenside (1721–70), and other physicians excelled as men of letters.

Some rose by virtue of bedside sagacity. William Heberden (1710–1801), who trained in Cambridge but practised in London, developed an impressive grasp, in the Hippocratic manner, of characteristic disease syndromes. Heeding Sydenham's advice that clinical symptoms should be described with 'the same minuteness and accuracy observed by a painter in painting a portrait', Heberden emphasised the importance of distinguishing symptoms that were 'particular and constant' from those due to accidental causes like age and constitution. His

Commentaries (1802), the fruit of 60 years' conscientious note-taking, debunked hoary errors (e.g. the supposed protective qualities of gout), described syndromes, and offered shrewd diagnostic and prognostic advice. The work contains original descriptions of angina pectoris, arthritic nodules in the fingers, and night-blindness. Samuel Johnson's description of Heberden as 'ultimus Romanorum, the last of our great physicians', pays homage to a creditable traditionalist, steeped in Classical learning and in old-school notions of the personal medical attendant, who lived into a new century when such skills would gradually be elbowed aside by the stethoscope and other diagnostic technology, the biochemical laboratory, and new ontological disease concepts.

Every court and capital had distinguished clinicians. Serving the French-speaking elite was the Geneva-born Théodore Tronchin (1709–81), Voltaire's favourite physician, perhaps the wealthiest and most fashionable practitioner of his time. An acute observer who vigorously advocated smallpox inoculation, Tronchin was one of many mid-century physicians to point out that the stomach disorder called Poitou colic was the product of lead poisoning. His *De colica Pictonum* (*On Poitou colic*; 1757) stands alongside the comparable observations (on the Devonshire colic) of Sir George Baker (1722–1809); physician to George III (1738–1820), it was Baker's unhappy lot to have to deal with the King during his first bout of insanity. In Rome, Giovanni Maria Lancisi (1655–1720) made a name for himself as physician to several popes.

DIAGNOSTICS

New bedside skills emerged. In his *Inventum Novum* (*New Discovery*; 1761), Leopold Auenbrugger (1722–1809), physician-in-chief to the Hospital of the Holy Trinity at Vienna, announced the technique of percussion of the chest, based upon his own extensive practice and verified by post-mortem experiences. An inn-keeper's son, Auenbrugger was familiar from childhood with the trick of banging casks to test their fullness. Moving from barrels to patients, he noted that when struck with a finger, a healthy subject's chest sounded like a cloth-covered drum; by contrast, a muffled sound, or one of uncommonly high pitch, indicated pulmonary diseases. Auenbrugger's percussion received, however, a muted reception from eminent contemporary physicians like Anton de Haen (1704–76), the most influential figure in Vienna. Only after Corvisart (1755–1821) recommended it in 1808 was percussion widely adopted.

In general, physicians rested content with the traditional diagnostic uses of the 'five senses'; they would feel the pulse, sniff for indications of decay, taste urine, listen for breathing irregularities, and observe skin colour. This time-honoured approach was almost exclusively qualitative. Thus, what standardly counted in pulse lore was not the number of beats per minute but their strength, firmness, rhythm, and 'feel'. Some attention was given to urine samples, but the traditional art of urine-gazing (uroscopy) was now dismissed as the trick of the quackish 'pisse prophet' and chemical analysis had barely begun. Qualitative judgments dominated, and the good diagnostician was he who, relying on acuity and experience, could size up a patient by close attention and familiarity.

In Britain at least – though not necessarily throughout the Continent – physicians rarely performed physical examinations. In contrast to a later era, when he would be expected to undertake a full 'physical' with the patient on a bed and clothing removed, the eighteenth-century British physician saw little need for direct physical contact. This was to some extent a matter of prudery. More importantly, traditional medical reasoning afforded no grounds for believing that physical examination would prove fruitful for diagnosing internal conditions. The *sine qua non* of traditional diagnostics was keen attention to the patient's recitation of his own 'history' (hence too the common and respectable practice of diagnosing by post). The sick person would tell the doctor what was wrong: when and how the complaint had started, what events had pre-cipitated it, the characteristic pains and symptoms, the periodicity of fever symptoms (a tertian ague, a quartan fever), and so forth. The patient would also inform his physician on life-style – eating and sleep-ing habits, bowel motions, emotional trauma, and so forth – not to men-tion the slightly indelicate matter of indulgence in quack medicines. Pugnacious patients might dictate to the doctors – though others went to the opposite extreme, complained William Buchan, treating 'physi-cians as conjurors, and think they need no information'. Armed with a fine memory, the expert clinician was thus to be a good listener, doing his detective work by astute questioning. Erasmus Darwin 'often disre-garded the accounts his patients gave of themselves, and rather chose to collect his information by indirect inquiry and by cross-examining them, than from their voluntary testimony. That distrust and that habit were probably favourable to his skill in discovering the origin of diseases, and thence to his pre-eminent success in effecting their cure'.

THE STUDY OF DISEASES

The good clinician knew his circle of patients, often treating them for several decades. But he also knew his diseases. Eighteenth-century practitioners trod in the 'Hippocratic' footsteps of Thomas Sydenham, amassing extensive empirical records, particularly of the epidemic disorders they saw especially virulent in their own times. Sydenham's works achieved a particularly wide circulation and high prestige among eighteenth-century physicians, who found many attractions in his recommendation of a natural history approach, in which diseases would be understood 'botanically', as discrete entities. Sydenham's awareness that Peruvian bark acted as a specific against intermittent fevers (malaria) encouraged the urge to identify other particular diseases for which specific remedies might be discovered.

The Plymouth doctor, John Huxham (1692–1768) displayed extensive knowledge of disease profiles in his *On Fevers* (1750); the Chester practitioner, John Haygarth (1740–1827), undertook analysis of smallpox epidemics, as well as typhus and rheumatic fever. William Withering (1741–99) investigated tuberculosis and scarlet fever, describing the severe outbreaks of scarlatina in 1771 and 1778. John Fothergill (1712–80), a Yorkshireman and Quaker who built up a lucrative London practice, was an avid follower of Sydenham. In his *Observations of the Weather and Diseases of London* (1751–54), he surveyed the urban disease environment and gave a valuable description of 'epidemic sore throat' (diphtheria), then growing more widespread as an often fatal malady of the urban poor. His friend and fellow Quaker, the philanthropist, John Coakley Lettsom (1744–1845), was the driving-force behind the clinical investigations pioneered by the Medical Society of London, founded in 1773. Such medical gatherings, common also in the provinces, collected clinical data and exchanged news. Also important for clinical science was the development of medical journalism. Doctors had always corresponded with each other, but hitherto the formal channels available for medical exchanges were distinctly limited. Things changed with the spread of medico-scientific societies and their publications. In the English-speaking world, Fothergill, Lettsom and other élite practitioners sent items of medical information to the *Gentleman's Magazine*, founded 1731, a general-interest periodical with a circulation touching 10,000, which carried essays on disease prevention, drugs, first-aid, epidemics and the new charity hospitals. Specific medical productions developed: in Britain, for instance, there were the *Medical Essays and Observations, Produced by a Society in Edinburgh*, which appeared in six volumes between 1733 and 1744; their successor, the *Essays and Observations*, published in Edinburgh in three volumes between 1754 and 1765; the *Medical Observations and Inquiries*, issued by a 'Society of Physicians' in London, appeared in six volumes between 1757 and 1784; the *Medical Transactions*, published in six volumes by the Royal College of Physicians of London from 1768 to 1820; the *Memoirs of the Medical Society of London* first appeared in 1787, continuing through six volumes till 1805; and so forth. Thanks to the energetic John Haygarth, the Chester Society for Promoting Inoculation put forth its own *Proceedings* from 1778–82. An extensive medical press was operating by 1800. As well as putting members of the profession in touch with each other, journals also generated *esprit de corps*, a zest for investigation and agenda for clinical research.

Systematic research programmes did not develop till the nineteenth century, yet many original observations upon diseases were made earlier. Notable were Friedrich Hoffmann's descriptions of rubella (1740); William Hunter's and Lancisi's delineations of aneurysm (1757); Robert Whytt's clinical picture of tuberculous meningitis (1768); Matthew Dobson's (d. 1784) demonstration that the sweetness of the urine in diabetes is due to sugar (1776); Lettsom's characterisation of alcoholism (1786); and so forth. Many valuable disease surveys were published, including Astruc's (1736) and Benjamin Bell's (1749–1806) studies of venereal diseases; François Emmanuel de Fodéré's (1764–1835) account of cretinism and goitre (1792); and the depictions by Thomas Beddoes and others of the worsening scourge of tuberculosis. Children's diseases attracted attention from William Cadogan (1711–97), Rosén von Rosenstein (1706–73), George Armstrong (1719–89), Michael Underwood (1737–1820), and Christoph Girtanner (1760–1800) – historians have spoken of the 'new world of the children' in the eighteenth century, and the age was certainly marked by burgeoning interest in paediatrics. George Cheyne's (1671–1743) *The English Malady* (1733) was only the most striking of many works addressing 'nervous diseases'; like various contemporaries, Cheyne also wrote on gout and digestive disorders, while James Lind (1736–1812), Thomas Trotter (1760–1832), and other naval practitioners studied scurvy. Robert Willan's (1757–1812) publications on skin diseases advanced dermatology. Various 'new diseases' attracted interest – the Swiss, Tissot, for instance, wrote extensively on onanism

405

(1762). The list of significant epidemic and clinical studies of disease attests growing practical observational skills and an emancipation from sterile book-learning and hide-bound authority.

Bedside acumen and an alert eye for the seasonality of epidemics nevertheless took understanding of ailments only as far as an appreciation of symptom clusters. Questions of the real nature and true causation (*vera causa*) of disease remained highly controversial. In an intellectual heritage derived from the Greeks, much sickness was still attributed to personal factors – poor initial physical endowment, neglect of hygiene, over-indulgence. What may be called the 'constitutional' concept of disease made good sense of uneven and unpredictable sickness scatter – even with rampant infections like smallpox, some individuals were afflicted, some were not, even in a single household. It also drew attention to individual moral responsibility and pointed to strategies of containment through self-discipline. This personalisation of illness had undeniable merits and attractions.

Theories of contagion also circulated. Belief that disease was spread by contact had unmistakable experience in its favour. Certain disorders, for instance, syphilis, were manifestly transmitted directly, person-to-person. Smallpox inoculation offered ocular proof of contagiousness. But contagion hypotheses had their difficulties as well. There were evident counter-experiences. If contact spread disease, why did not disorders spread exponentially – why were not all family members, all physicians, and nurses laid low? Why were some people stricken and others spared? And what was it that was actually being transferred in cross-infection? Was it some tangible thing, some 'seed of disease' or poison? The question of the objective existence of morbific matter had long been vexed. To many, the notion of disease being conveyed person-to-person smacked of obsolete vulgar doctrines of 'influence' or witchcraft maleficium (casting a spell), and so was liable to be ridiculed as a throwback to bygone superstitions.

Such misgivings explain the popularity of miasmatic thinking, the conviction that sickness typically spread not person-to-person but from environment to individual, for intelligent scrutiny revealed the differential dangerousness of locations. With intermitting fevers like 'ague' (malaria), it was common knowledge that those living in estuarine areas, near marshes and creeks, were especially susceptible. Low and spotted fevers –

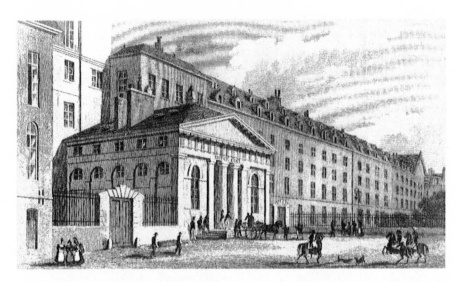

Fig. 53. Hôtel Dieu, Paris, early nineteenth-century view. The Hôtel Dieu was Paris's
main general hospital. (The Wellcome Institute, London. L4302.)

among them conditions we would now identify as typhus – were recognised as infecting populations in the overcrowded, ill-ventilated slum
quarters of great towns, just as they also struck the occupants of gaols,
barracks, ships, workhouses, and other congested and filthy institutions.
There was an obvious plausibility in the supposition that disease lay in
poisonous exhalations carried in the atmosphere, exuded by putrefying
organic material, waterlogged soil, rotting vegetable and decomposing
animal remains, stagnant water, and other noisome properties of the
milieu. Bad environments, the argument ran, generated bad air (signalled
by stenches), which in turn triggered disease. Energetic investigators set
about tracking down the 'miasmata' held responsible for the waves of
epidemic and endemic fevers sweeping Europe – measles, scarlatina,
typhus, typhoid and malaria. After 1750, reformers directed attention to
the rise of 'septic' diseases – gangrene, septicaemia, diphtheria, erysipelas,
and puerperal fever – especially rampant in slum quarters and institutions like gaols and hospitals. Paris's general hospital (the Hôtel Dieu)
had an atrocious reputation as a nest of infection.

It has been tempting for historians to split disease theories into two
rival camps: 'miasmatists' against 'contagionists'. It seems a convenient
division, because each doctrine had a destiny ahead of it. Miasmatic
doctrines supposedly fuelled the great later public health movements,
enshrined in the conviction of Edwin Chadwick (1800–90) that 'all

smell is disease': a theory which, though wrong, nevertheless secured sanitary reform. Contagionism for its part might be seen as the forerunner of the Pasteurian germ theory of disease.

But such a polarity is anachronistic and simplistic. Medical thinking on the causes of epidemics was many-faceted, and eclectic. There were no rigid party-lines, no heroes and villains. Investigators did not see the aetiology of epidemics as requiring a choice between blaming either the individual or the environment. Analyses typically accepted that aetiology was multifactorial – one common way of expressing this was to speak of a combination of 'predisposing' and 'precipitating' causes. In any case, it was widely understood that different disorders – smallpox, malaria, gout – had distinctive causative patterns.

Indeed, investigators were less interested in ascertaining the root causes of disease than in documenting its nature, manifestations and configurations. That is why the umbrella-term 'fevers' was so convenient and widely utilised. Fevers could be recognised as epidemic. Yet they could also be interpreted in terms of classic humoral theories of a febrile 'crisis' within the body, involving 'coction' of morbific matter, to be resolved by the expulsion of peccant humours through orifices and pores. Physicians still widely accepted the Hippocratic view that fever was a natural process requiring to be 'supported' rather than suppressed. The good physician was the capable manager of fevers, understanding their natural pattern and knowing how best to bring them out. For the risk with too drastic intervention was that fevers would 'turn in' and pose a yet more serious threat to the constitution. This Hippocratic view of fevers, mediated through the influential Thomas Sydenham, permitted eighteenth-century clinicians to view major diseases in terms of a social epidemiology while also insisting on the unique features of the individual case.

Energetic attempts were made to prevent or contain epidemics. Milieus responsible for severe febrile disorders – slums, camps, ships, gaols – were identified and experiments conducted upon the causes and the control of putrefaction, widely assumed to be the root cause of septic fevers. As is shown by the endeavours of gaol reformers like John Howard (1726–90) and enlightened naval captains, notably James Cook (1728–79), the preference was for a comprehensive 'managerial' strategy of cleanliness – washing, fumigation, whitewashing, sprinkling with lemon juice or vinegar (considered 'antiseptic'), abundant ventilation, good morals and discipline among ships' crews or institutional inmates. The value of citrus fruits in combating scurvy was recognised within a wider cleanliness package.

Such practical measures commanded wide assent, regardless of theoretical underpinning. True, 'contagionists' had been strong supporters of the system of lines and cordons sanitaires (p. 220f.) enforced on the borders of the Habsburg Empire and at Mediterranean ports, designed to stop bubonic plague spreading from the Levant. In the English plague scare of the early 1720s, sparked by the Marseilles outbreak, the orthodox medical view was formulated by Dr Richard Mead, who had been commissioned by the Government to investigate the question. In his *Short Discourse Concerning Pestilential Contagion, and the Methods to be Used to Prevent it* (1720), Mead plumped for the traditional package of contagion theory plus quarantine, measures opposed by those who denied the specific contagiousness of plague and feared that quarantine – a so-called 'French measure' – would ruin British trade. Once the perils of plague receded, rigorous isolationist policies lost their advocates. Rather, a broad mix of 'hygiene' measures found favour, designed to cleanse and improve conditions in institutions and among vulnerable social groups. Urban improvement and personal hygiene were widely implemented in Hanoverian London, and they had an acknowledged success. 'In the space of a very few years', declared John Coakley Lettsom in the 1790s:

> I have observed a total revolution in the conduct of the common people respecting their diseased friends. They have learned that most diseases are mitigated by a free admission of air, by cleanliness and by promoting instead of restraining the indulgence and care of the sick.

Gilbert Blane (1749–1834) similarly believed that the living conditions of the metropolitan poor had improved as a result of greater use of cotton clothing, soap, water, and cheap fuel, and heightened public awareness of the value of ventilation.

NOSOLOGY

Two further developments in disease theory should be mentioned. Many were attracted by the idea of classifying maladies nosologically, sorting diseases into classes, species, and varieties, as in botany and zoology, with a view to a firmer grasp of affinities and differences. Built on Sydenham's notion of a 'natural history of disease', a disease taxonomy would hopefully establish diseases as real entities, governed by natural laws that could serve as tangible objects of inquiry, as in

François Boissier de Sauvages's *Methodical Nosology* (1771). Symptom clusters would provide the basis for disease classification. For William Cullen, nosology served as a useful teaching-aid, a filing system for data, a compendium for the busy young doctor. Take fevers. Fevers were labelled by Cullen as pyrexiae or febrile diseases, differentiated by local inflammations. Within the pyrexiae, diseases well-defined and spreading by contact, like smallpox, were attributed to specific contagions (and were also known as 'strictly contagious' diseases).

Did such nosological systems prove valuable? Perhaps not. For many of Cullen's students, to say nothing of his critics, appear to have believed that such grand nosological structures were more trouble than they were worth, and nosology was widely ridiculed as a house of cards.

PATHOLOGY

Of infinitely greater long-term significance was pathological anatomy. Since Vesalius, the idea had grown that the good practitioner must be proficient in gross anatomy. An inevitable consequence was that increased attention began to be paid to the connexions between the sick body and the disease signs afforded by the corpse. Anatomy, in other words, paved the way for morbid anatomy and new skills in reading pathological signs in the cadaver. Post-mortem investigation would show the changes brought about within the body by disease (not least, cause of death), and give insight into the sources of the deceased patient's symptoms and signs.

The trail was blazed by the illustrious Italian, Giovanni Battista Morgagni (1682–1771), professor of anatomy at Padua. Building on earlier necropsy studies by Johann Wepfer (1620–95) and Théophile Bonet (1620–89), Morgagni, almost 80, published in 1761 his *De Sedibus et Causis Morborum* (*On the Sites and Causes of Disease*). This work surveyed the findings of some 700 autopsies. Morgagni's book quickly became famous; it was translated into English in 1769 and German in 1774.

In *De Sedibus*, Morgagni demonstrated that diseases are located in specific organs, that disease symptoms tally with anatomical lesions, and that pathological organ changes are responsible for most disease manifestations. It was Morgagni who thus finally clinched the direct relevance of anatomy to clinical medicine. Morgagni followed a largely empirical method in morbid anatomy, believing that repeated observations improved the reliability of the results. He laid bare divers disease conditions, includ-

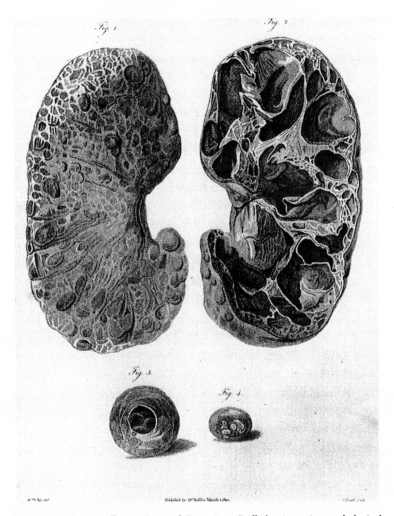

Fig. 54. Matthew Baillie, *A Series of Engravings*. Baillie's pioneering pathological work was exquisitely illustrated. Here polycystic kidney disease is displayed. (The Wellcome Institute Library, London. L15609.)

ing syphilitic aneurysm, acute yellow atrophy of the liver, and tuberculosis of the kidney. He showed the clinical features of pneumonia, and demonstrated that intracranial suppuration is a sequel of discharge from the ear (and not vice versa). Morgagni established the dictum of his teacher, Antonio Maria Valsalva (1666–1723), that, in stroke, the cerebral lesion is on the opposite side from the resulting paralysis.

But if he was concerned with general disease phenomena, Morgagni also recognized the importance of unique manifestations in the individual instance, and his case-reports took note of such factors as age, sex, marital status, and occupation. In the time-honoured manner, he inquired after previous illness, family history (to identify possible hereditary factors), and environmental conditions. The vast scope of Morgagni's observations of diseased viscera and his valuable new disease descriptions set pathological investigation on the map.

Others continued his work. In 1793, Matthew Baillie (1761–1823), a Scot and a nephew of William Hunter practising in London, published his *Morbid Anatomy* (1793). Illustrated with superb copper-plates by William Clift (1775–1849) – it depicted, amongst other things, the emphysema of Samuel Johnson's lungs – Baillie's work was more of a textbook than Morgagni's; thus it described in succession the morbid appearances of each organ. Typically of the times, Baillie made little use of the microscope, and did not attempt to deal with the nerves or the spinal cord. He offered numerous new descriptions, including ovarian cysts and gastric ulcers, and provided the first faithful definitions of cirrhosis of the liver and of hepatisation of the lungs in pneumonia. He showed that death from polypus of the heart was really due to a clot of fibrin, and in his second edition (1797) developed the idea of 'rheumatism of the heart' (rheumatic fever).

Pathology became more fully systematised with the publication in 1800 of the *Traité des Membranes* (*Treatise on Membranes*) by Marie François Xavier Bichat (1771–1802), who focused particularly upon the histological changes produced by disease. As developed by Morgagni, pathology had dealt with organs. Bichat changed the focus. 'The more one will observe diseases and open cadavers', he declared, 'the more one will be convinced of the necessity of considering local diseases not from the aspect of the complex organs but from that of the individual tissues'. Bichat's work heralded the patho-anatomy of the nineteenth century.

Around 1800 clinical judgment was still drawing upon the threads and patches of humoralism. Disease theories remained multifactorial (later critics would say confused). Yet, thanks to developments in pathology, attention was newly being paid to normal and abnormal structures and functions, a trend that would come to fruition in the nineteenth century.

Therapeutics

If no theories revolutionised concepts of aetiology and epidemiology, did the eighteenth century see improved prospects of relief and recovery? If disease remained a shadowy enemy, was it, nevertheless, one that could be defeated?

These questions admit of no final answers, because therapeutics is multiform. The potency of disease, the hazards of life, and the imperfections of medicine dictated recourse to varied healing methods, old and new, professional and lay. Therapeutics took many forms, which often made strange bedfellows. The profession deployed a battery of weapons, ranging from dietetics to drugs, from regimen to surgery, aided, tacitly at least, by the placebo effect of a good bedside manner. And alongside doctors, regular and irregular, myriad other modes of healing were utilised, some primarily medical, others ritualistic, community or family-based. The sick largely initiated and often conducted their own treatments – the bureaucratised 'healing machines' of state medicine are of twentieth century origins. And we must avoid anachronistic judgments upon the success (or more commonly shortcomings) of the therapeutic strategies of the past. Today medicine promises and patients anticipate 'cure' for most ailments. In former days, expectations were more modest, and recourse was had to medicine in the hope of obtaining relief, resuming work, or simply gaining reassurance that the malaise, though uncured, was under supervision.

RELIGION AND MAGIC

Not only 'ignorant peasants' looked to religious healing. Physic and faith still criss-crossed at innumerable points. In southern Europe and throughout Latin America, the Catholic Church continued to promote authorised healing procedures – holy waters and wells, shrines, relics, pilgrimages, ex-voto offerings, processions, masses, and the invocation of saints. And, even in Protestant nations where such 'superstitions' were censured, individual quacks, itinerant healers, seventh sons of seventh sons, and 'strokers' claimed the divine gift of miracle cures. Bourbon and Stuart monarchs, of course, paraded their theocratic powers by touching for the 'king's evil' or scrofula; in England such thaumaturgical healing lapsed with the Hanoverian succession in 1714 (the infant Samuel Johnson was one of the last to be touched by Queen Anne), but the rituals long continued in France, being revived at the Bourbon restoration in 1815. So long as rural communities believed in *maleficium* (evil) and witchcraft edicts remained on the statute book, it is hardly surprising that therapeutic activity also wore a supernatural hue.

Magic still underlay certain kinds of healing. Although the mechanical philosophy won favour among the Enlightenment elite, in rural and plebeian communities ailments continued to be treated with charms, spells, sigils, and ritual incantations. The touch of a hanged man's hand, for instance, or the rope that launched him into eternity, were popularly credited with curative powers. Medical magic rarely possessed a distinctive cosmology of its own. Rather it comprised a potpourri of ad hoc practices that invested curative objects and healing rituals with special powers: a herb, a formula repeated to the letter, ceremonial gestures or objects involving displacement, expulsion, or sympathy. It was thus believed by association that springs or corn dollies would aid fertility.

Some cures were indisputably magical. Back in the seventeenth century, the antiquarian and Fellow of the Royal Society, John Aubrey (1626–97), recorded numerous formulae along these lines: 'write these characters + Zada + Zadash + Zadathan + Abira + in virgin paper, I beleeve parchment, carry it always with you, and no gun-shott can hurt you'. But where did indisputably 'magical' healing practices end, and natural ones begin? In case of a stye, it was common to stroke the affected eye with a black cat's tail – was that a natural remedy or an echo of black magic? A much-touted cure for inflammation of the brain, still cropping up in family medicine books as late as the 1770s, was to 'cut open a live Chicken or Pigeon, and apply it to the Head' – was this a medical therapy, or did the supposed efficacy lie in the sacrifice? Similarly with the doctrine of signatures in herbal lore. The fact that the plant eyebright (*Euphrasia officinalis*) had a bloom resembling an eye showed it to be a specific for eye disease; the yellow of saffron signified it was good for jaundice, and the leaves of the lungwort plant, which vaguely resembled the lungs, announced it alleviated pulmonary disease. As is revealed by the dozens of plants used to cure warts, it would be anachronistic rigidly to demarcate herbal remedies used magically from those deployed empirically. Surviving family recipe books show heaps of healing salves, prophylactics, and remedial practices, some of which – the use of dead toads or vipers' blood, for example – were surely rooted in the occult, even if, in course of time, they became disengaged from their original principles. The *éclat* of Enlightenment unorthodox healers, notably Franz Anton Mesmer (1734–1815), pioneer of hypnotherapy, reveals the enduring appeal of spectacular healing practices. Charismatic figures like Mesmer may be viewed as transitional figures on a path leading from sorcery to psychoanalysis.

Alongside and gradually supplanting religico-magical approaches to healing were therapeutics of a physical kind, built upon Greek foundations but incorporating the new theories of the Scientific Revolution. Though many treatments wore an ad hoc appearance, such therapeutic strategies depended upon entrenched concepts of bodily functions and disease aetiology stemming from humoralism. Holistic and constitutional in their reasoning, healers naturally had recourse to regimen and diet, both as preventive and as curative measures. The enduring popularity, likewise, of purging and phlebotomy hinged on the old conviction that sickness followed plethora (excess) or the build-up of peccant humours in the system, requiring periodic discharge.

Eighteenth-century mechanistic approaches, with their vision of a body governed by universal laws of matter in motion, produced new physiological and pathological concepts. Yet, as so often in medicine, treatments changed less than the theories rationalizing them. As may be seen from *An Essay on Regimen* (1740), *The Natural Method of Cureing Diseases of the Body and the Disorders of the Mind* (1742), and other writings by the highly influential Scotsman, George Cheyne (1671–1743), the new mechanical physiology by no means undermined traditional holistic methods. Cheyne touted the nervous system as the locus of most disorders, but prescribed conventional dietary regulation.

Yet certain changes were in the air, sanctioned in part by Thomas Sydenham's notion of a natural history of disease, and by the structure/function orientation of the mechanical philosophy. These prompted the idea that complaints were not particular to the constitution of the particular sufferer but 'specific' to the disorder, by analogy with botanical or zoological types. Such shifts had long-term therapeutic implications, especially in the light of changes in matter-theory and chemistry. Developments from Paracelsus to Boyle had already cast doubt on the Classical idea of the four elements as the universal building blocks of reality, prompting the notion of distinctive chemical affinities. The Paracelsan and Van Helmontian tenet that specific diseases needed specific remedies (e.g. mercury for syphilis) had been boosted by the growing popularity of iatrochemistry, and was further strengthened by popular medico-chemical writers like Nicholas Lemery (1645–1715) and Peter Shaw (1694–1763). Once scorned as quackish by orthodox physicians, specific chemical remedies grew more acceptable.

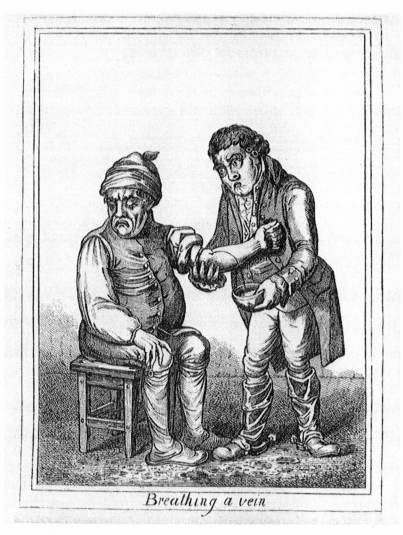

Breathing a vein

Fig. 55. Gillray, 'Breathing a Vein'. A comic illustration of blood-letting (also known as venesection or phlebotomy). (The Wellcome Institute Library, London. V11197.)

HUMANIST HEALING: THE OLD WAYS

Thus different traditions sanctioned various healing approaches. Wielding consumer power and also driven by desperation, the sick had a choice of practitioners. They also engaged in self-healing. It is against these backgrounds – environmental hazards, dangers of infection, fears of contagion and contamination, and a salutary concern with purity – that therapeutic strategies must be assessed.

Humanist medicine remained prestigious among traditional clinicians and their upper-crust patients. It recommended a many-faceted approach, tailored to the needs of the individual whose disorder was being monitored by a physician who would devise plans of recovery and healthy living. Traditional medicine stipulated courses of action centred upon temperance and hygiene, requiring prudent attention to such desiderata as good air, diet, evacuations, sleep, exercise, and peace of mind. These factors, called the 'non-naturals', were regarded as essential in avoiding – or, if too late, remedying – what physicians called the 'contra-naturals', in common speech, disease. Therapeutic means were to supplement the healing power of nature operative in all sound constitutions. There are, however, signs that healing was now growing increasingly medication-centred, and prescription of drugs was to become the chief outcome of medical encounters. But routine dispensing of medication, rather than the formulation of a comprehensive regimen, was frowned upon in best circles, as resembling the short-cut of nostrum-mongers who (according to Cheyne's gibe) 'never dare order a Regimen, and who are continually cramming their Patients with nauseous and loathsome Potions, Pills and Bolus's, Electuaries, Powders and Juleps'.

Viewing health as natural balance and harmony, tradition thus sanctioned the use (both preventive and therapeutic) of various physical strategies, including dietetics, bathing, and blood-letting. These were thought to lie within the power of the health-conscious layman. It was not unusual for sick people to 'breathe a vein' (let blood), even without the attendance of a barber or surgeon. Blood-letting was popular. 'There were not a few, especially among the country working-people, who deemed bleeding once or twice a year a great safeguard, or a help to health', was Sir James Paget's (1814–99) recollection of popular practices in early-Victorian rural England:

> [Countryfolk] came frequently on market-days at the times of spring and fall, and generally did their work in the market and then walked to the surgery. There they were at once bled, and usually were bled till they fainted, or felt very faint and became pale; then a pad was put over the wounded vein, and a bandage round the elbow; and they went home, often driving three or four miles into the country. I have no recollection of any evidence that either good or harm was ever done by this practice.

Phlebotomy lasted well into the nineteenth century, though it waxed and waned in favour. Benjamin Rush (1746–1813), the so-called 'American Hippocrates', had exorbitant faith in blood-letting, and

American regulars followed his example and bled copiously. Venesection also became established as a treatment of choice for tropical diseases.

DIET

Other physical methods remained popular. Dietary regulation was always prominent – and 'diet' traditionally meant more than food, the Greek term *diaita* implying a way of life. Dietetics thus concerned not only food and drink, but choice and direction of everyday conduct. Building on classical thinking, a huge dietary lore circulated in works like John Arbuthnot's (1667–1735) *An Essay Concerning the Nature of Aliments* (1731), explaining the health-giving or – threatening qualities of edible and medicinal herbs. Socio-cultural biases shaped judgments: identified with aristocratic tables, butcher's meat was widely praised as nourishing and healthy – though attacked by others as 'luxurious'. Black bread, rye bread and pot-herbs, those staples of the poor, were traditionally disparaged as indigestible. Victuals were thought to have hot or cooling, moist or dry qualities that would affect fluid balance. Maladies like chills, inducing excessive phlegm, thus required hot or tangy foods – red meat, spiritous liquors, spices, and savouries. For hot, dry fevers, by contrast, cooling fluids like barley water were what the doctor ordered.

Debates flared over the morbific and therapeutic qualities of foodstuffs. Physicians like Cheyne and Tissot, who condemned high society high-living for causing hypochondriacal and nervous disorders, pointed an accusing finger at the favoured 'high diet', with its abundance of game and piquant sauces, all washed down with wines, brandy, and port. Such 'diseases of civilization', they argued, could be combated by the simple, digestible diets of rustics, with their whole grains and greens, milk and water. The Enlightenment sowed the seeds of the moral and medical vegetarianism that blossomed in the nineteenth century.

A further factor in well-being lay in choice of abode. Harking back to the Hippocratic *Airs, Waters, and Places*, environmentalist theories attributed fevers and agues to injurious soils, vapours, fogs, exhalations, standing water, and other miasmata, and taught that the road to recovery required change of air or location. Collapsing in 1753 from various constitutional maladies, above all gout and dropsy, the novelist Henry Fielding (1707–54) quit his London town house and moved to Ealing, then a country village some miles out of town, because, he wrote, it had 'the best air, I believe, in the whole kingdom, [being] ....

418

open towards the south, whilst it is guarded from the north wind by a ridge of hills, and from the smells and smoke of London by its distance'. When Fielding did not improve, however, his physician urged him to winter in the mild surroundings of Aix-en-Provence in the South of France; eventually he set sail, as he records in his posthumously published *Voyage to Lisbon* (1755), on a last, forlorn trip to mild Portugal. Tobias Smollett (1721–71), a medical practitioner though now more famous as a novelist, spent much of the 1760s scuttling round the Italian Riviera trying to 'recruit his lungs' (as the phrase was), racked by respiratory troubles, probably tuberculosis. Delicate gentlefolk from Northern Europe, especially the 'pthisical' or consumptive, were commonly following the birds south in winter, making pilgrimages to Montpellier or Livorno in search of pure, balmy air.

EXERCISE

Another strategy for health lay in exercise, above all, travel. No prescription, perhaps, was touted more enthusiastically – and, maybe, more desperately. Riding – colloquially 'Dr Horse' – was best for recuperating a sound system, but even a smart outing in a chaise would do. The brisk, rhythmic motion would settle dyspepsia, restore appetite, and brace the solids. 'I must be on horseback for life, if I would be healthy', claimed John Wesley (1703–91), who combined riding for health with itinerant preaching. On one occasion the actor, David Garrick (1717–79), attributed recovery to 'that excellent physician, a horse'. When Samuel Johnson heard his acquaintance John Perkins, the brewer, was sick and needed a break from business, he dispatched him a plan of health advice. 'I am much pleased that You are going on a very long Journey', he announced, a trifle ambiguously, 'which may by proper conduct restore your health and prolong your life':

> Observe these rules
> 1. Turn all care out of your head as soon as you mount the chaise.
> 2. Do not think about frugality, your health is worth more than it can cost.
> 3. Do not continue any day's journey to fatigue.
> 4. Take now and then a day's rest.
> 5. Get a smart seasickness if you can.
> 6. Cast away all anxiety, and keep your mind easy.

The benefits of travel could be combined with taking the waters, the most stylish therapeutic strategy. Spas abounded all over Europe, but it was in England's burgeoning consumer culture that spas first became big business, offering healing rituals, social, elegance, and fat profits for hoteliers and doctors. Pre-eminently Bath, but also Tunbridge Wells, Buxton, Scarborough and Cheltenham provided concerts, balls, gambling, diversions, and assignations, to accompany dipping and taking the waters. By 1801, Bath, a city whose *raison d'être* lay in mixing medicine and merriment, had astonishingly become the seventh largest city in the United Kingdom.

SPAS

Taking the waters assumed many forms. It could mean immersion in public baths, hot or cold, or having water pumped over one's body. But thanks to developing interest in mineral chemistry, attention was now given to drinking the waters, as particular chemical properties were claimed for specific springs: chalybeate waters were widely touted as purgatives, while Bath waters had a name for curing barrenness – at least, lots of women left Bath pregnant. Resorts began to bottle their waters and dispatch them to far-flung parts. Gaggles of mercenary physicians and quacks settled in spa towns, and balneological pamphlet wars were waged, contesting the therapeutic properties of various springs. Ever sceptical of what he dubbed 'the sick trade', Thomas Beddoes, who lived near the Bristol 'Hotwell', renowned as a consumption cure, suggested that because such resorts were frauds, little better than 'charnel houses', a sign should be fixed upon Temple Gate, Bristol warning visitors: '*Lasciate ogni speranza, voi ch'entrate*' (Abandon hope all who enter here).

After 1750, with England leading the field, taking the waters was linked to the supposed therapeutic virtues of the seaside. A few physicians, like Dr Richard Russell (1687–1759) of Brighton, contended that sea water should preferably be *drunk* (the salts were assumed beneficial). But most recommended the seaside for bathing with the additional boon of sea air, whose properties were vaunted, especially for the tubercular. The virtues of fresh air had long been recommended; the Philadelphia polymath, Benjamin Franklin (1706–90), extolled air bathing, sitting unclothed in front of an open window each morning; while his Scottish contemporary, James Graham (1745–95), quack, sex therapist, and religious enthusiast, promoted bracing air combined with mud-bathing.

From mid-century, coastal resorts developed as therapeutic centres, till, by 1800, they were big business enough to be the target of a satirical novel by no less than Jane Austen (1775–1817). The title of *Sanditon* refers to its 'hero', a new (fictional) Channel health resort, whose chief booster,

> held it as certain, that no person could be really well, no person ... could be really in a state of secure and permanent health without spending at least six weeks by the sea every year. – The sea air and sea bathing together were nearly infallible, one or the other of them being a match for every disorder, of the stomach, the lungs or the blood; they were anti-spasmodic, anti-pulmonary, anti-sceptic, anti-bilious and anti-rheumatic. Nobody could catch cold by the sea, nobody wanted appetite by the sea, nobody wanted spirits, nobody wanted strength. They were healing, softening, relaxing – fortifying and bracing – seemingly just as was wanted – sometimes one, sometimes the other. – If the sea breeze failed, the sea-bath was the certain corrective; – and where bathing disagreed, the sea breeze alone was evidently designed by nature for the cure.

Habits like taking the waters had many critics. But it was not just a fad of the fashionable. It is easy nowadays, with the Anglo-American 'pill for every ill' healing dogma, to forget the great assortment of physical methods formerly recommended. Yet there is no denying that the apex of therapeutics was the prescription of drugs. For one thing, humoralism highlighted the operations of the stomach, implying that orally-taken medicines would permeate the whole system. For another, drugs were saleable commodities. With private medicine, it was easier for medical practitioners to extract payment for pills, ointments, lotions, and salves than simply for attendance or advice.

DRUGS

As herbals and home recipe-books show, there was a widespread drug lore, passed down from Antiquity. Whether used simply or in compound mixtures, distilled, dried, ground, decocted or otherwise blended and amalgamated, herbs still constituted the bulk of the drugs employed both by villagers and by apothecaries. Most herbal remedies were designed to act as purges and emetics, although learned medicine also made a fancy parade of alteratives, bitters, diluents, deobstruents, and similar hifalutin categories, each with its own rationale and action. Alteratives, for example, were supposed to strengthen the system, without necessarily possessing any disease-combating properties; bitters were meant to brace the solids (e.g. clear the head after a hangover and create an appetite).

Pharmacy changed slowly, and no radical breakthrough came until nineteenth-century French pharmaceutical chemists undertook laboratory analysis of the traditional *materia medica*, isolating compounds like morphine, codeine, and quinine. Regular doctors claimed there was a subtle art to drugging that transcended the pill-popping habits encouraged by quacks and indulged in by laymen like Samuel Johnson who, scornful of 'popgun remedies', obstinately doubled or trebled the recommended dose. Medications must be regarded, learned physicians emphasised, not as cures in themselves, but as single items in carefully-structured therapeutic regimes. Dosage and frequency had to be precisely tailored to the individual patient's needs, being modified even on a day-to-day basis, thus explaining the practitioners' habit of prescribing only a few measures at a time but prescribing extremely frequently – customs alleged by sceptics to promote profiteering. Whether or not they believed implicitly in all the elaborate rituals and rationalizations for drug administration devised by physicians, patients certainly showed interest in the complexities. When his niece, Nancy, had a touch of 'ague', probably malaria, James Woodforde (1740–1803), a Church of England parson in Norfolk, attended meticulously to the course proposed by his general practitioner:

> Dr. Thorne's Method of treating the Ague and Fever or intermitting Fever is thus – To take a Vomit in the Evening not to drink more than 3 half Pints of Warm Water after it as it operates. The Morn' following a Rhubarb Draught – and then as soon as the Fever has left the Patient about an Hour or more, begin with the Bark taking it every two Hours till you have taken 12 Papers which contains one Ounce. The next oz. etc you take it 6. Powders the ensuing Day, 5 Powders the Day after, 4 Ditto the Day after, then 3 Powders the Day after that till the 3rd oz. is all taken, then 2 Powders the Day till the 4th oz. is all taken and then leave of. If at the beginning of taking the Bark it should happen to purge, put ten Dropps of Laudanum into the Bark you take next, then 4, then 3, then 2, then 1 and so leave of by degrees.

Here we see the standard recourse to purging, but in an elaborate context. The initial purge would evacuate the system and thus pave the way for the truly effectual medicine, the 'bark' (Peruvian bark or quinine). If the purge produced unwanted side effects, laudanum (i.e., liquid opium) would counteract them. (Often the reverse was the case: opium used as a painkiller produced constipation, needing to be countered with senna.) Thus, though Woodforde probably kept at home stocks of all the drugs deployed by Dr Thorne, the secret lay in the art of dosing. In other words, the physician made it his business to convince clients that drugs were not sufficient in themselves, but efficacious only as part of a wider regime, understood by the doctor alone.

Hindsight suggests that the art of prescription was a fancy palaver to disguise the fact that few drugs actually cured. Nevertheless, certain improvements were made in the medical armamentarium. Thanks to chemical advances, mineral and metallic drugs gained wider use. Mercury was a favoured treatment for syphilis; antimony-based medicines achieved wide circulation as febrifuges (in England, patented as Dr James's Powders); and calomel, used as a purge, enjoyed a lasting vogue from the late eighteenth century. More importantly, trade with the New World and the Orient brought new drugs and improved supplies of old ones, above all, opium, imported mainly through the Levant. It was used to soothe the respiratory tract (and especially to reduce coughs associated with the rising 'white plague' of tuberculosis), to manage diarrhoea, and as an analgesic. Guaiac bark was imported from Spanish America and used against syphilis, and the New World also yielded Peruvian or Jesuit's bark (cinchona), a genuinely effective specific against malaria. Imports like tea, cocoa, tobacco, and coffee also had their medical champions, though opinion increasingly condemned them as deleterious and habit-forming.

Spurred by new drugs, pharmacy grew more organised, and guilds and companies were formed. Large manufacturing druggists emerged, dealing wholesale with hospitals and the colonies. The London chemist, Thomas Corbyn (1711–91), like many others in the trade a Quaker, stocked over 2500 different items of materia medica, employed around 10 employees, and, by the 1780s, was running a business with a capital of some £20,000. He traded extensively with the Americas, from Nova Scotia to Jamaica, and with France, Spain, and Portugal, where pharmaceutical manufacturers were less well established. Businesses like Corbyn's – there were several in London – point to the emergence of a pharmaceutical industry. The standardisation of medications was aided, throughout Europe, by the sponsoring of official pharmacopoeias. That of the Royal College of Physicians of London had a wide circulation, even if its contents do not, in retrospect, inspire confidence. Exotica like crabs' eyes, viper's fat and coral were still listed, alongside such mainstays as senna and sarsaparilla. The fifth *London Pharmacopoeia* (1746), revised by Mead, Heberden, and John Freind (1675–1728), eliminated human fat, spider-webs, moss from human skulls, unicorn's horn, virgin's milk (not the literal liquid but an alchemical remedy), bones from the stag's heart, and the like, but still retained mithridate, wood-lice, pearls, bezoars, vipers, and coral. Most of the animal *materia medica* had disappeared from the sixth *Pharmacopoeia* (1788), and among the new drugs and compounds appearing were aconite, castor oil, quassia, magnesia, ether, tartrate of iron, oxide of zinc, Dover's powder, Hoffmann's anodyne, Huxham's tincture, James's powder, sarsaparilla decoctions, and paregoric (liquid opium).

A few breakthroughs were achieved. It became recognised that willow bark was effective in treating ague, though less effective than Peruvian bark. In 1785, William Withering (1741–99), an Edinburgh-trained Birmingham practitioner and fellow-member with Erasmus Darwin of the Lunar Society, produced *An Account of the Foxglove and Some of its Medical Uses etc; With Practical Remarks on Dropsy and Other Diseases*, which demonstrated that digitalis had a powerful stimulant action on the heart, increased urine flow and was effective in reducing oedema. An ardent medical botanist and follower of Linnaeus, Withering had heard from a country woman of a herbal concoction useful in treating swollen hands, feet, and legs. He recognised that the effective ingredient in the dropsy medicine was foxglove, whose leaves yielded digitalis, and carefully monitored use of the drug, to ascertain the safest and optimal dosage, for treating both dropsy and heart disease. (Foxglove was effective against cardiac dropsy though not renal dropsy, but the distinction was not grasped until the work of Richard Bright, 1798–1858.) It was not until 1809 that digitalis appeared in the *London Pharmacopoeia*.

Growing use of opium is worth noting, for it signals concern with pain-relief. For millennia, sick people had to bear suffering unimaginable nowadays. They had recourse to prayer and philosophy, alcohol too. But traditional Western medicine lacked effective pain-killers; indeed, pain-relief was marginal to its rationale. Enlightenment thinkers, notably the Utilitarians, with their accent upon pleasure and pain, began to be more sensitive to pain as an evil meriting alleviation. A remedy was to hand, in opium. 'Providence has been kind and gracious to us beyond all Expression', wrote Cheyne, 'in furnishing us with a certain Relief, if not a Remedy, even to our most intense Pains and extreme Miseries'. Commonly taken in the more palatable liquid forms of laudanum and paregoric or in nostrums like 'Gregory's Cordial', opium was openly on sale, and bought in penny paperfuls by common people to manage routine pains – especially in fenland areas where it countered 'marsh fever' (malaria). And it was widely touted by doctors. Erasmus Darwin's *Zoonomia* (1794–96) recommended opium for anorexia, impotence, gallstones, epilepsy, sleepwalking, and tetanus ('very large doses'). Doctors remained confident that opium was not seriously habit-forming, although it is now clear that prominent figures, including several of Darwin's patients, became hopelessly addicted.

Overall, pharmacy left much to be desired. Quack nostrums were often unsafe. Polypharmacy – complex drug cocktails, in which certain ingredients were supposed to counter the deleterious effects of others – was open to glaring abuses. Violent purgatives and lead – or mercury-based medicines caused spasm and colic, often relieved by belladonna or other concoctions that induced further poisoning. Physicians like the Scottish naval doctor, Thomas Trotter, warned that modern society was over-indulging in a smorgasbord of potentially lethal sedatives, drugs, tonics, sedatives, and narcotics, alongside stimulants like tea, tobacco, and carbonated waters. At the close of the century, the German physician, Samuel Hahnemann (1755–1843), reacted against such abuses by developing his 'homoeopathic' system, which, alongside the celebrated dictum of *similia similibus curantur* (like cures like), also stressed the need for the absolute purity of drugs and for minimal dosage. The age of pharmaceutical reform was dawning.

MADNESS AND ITS TREATMENTS

Other forms of treatment deserve mention. The handling of the insane was transformed in the more advanced parts of Europe. Lunacy had traditionally been viewed through various lenses. In the Reformation era, it was often diagnosed as praeternatural in origin, but by the eighteenth century the theory of insanity as demonic possession was discredited amongst all except religious sectaries. The regular, law-governed world portrayed by the mechanical philosophy discounted the possibility that Satan possessed people's bodies and minds. In any case, after the carnage of the witch-craze and the Thirty Years' War, responsible public opinion turned against 'Convulsionaries', 'Ranters', and the rest of the religious lunatic fringe. Conservative interests and enlightened minds discredited the 'revelations' of visionaries, and declared that the 'possessed' were crackbrained, afflicted by the spleen, vapours, hysteria, or other morbid conditions.

The time was ripe for new theories of insanity, promoted by the medical profession. Mania and melancholy, Enlightenment physicians argued, derived not from the Beyond but from the body; insanity was physical, organic. Here they were able, of course, to build upon a humoral interpretation of mental disorder, that emphasised the role of yellow bile ('choler') in precipitating mania and black bile (melancholy) in producing dejection, and attributed hysteria to the erratic movements of the wandering womb.

But such humoral explanations also lost credit as the New Science pictured the body as a machine. Study of the nervous system made progress; and Descartes, Thomas Willis, and the iatro-mathematicians associated with Archibald Pitcairn (1652–1713) and George Cheyne maintained the interaction of the vascular and nervous systems with the brain. Hypotheses of the nerves as hollow pipes, or as wires conveying waves or impulses, led to competing theories in which disordered thought, moods and behaviour were ascribed to some defect of the gut or nervous organisation, resulting in tension, slackness, obstruction. The concept of neurosis was devised, as was the condition colloquially called 'nerves'.

The new neuro-anatomy associated with Haller, Whytt, Cullen, and others held promise for psychotherapeutic interventions. If insanity was a bodily disease, it would surely be responsive to physical treatments. Hence, an arsenal of medical 'cures' like camphor came into vogue, some designed to sedate maniacs, others to invigorate melancholics (opium was freely prescribed for both purposes!). There were physical treatments like blood-lettings, emetics, and violent purges to discharge gastric toxins; shock treatments like cold showers; new technologies like electric shocks (common from this time), rotatory chairs or mechanical swings, designed to disrupt *idées fixes*; and, when all else failed, mechanical restraints like shackles and straitjackets. With many such devices, treating the body was intended to restore the mind. Thus, William Perfect (1740–89), a private madhouse keeper in Kent, deployed upon his patients a veritable battery of physical techniques, designed to tranquillise the frenzied. He had recourse to drugs (opium for example), solitary confinement in darkened rooms, cold baths, a 'lowering' diet, blood-letting, purgatives, etc. These would pacify the body, thereby sedating the mind and rendering it receptive to sweet reason.

Disciplining the system through drugs and mechanical interventions played a large part in Enlightenment techniques. Above all, the age vested its hopes in the madhouse. The asylum's segregative environment suited 'psychiatric' techniques of mastering madness that would directly command the mind, the passions and will, and thereby rehabilitate. In particular, as the failure of medications became clear and humanitarian critics condemned manacles and straitjackets as cruel and counter-productive, the well-run asylum commended itself as the preferred form of therapy.

A new outlook arose after 1750, voicing late Enlightenment ideologies. Madness, it was now claimed, was not an organic disorder requiring medication. It was distinctive, because it was *psychological*, the consequence of bad habits and misfortunes; hence it needed a psychotherapeutics. The solution lay in 'moral therapy', acting upon the mind. These new psychological approaches drew on earlier philosophical foundations. Descartes's *cogito ergo sum* ('I think, therefore I am') had highlighted the role of consciousness in shaping identity; his English successor and critic, John Locke, had viewed madness as the child of uncontrollable imagination or illogical thought-processes; and the *enfant terrible* of the Enlightenment, Jean-Jacques Rousseau (1712–78) suggested that artificial urban high-life alienated man from his soul, creating a divided self – a line of thought developed by Romanticism and culminating in Freud's *Civilization and its Discontents* (1930). By 1800, influential figures – Philippe Pinel (1745–1826) in France, Vincente Chiarugi (1759–1820) in Tuscany, William Tuke (1732–1822) in England, and Johann Christian Reil (1759–1813) in Germany – had formulated a psychological model of lunacy. Insanity could therefore best be corrected, they thought, by interpersonal psychodynamics between patient and doctor, accentuating 'moral' methods – kindness, reason and humanity. The right site for these close encounters was the asylum, homely, secluded, tranquil.

These pioneers did not invent the asylum, they wanted it reformed. In medieval times, crazy people had rarely been sent to special institutions, being mostly allowed to wander or looked after – often a euphemism for neglected or brutalised – by the family or village. From the seventeenth century, notably in France, policy-makers recommended sequestrating lunatics under lock and key in special madhouses. The rise of bureaucracy and absolutism, the labour discipline required by capitalism, the growing authority of science, the rule of law and the spread of literacy and education – all these aspects of 'progress' in the age of reason may have undermined an older tolerance for strange folks and their ways. In what Foucault called – many scholars

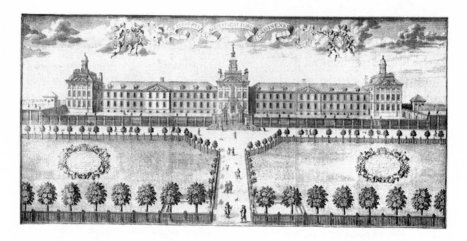

Fig. 56. Bethlem Hospital, London (engraving *c.* 1700). Bethlem was long Britain's main lunatic asylum. Its building was designed by the scientist Robert Hooke. The splendour of the architecture may have contrasted with the rather traditional regime within. (The Wellcome Institute Library, London. M19150.)

think exaggeratedly – 'the great confinement', the irrational were to be routinely locked away, from the mid-seventeenth century in institutions known as Hôpitaux Généraux situated in Paris and other major French cities. In France, most institutions for the insane were run by public authorities or by the Church. In England, by contrast, the scene was dominated by private madhouses in what was called the 'trade in lunacy'. Confinement of the insane expanded in eighteenth-century England, though not nearly as rapidly as after 1800. Up to 10,000 lunatics were under sequestration in England in 1800, in asylums, workhouses and other places of detention, whereas by 1900, the total was verging on 100,000.

In this drive to institutionalise lunatics lies a rich irony: for the impetus sanctioning this massive corralling came from high-minded, well-meaning reformers. Loathing the heartlessness of neglect and the brutality of old madhouses like London's Bedlam (Bethlem Hospital), progressive mad-doctors argued that care and cure would best be promoted by transferring the insane, under due legal protection, to purpose-built, fully-provisioned, well-staffed institutions. Given personal attention and occupational therapy in a supportive environment, their faculties would be repaired and their behaviour rectified. Once cured, they could be restored to society. Espousing a 'moral therapy' designed to revive the dormant humanity of the mad, optimistic 'mad-doctors'

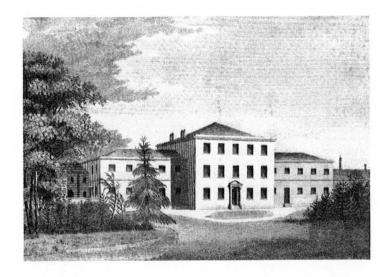

Fig. 57. The York Retreat. Opened in 1796, the York Retreat was prominent amongst the new lunatic asylums which inaugurated a reign of reason, kindness and psychological management. (The Wellcome Institute Library, London. L811.)

like Pinel and the Tukes aimed to re-educate their charges like children, in asylums that would be havens in a heartless world. Aspirations, however, outstripped achievements, and by the latter part of the nineteenth century the lunatic asylum was becoming one of the more problematic features of modern medicine.

CHILDBIRTH

Alongside madness, another aspect of medical intervention undergoing rapid change, at least in certain nations and the more affluent social classes, was the management of childbirth. Birthing was traditionally an event exclusive to women (the mother, her female relatives and friends, and a midwife), conducted according to folk and religious rituals. But, first within polite and bourgeois society in England, and, by the nineteenth century in North America, the traditional 'granny midwife' became widely displaced by a male operator, the 'man-midwife' or accoucheur. This new obstetrician claimed superior expertise. As a qualified medical practitioner, armed perhaps with a degree from a prestigious medical school, his anatomical expertise made him confident that he could let Nature take her course in case of normal deliveries. Contrary to some feminist historians' claims, leading man-midwives

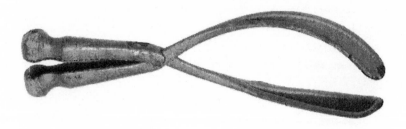

Fig. 58. Obstetric forceps 1746. After long being the preserve of the Chamberlen family, forceps became common after about 1730. These are the straight forceps preferred by William Smellie. (The Wellcome Institute Library, London. M1487.)

like William Hunter prided themselves upon being less interventionist than traditional midwives.

Yet accoucheurs also possessed, unlike the midwife, surgical instruments, above all, the new forceps, for use in difficult labours and emergencies. Introduced in the seventeenth century as the secret of the Chamberlen family, forceps became common property by 1730. Accoucheurs could claim distinctive expertise, since they were frequently attached to the newly-founded lying-in hospitals and charities sprouting in large towns, or directed obstetric schools. In London the leading instructors were Scots: William Smellie (1697–1763), and his pupil, William Hunter (1718–83). Smellie mastered obstetrics in Paris before teaching it in London in the 1740s. He devised models for student practice, including a leather-covered manikin. After introducing the steel-lock forceps in 1744, he developed the improved curved and double-curved forceps. His *Treatise on the Theory and Practice of Midwifery* (1752) proved a leading text, establishing safe rules for forceps use. For his part, William Hunter had five years' training at Glasgow University, three as Cullen's pupil, before beginning in 1746 to give private lecture courses on dissecting, surgery, and obstetrics. His *The Anatomy of the Human Gravid Uterus* (1774) offered outstanding illustrations of the foetus and womb.

In America, medical midwifery developed under the influence of William Shippen (1736–1808), who had studied in London with William and John Hunter, and under Cullen and Alexander Monro II (1733–1817) in Edinburgh. Shippen taught anatomy and midwifery in

Philadelphia from 1763, helping establish the domination of male operators that became so conspicuous in the USA.

Where male accoucheurs flourished, childbirth was transformed from
a women-only rite. Fashionable ladies now had their husbands present at
labour. They gave birth in rooms into which daylight and fresh air were
admitted. Delivered safely, their newborns would no longer be swaddled:
according to new theories, allowing freedom to infant limbs would
strengthen bones and promote healthy development. On medical advice,
such modern ladies also now breast-fed their babies: surely mother's milk
was best and would encourage good mother–baby bonding.

Thus Enlightenment values promoted dramatic changes in the theory and practice of baby and infant care. But the changes just described
were by no means universal. In France, for instance, wet-nursing
remained common. And the medicalisation of childbirth through male
practitioners was a local phenomenon. Sir Fielding Ould (1710–89)
taught the techniques in Dublin, Charles White (1728–1813) in
Manchester, Pieter Camper (1722–89) in the Netherlands, and other
pioneers spread the message in Paris, Vienna, and Copenhagen. But in
the German principalities, midwives were not challenged by male operators; rather they secured improved training, receiving lectures and
gaining medical licences. Male practitioners made no headway in
staunchly Catholic countries like Italy. In thinly-populated Sweden the
medical profession did not attempt to supplant midwives but gave them
training and used them as their subordinates. In short, though medical
developments were in many respects international, cultural differences
ensured irregular, uneven, and distinctive patterns of change.

INOCULATION

The most astonishing improvement in practical medicine at this time
related to smallpox: the introduction, first of inoculation and then of
vaccination – not, strictly, of course, a therapeutic but a preventive
measure. 'The speckled monster' was intensely virulent, responsible in
some years for perhaps a tenth of all deaths. Queen Mary of England
(1662–94) died of it. There had long been some folk awareness in
many parts of Europe of the immunising properties of a dose of smallpox; but it was not till around 1700 that the medico-administrative
elites took notice. The first notable account of artificial inoculation was
published in the *Philosophical Transactions* of the Royal Society of
London in 1714; but widespread publicity was achieved thanks to the

observations of Lady Mary Wortley Montagu (1689–1762), wife of the British consul in Constantinople, who reported how Turkish peasant women performed inoculations. To 'graft' the disease, fresh lymph or dried crusts were introduced into the skin of healthy individuals, the aim being to induce a mild dose, so as to confer lifelong protection, hopefully without permanent pock-marking.

Back in Britain, Lady Mary had her five-year-old daughter inoculated in 1721 by the Scottish surgeon, Charles Maitland (1677–1748). Experiments with condemned felons followed, and the soon-to-be George II (1683–1760) arranged for the operation to be performed on his two daughters. Thereafter inoculation secured respectability and spread, if sporadically – partly because of set-backs, partly because fashionable physicians turned inoculation from a simple, quick, and cheap procedure into an elaborate and expensive rigmarole, involving lengthy patient preparation and a recuperation period of isolation in an inoculation residence.

Simpler techniques were pioneered in the USA in Charleston, South Carolina in 1738 by a local physician, James Kirkpatrick (c. 1696–1770), involving an arm-to-arm variolation method that proved safe. But the real breakthrough, leading to mass inoculation, came in Britain with the work of the Sutton family, Robert (1707–88) and his sons, especially Daniel (1735–1819). The Suttons, humble surgeons from East Anglia, devised an easy, safe and cheap technique, involving application of a small quantity of material to a scratch on the arm. They bulk-inoculated whole villages at a time, up to 500 people a day, to minimise risks of accidental spread of the infection to uninoculated parties. Between them, the Suttons claimed to have inoculated around 400,000 people, with a minuscule death-rate. Inoculation dispensaries were later founded in towns like Chester, where the public health activist, John Haygarth (1740–1827), took the lead, hoping for eventual blanket inoculation.

Smallpox inoculation caught on first in England (there was some resistance from predestinarian Calvinists in Scotland) and spread gradually to other countries, being supported in France by the *philosophes*, endorsed by the Académie Royale des Sciences, and spurred by the death of Louis XV (1710–74) from the disease. In Prussia, Austria, and Russia, variolations of members of the royal household helped publicise the measure. Catherine the Great (1729–96) had her family inoculated by Thomas Dimsdale (1712–1800), an English surgeon who was

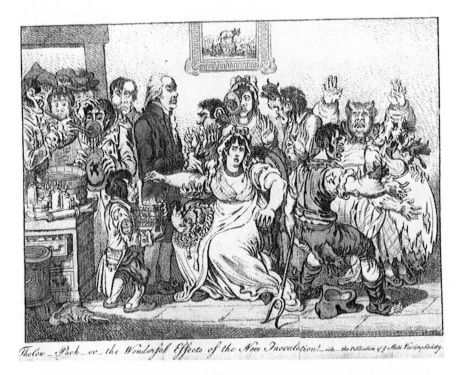

Fig. 59. Gillray, Edward Jenner among his patients. Gillray humorously played on
fears of the dangers of smallpox vaccination involving the injection of cowpox. (The
Wellcome Institute Library, London. V11072.)

awarded £10,000 for his services. Nevertheless, inoculation was slow
to spread to much of the Continent – there was notable opposition from
leading Austrian physicians and only lukewarm support in the German
principalities – and it proved almost impossible to perform safely in
cities, where the risks of cross-infection were grave. The consequence
was that smallpox mortality remained high.

Therein lies the huge significance of Edward Jenner's introduction of
vaccination at the end of the eighteenth century. Vaccination involves
artificial grafting not of smallpox virus, but of cowpox, a far less dangerous disease but one conferring comparable immunity. A retiring
West Country practitioner who had been John Hunter's star pupil,
Jenner (1749–1823) had witnessed the immunity that the bovine disorder, caught from cattle, gave to milkmaids, and had the sagacity to
transform it into a medical technique. On May 14, 1796, Jenner performed his first vaccination, upon a country boy, James Phipps, using
matter from the arm of a cowpox-infected milkmaid, Sarah Nelmes. *An*

Inquiry into the Causes and Effects of the Variolae Vaccine (1798), argued the case for vaccination. The Royal Jennerian Society for promoting vaccination was founded in London in 1802, and Parliament voted him a grant of £10,000. Vaccination later became compulsory in various states (Sweden came first, where the village bell-ringer was sometimes appointed official vaccinator), though in Britain powerful lobbies contested state-imposed vaccination on libertarian grounds. Smallpox immunisation saved tens and perhaps hundreds of thousands of lives (and misery as well; for smallpox commonly disfigured, and could cause blindness and sterility). It was a tangible mark of medical progress.

Surgery

The therapeutic scope and occupational status of surgery changed considerably in the eighteenth century. Often called 'the cutter's art' and seen as a manual skill rather than a liberal science, it was traditionally regarded as inferior to physic in the medical hierarchy. Normally, surgeons passed through not an academic, but a practical, education; they were aligned with barbers and scathingly compared to butchers. Organised in guilds, surgery typically carried modest prestige. The business of surgery could be represented as demeaning and contaminating. Unlike the clean-handed physician, the surgeon was habitually dealing with the diseased and decaying body rather than with health maintenance. He had to handle corruptions of the flesh – tumours, wens, gangrene, syphilitic chancres. His means were invasive – the knife, cauterising instruments, the amputating saw.

THE TRADITIONAL SURGEON

Frequently butts of satire, old-style surgeons have traditionally received scant credit from historians. A standard historiography represents surgery as a crude and bloody art, at least prior to anaesthesia and antisepsis in the mid-nineteenth century, whereafter it could become more exact, scientific, and successful. The caricature, however, tells but a partial truth. For one thing, recent studies of the traditional surgeon's day-to-day work have demonstrated that his craft did not revolve around bloody, spectacular, and frequently lethal operations like amputations or trephining. The business of a surgeon like the Londoner, Daniel Turner (1667–1741), was a round of minor running-repairs – bloodletting, lancing boils, dressing skin infections, pulling teeth, delivering babies in

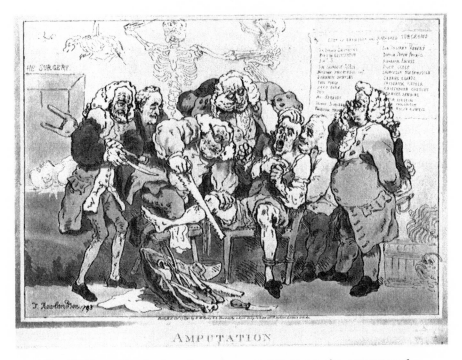

Fig. 60. Thomas Rowlandson. Five surgeons participating in the amputation of a man's lower leg, 1793. Humorous cartoon suggesting the brutality of eighteenth-century surgery. Note the image of Death in the background. (The Wellcome Institute Library, London. V11038.)

difficult labours, managing whitlows, trussing ruptures, treating leg ulcers, patching up fistulas, medicating venereal infections, and so forth. The traditional surgeon had to minister to scores of external conditions requiring routine maintenance through cleansing, pus removal, ointments, and bandaging. The conditions he treated were mostly not life-threatening, nor were his interventions glamorous. Recent studies of ordinary surgeons have shown their fatality rate was low. Surgeons learned their limits. The range of internal operative surgery they would undertake was narrow, because of the risks of trauma, blood-loss, and sepsis. A dextrous surgeon would extract bladder-stones or extirpate cancerous tumours from the breast; but exploration into the abdominal cavity was strictly for the future. Malfunctions of the heart, liver, brain, and stomach were treated not by the knife but by medicines and management, for major internal surgery was not feasible before the advent of anaesthetics and antiseptic procedures. A surgeon would occasionally slit open the belly of a dying woman in labour to deliver a baby that could not be born naturally, but that was a desperate measure and there is no record of a mother surviving a Caesarian operation in Britain till the close of the eighteenth century.

Tangible improvements arose, however, in certain surgical techniques. Take the treatment of bladder-stones. A popular seventeenth-century procedure, known as the 'apparatus major' had involved dilating and incising the urethra to allow the introduction of instruments to extract the stone. A superior method was instituted by the itinerant practitioner, Jacques de Beaulieu ('Frère Jacques', 1651–1719). Known as lateral cystotomy, it involved cutting into the perineum and opening up both bladder and bladder neck. The distinguished surgeons, Johannes Rau (1688–1719) in Amsterdam and William Cheselden (1688–1752) in London, deployed the method with significant success, Cheselden describing the operation in his *Treatise on a High Operation for Stone* (1723). Cheselden won fame for performing lithotomy with exceptional rapidity – he could complete the excruciatingly painful knife-work in a couple of minutes, whereas other surgeons might take 20. His became the most popular technique. This example shows a pattern common in early modern medicine, whereby innovations first introduced by itinerants or quacks found their way into regular practice. The same applies to hernia; traditionally the domain of travelling itinerants, hernia was increasingly dealt with by regular surgeons, aided by truss-making improvements.

Other operations also underwent refinement. The distinguished French surgeon, J. L. Petit (1674–1750), developed new practices with amputations at the thigh. Military surgery advanced markedly, in particular management of gunshot wounds, and army surgeons contributed much to investigation of the complaints that typically followed wounds, including hospital gangrene, tetanus, and erysipelas. The military proved the best school of surgery, because warfare and colonial expansion created insatiable demands for junior surgeons willing to serve abroad or aboard ship. By 1713, the British fleet had 247 vessels, each carrying a surgeon and mate. For those with strong stomachs, like the surgeon-hero of Tobias Smollett's (1722–71) novel, *Roderick Random* (1748), naval or military service provided boundless experience and a valuable leg-up into the profession.

Specialist surgeons also pioneered new techniques. By 1700 it was recognised that cataract involved a hardening of the lens. The French oculist, Jacques Daviel (1696–1762), found a way to extract the lens of the eye once it had become opaque through cataract, performing the operation several hundred times with good results. Also skilled at the same operation was the British 'quack' oculist, John ('Chevalier') Taylor (1703–72), who practised with immense razzmatazz at many of the courts of Europe (allegedly contributing to the blindness of both Bach and Handel).

Other surgeons achieved fame for their dependable skill or innovations. A humane operator, Percivall Pott (1714–88), surgeon at St. Bartholomew's Hospital in London, published on hernia, head injuries, hydrocele (swelling of the scrotum), fistula in ano, fractures, and dislocations, as well as being the first to observe that chimney sweeps suffer from cancer of the scrotum. Pierre-Joseph Desault (1744–95), Bichat's teacher and founder of the first important surgical periodical, the *Journal de Chirurgie* (1791–92), improved treatment of fractures, and developed methods of ligating blood-vessels in case of aneurysm. Orthopaedics advanced, especially thanks to Nicholas André (1658–1742) and the Genevan, Jean-André Venel (1740–91). Venel advocated mechanical devices to correct lateral curvature and torsion of the spine. Various spinal braces were developed, and Jean-Pierre David (1737–84), a Rouen surgeon, produced an influential description of spinal deformity from caries, alongside wider studies of bone necrosis. Improved obstetrical skills have already been discussed.

Thanks to these technical improvements, surgery rose in professional standing. This occurred first in France. As elsewhere, French practitioners were originally barber-surgeons, but they gradually succeeded, thanks to royal favour, in emancipating themselves from their ties to the barbers. In 1672, the Paris surgeon Pierre Dionis (1643–1718) was appointed to lecture in anatomy and surgery at the Jardin du Roi. Then, in 1687, Louis XIV's anal fistula proved a blessing in disguise. A successful operation on the Sun King by C. F. Félix (1650–1703) contributed to surgery's growing prestige. From the early-eighteenth century, surgery was widely taught in Paris through lectures and demonstrations, leading to the abolition in 1768 of conventional surgical training by apprenticeship. Thereafter, surgeons began to vie with physicians in status, claiming that surgery was no mere empirical craft of the hand but that it possessed an independent theory of its own, and so constituted a separate science. This view of surgery as a science squared with the Enlightenment accent upon practical not bookish learning and with moves to conceptualise disease in a localised manner. It became possible to commend surgery as the most experimental and therefore progressive branch of medicine. The breakthrough came in 1731, when a royal charter established the Académie Royale de Chirurgie; 12 years later, Louis XV formally dissolved the link between the surgeons and barbers.

THE EMERGENT SURGICAL PROFESSION

Thanks to these developments, France led the world in surgery for most of the century, drawing students from all over Europe. This pre-eminence was embodied in the dominating figure of J. L. Petit (1674–1750). In Paris, hospital teaching was fostered. The surgeon P. J. Desault (1744–95) at the Hôtel Dieu introduced bedside teaching of surgery as part of a new accent upon clinical medicine. Concentrating medical education at the hospital reinforced the links growing ever since Vesalius between surgery and anatomy, and helped establish the 'anatomico-localist' perspective on disease that became so prominent in the hospitals of post-Revolutionary Paris, stimulated further by Bichat's work on tissues. By Bichat's day, the radical reform of French medical education imposed in 1794 had led to surgery being taught alongside medicine to all students. The prominence of the hospital in the post-1789 medical system and the prestige of patho-anatomy elevated the status of French surgery.

Parallel developments occurred elsewhere. It is significant that the professional identity of Alexander Monro (primus) (1697–1767), first incumbent of the chair of anatomy and surgery in the Edinburgh medical school, was surgical. Monro taught anatomy, but he also gave instruction in surgical operations, to both medical students and surgical apprentices. The development of Edinburgh medical education was to erode the divisions between physic and surgery. From 1778, the Royal College of Surgeons of Edinburgh awarded its own diplomas, which were almost as valuable as a university degree. It made sense to Edinburgh medical students to equip themselves to practise both skills, particularly if they were expecting to become general practitioners.

The rise of the hospital proved fortunate for surgeons. For one thing, the hospital became a major site for accident and emergency cases – treated by surgeons rather than physicians. Moreover, hospitals typically provided supplies of unclaimed dead bodies, primarily of the poor, whom surgeons could dissect post mortem. Hospitals offered venues for surgeons to lecture to students. In 1743, in London, William Bromfield (1713–92) and Frank Nicholls (1699–1778) gave courses of nearly 40 lectures each at Guy's Hospital, including anatomy, surgery, physiology, pathology, and midwifery.

Not least, the spread of anatomy schools, first in Paris, and then in London, boosted surgery's prestige. Among the most illustrious, the school established in Great Windmill Street, Piccadilly, by William Hunter (1718–83), also offered instruction in surgery, physiology, pathology, midwifery, and diseases of women and children. William Hunter and his younger brother, John, were principally surgeons, but running an anatomy school permitted them to link surgery with experimentation. John Hunter (1728–1793), the leading surgeon-physiologist of his age, became a prolific dissector of both human and animal material. Whereas William was a fashionable accoucheur and teacher, John devoted his energies and income to research, focusing on comparative studies of relationships of structure and function throughout the animal kingdom. Addressing surgical topics such as inflammation, shock, disorders of the vascular system and venereal disease, John Hunter's four main treatises, *Natural History of the Human Teeth* (1771), *On Venereal Disease* (1786), *Observations on Certain Parts of the Animal Oeconomy* (1786) and *Treatise on the Blood Inflammation and Gunshot Wounds* (1794), mark the rise of surgery from manual craft to scientific discipline. Omnivorous for scientific knowledge, John Hunter amassed a huge series of anatomical and biological specimens, about 13,000 of which became the basis of the Hunterian Museum of the Royal College of Surgeons. He trained many eminent pupils, including Jenner, Astley Cooper (1768–1841), John Abernethy (1764–1831), Henry Cline (1750–1827), William Clift (1775–1849), and Philip Syng Physick (1768–1837), the American who imported Hunterian surgery into the New World.

By 1800 surgery's reputation had definitely risen. The surgeon had distanced himself from the traditional barber and bleeder (in London, the Company of Surgeons split from the barbers in 1745). Surgery achieved its own voice through such journals as the *Mémoires de l'Académie Royale de Chirurgie* (1743–73). Within a century, the surgeon had further risen in status to become, perhaps, the most fashionable of all the medical practitioners.

Popular medicine

The discussion so far has focused upon medical men, their knowledge and skills. But trained medical personnel comprised only the tip of the healing iceberg. From peasants to princelings, everyone held deeply-entrenched views about living and dying, health and sickness, healing and treatments. Across most of Europe and her empires overseas, medical professionals were still few and far between, mainly serving affluent court and city clienteles; suspicion of doctors was, in any case, rife. Under such circumstances, ordinary people felt driven to take steps to protect their health, and, upon falling sick, largely treated themselves, at least in the first instance. For disease and death were ever threatening in a biological *ancien régime* in which life expectations might be little more than a third of today's – around 1750 an Englishman had a life expectancy of about 36 years, a Frenchman around 27. Christianity revolved around the great mystery of death; artists symbolised it with their skulls, death's heads and *memento mori's*; funerals were celebrated with solemn pomp; and with the invention of the newspaper came the obituary column. Small wonder that popular culture boasted a comprehensive medical lore.

Journals, sermons, letters, and diaries confirm the grip of illness and death upon people's minds. Such documents give glimpses of wider 'sickness cultures', revealing beliefs about the meaning of life and death, the causes and purposes of sickness, its prevention and cure, the relations between body and soul, suffering, and sanctity. The body's condition in health and sickness provided the basis for wider ideas of identity and destiny, of social, moral and spiritual well-being, that were handed down in families, droned from the pulpit, gleaned in works of piety, or picked up from health-care manuals.

Nowadays good health is a normal expectation, while disease is widely regarded as alien and invasive. None of this would have rung true to sufferers in the world we have lost. Illness was widely viewed not as a random accident but as providential. Individuals were expected to exercise control over their constitution, their internal humoral balance. One's life was, in principle at least, in one's own hands (and in God's). Worlds apart from modern 'doctor dependence', such views made good sense at a time when curative medicine was a weak reed and the doctor often a day's ride away or unaffordable. For many, 'medicine without doctors' was both necessity and choice. People coped with the fact that doctors were not miracle-workers by viewing health as ultimately their personal responsibility and the decree of the Almighty.

POPULAR IMAGES OF THE BODY

Taking care of one's health meant understanding one's body. This was both simple (it was directly experienced) and appallingly difficult (the interior was hidden). Unable to peer directly inwards, to inspect food being converted into energy and excrement or to check the causes of pain, people relied upon analogy, drawing inferences from the natural world. Cottage economies in rural societies offered prompts for body processes: the curdling of milk into cheese suggested the transformation of semen into a fleshy foetus. Similarly, food simmering on the hob became a natural symbol for its softening and decomposition in the stomach; in kitchen chemistry, the gut merely completed the work of the fire, the stock, and the stirring-spoon. Homely views were entertained of the insides. 'The Generality', remarked the surgeon, Daniel Turner (1667–1741), had the 'Notion of their Stomach ... as a Bason to Receive' and their 'Bowels ... as a Pipe .. to convey off what is left'. Peasant mentalities thus mapped internal body events onto the wider environment; magic, folksong, and fable explained conception and childbirth; and growth, decay, and death found mirrors in the seedtime and the harvest. Natural symbols were called upon; hoping to assist conception, country women treated springs as fertility shrines. To fathom abnormalities and heal ailments, peasant thinking enlisted the suggestive qualities of strange creatures like toads and snakes (hibernation, the shedding of skins), and the evocative profiles of natural features like valleys, caves, and, above all, the Moon. A sapling with a cleft trunk suggested wounding and recovery, and would by consequence be used in healing rituals. In the traditional living world of Mother Nature, analogies implied efficacy and rural experience sustained a symbolic physiology, whose accent was on organic wholeness, rhythmic flow, and change.

The explanatory potential of living nature for imagining the body's interior has been superbly elucidated in a study by the German medical historian, Barbara Duden, of nearly 2000 women from Saxony, whose experiences were documented in the casebooks of their physician, Johann Storch (1681–1751). As Storch's medical records show, no physician ever probed inside these women's bodies (even post-mortems were exceptional); their bodies were opaque and known only by what was taken into them and what was evacuated. It was possible to form inferences about the interior only thanks to their own testimony and to signs emanating from the body. Storch's patients clearly regarded their insides as theatres of ceaseless change. The maladies registered – complaints presented to the doctor by the women themselves – reflected convictions that the innards were involved in constant transformations. Patients might claim, for example, that their sweat sometimes stank of urine; that if they failed to menstruate, they developed diarrhoea or that the delayed monthly discharge was finally expelled as bloody sputum. The interior was a magic mixer, a source of limitless metamorphosis, and almost any element could turn into any other. The healthy body had to flow. In an agrarian society preoccupied with the weather and with changing seasons, the system operating beneath the skin was naturally viewed as fluid, a succession of transactions – digestion, fertilisation, growth, expulsion. Not structures but processes counted.

Storch had no difficulty in making sense of his patients' images. For the fluid body image was also held by traditional learned medicine, and maladies were thought to migrate round the body, manoeuvering, probing weak spots, and, like marauding bands, being at their most perilous when they targeted central zones. Therapeutics, it was argued, should counter-attack by forcing or luring ailments to the extremities, like the feet, where they might be expelled in the form of pus or scabs. In such a view a gouty foot might even be a sign of health, since the big toe typically afflicted was an outpost far distant from the vital organs – disease in the toe was disease held at bay.

Holding similar beliefs about the complicated processes going on in their insides, the Saxon women offered Dr Storch very 'subjective' accounts of their maladies. They complained, Duden notes, of the following ailments:

> Slight headache, darkness of the eyes, a feeling that their hair was falling out or sight was fading or hearing was disappearing, a tearing in the jaw, a dizzy and dull headache, heavy tongue and speech, toothache, nosebleed, a flux in the ear, hiccups, a sore throat, a rising in the throat and constriction of the same, contraction of the throat, withdrawing of the gum, bilious vomiting, choking, hoarseness and coughing, phlegm dripping from the head onto the throat, neck pains, tightness of throat, sweating of the head, gloominess of thoughts,

– and hundreds more similar conditions. It is an exhausting list, but that is the point. These women experienced practically no 'diseases' that match the diagnostic categories of modern scientific medicine. Rather, changes were happening to their bodies that they could feel but not control, and which, being strange and painful, incommoded and frightened them.

In this milieu of unseen bodily processes, how was the prevalence of sickness and death explained? Above all, how did people cope with the question: why did it happen to me? Facing that dilemma, popular culture tended to see sickness as the finger of Providence. God used illness for higher purposes. It could, for example, be a test of the righteous or an affliction to smite the ungodly, like the Old Testament plagues hurled against the Egyptians. The notion of suffering as a spiritual education was widely endorsed by Pietist followers of Stahl in Prussia. Belief that disease had divine meanings did not, however, contradict the idea that it also had natural causes to be treated medically; few anticipated later Christian Scientists in thinking that faith was at odds with medicine.

SELF-CARE AND DOMESTIC MEDICINE

Self-reliance was both necessary and prized. Diaries show that when people fell sick, they frequently framed their own diagnosis. Explaining symptoms was reassuring – it quelled anxiety. But it also helped sufferers to make their next decision – whether to summon professional help. Many still had recourse, as discussed earlier, to folk or magical means, and Robert Southey (1774–1843) noted in 1807 that 'a cunning man, or a cunning woman, as they are termed, is to be found near every town'. But magic was losing its place in lay healing. Its decline, at least among the literate, was one facet of what Max Weber called the 'demystification of the world' and also of the withdrawal of elite from vulgar culture. Other expedients took its place. The aid of friends, family, wise-women or the priest was widely sought. 'Agues are much about', wrote an English country parson in the mid-eighteenth century, 'and my wife being a professed Sangrado [a bleeding doctor] for that distemper, has a multitude of patients, that come to her three or four miles round, and great success she has with her powders'. Contemporary letters abound with recipes and treatments swapped among families and friends. Many households maintained manuscript recipe books, bulging with health advice. Family members cultivated healing skills. The American preacher, Cotton Mather (1663–1728), had a trio of daughters; he wanted one to grow up good at cooking, one at sewing, and one at home physic.

Families also had recourse to kitchen-physic, and increasingly there were shop-bought items: purges, vomits, pain-killers, cordials, and febrifuges (medicines to reduce fever). In mid-eighteenth century England, where medicine, like everything else, became highly commercialised, it was common for middle-class families to stock up with patent medicines like Dr James's Powders, the Georgian equivalent of aspirin. Ready-made medicine chests became popular. Overall, medicine was spreading as a commodity as part of the general triumph of the capitalist, service economy in Northwest Europe and on the Atlantic seaboard of America. In England above all, a national market developed for proprietary concoctions, centrally manufactured and distributed from franchised warehouses to retail outlets, including newspaper offices which served as advertisers and distributors. Some were respectable, though many were just swindles, like Solomon's Balm of Gilead, Brodum's Cordial, and similar best-selling 'restoratives' and 'rejuvenators'. Others were sinister, such as Hooper's Female Pills and other abortifacients. Where they flourished – mainly in urbanised regions with high literacy rates – proprietary medicines changed the face of lay healing. Those falling sick developed the habit of swallowing a pill or taking a dose from ready-made medicaments stored in home medicine-chests.

POPULARISING MEDICINE

Crucial to this more 'rational' domestic medicine was the spread of printed health manuals, supplanting a traditional, quasi-magical oral health culture with simplified versions of elite medicine. Scores of cheap texts poured off the presses in many European nations with titles like *The Poor Man's Medicine Chest* (1791). In his immensely popular *Primitive Physick* (1747), John Wesley, the founder of Methodism, taught the literate poor how to treat their ills with the aid of simple kitchen ingredients like onions, garlic, and honey. Because professional medicine was a scam, Wesley warned, each man should take health, as well as salvation, into his own hands. William Buchan's *Domestic Medicine* (1769) and Samuel Tissot's *Avis au Peuple sur la Santé* (1761) (*Advice to the People Regarding their Health*) ran to scores of editions, and were translated into numerous languages. Buchan's was to become the favourite health manual in Spain, Tissot's in France and Central Europe. A Swiss Protestant, Tissot hoped to impart medical education to peasants, suspecting that wretched health-care was contributing to rural decline. But he also wrote for all strata of society, penning works on the disorders of literary men (1766), and of the fashionable rich (1770), as well as a diatribe against masturbation (1760).

Buchan's work carried a more radical charge. Though an Edinburgh-trained physician, he denounced the medical profession as oligarchic and monopolistic, and stressed the capacity of ordinary people to treat their disorders, not just chills and fevers but major conditions like dislocated limbs and venereal disease ('in nineteen out of twenty cases, where this disease occurs, the patient may be his own physician'), trusting to the healing power of Nature. Buchan aimed to 'lay open' medicine to all, in later life advocating a kind of medical democracy as a fulfilment of the rights of man declared by the French Revolution. Like Wesley, Buchan set great store by simple treatments, regarding diet, hygiene, and temperance as more beneficial than pricy polypharmacy.

Buchan devoted attention to industrial and occupational accidents, which might need urgent treatment before expert aids were to hand. He popularised the new resuscitation techniques being developed by Humane Societies, concerned to halt the rise in deaths from drowning accidents. Prudent households, he advised, should possess a medicine chest, containing items like adhesive plaster, agaric of oak, cinnamon water, and so on.

Authors of many nationalities ploughed similar furrows. In his *Catechism of Health* (1794), the German physician, Bernhard Faust (1775–1842), used a question-and-answer format to impart his advice, and, like Wesley, portrayed healthiness as next to godliness. Embodying Enlightenment ideals, such writers made much of the duty of parents to minister to their children (infant welfare had long been disregarded by the medical profession, being left largely to mothers, nurses, and midwives). Not least, if common people were instructed to treat their own diseases, argued popular writers, they would no longer fall prey to cheating quacks.

Works like Buchan's proved immensely popular, giving medical instruction to literate people eager to improve themselves. Their authors expressed mixed feelings, however, about the idea of everyone being his own doctor, fearing that too many foolish practices retained credit among the people. 'Some try bold, or rather fool-hardy experiments to cure agues', noted Buchan, 'as drinking great quantities of strong liquor, jumping into the river, &c'. But Buchan deemed it best to drive out bad practices with better. Other, less sanguine, popularisers sought a compromise, aiming to teach readers how to preserve their health, but urging them, when sick, to consult a doctor.

What happened, then, once the sick person decided to call the doctor? Much depended upon rank and class. Affluent patients did not hold practitioners in awe; all but the boldest or most eminent physicians deferred to social superiors, and sick patients expected doctors to fall in with their self-diagnoses and favourite treatments. Samuel Johnson – a man who respected doctors, though he was a trying patient – bullied his medical attendants, on one occasion insisting against his physician's advice that his surgeon bled him. Dr Thomas Percival's (1740–1804) pioneering *Medical Ethics* (1803) advised physicians to accommodate themselves to the whims of moneyed clients – while, of course, denying any such indulgence to charity patients in hospital. Indeed, books of medical ethics began to appear in the latter part of the eighteenth century precisely as part of an attempt by members of the medical profession to develop codes of conduct that would increase professional leverage over their patients. Such works were not profound philosophical inquiries into the theoretical grounds of the duties of doctors, but rather supplements to the traditional gentlemanly codes of honour that had long dictated the proper behaviour of professional men.

The sick felt no compunction about shopping around for second and third opinions, and made free use of quack, family, and unorthodox remedies as well, adopting a try-anything mentality. They picked some healers because they were trained, others because they possessed great experience; some because they were orthodox, others because they promised something out of the ordinary; some because they had high status, others because they were close to hand, or charged nothing, or were family acquaintances, familiar, reliable, obsequious, or benevolent.

The medical profession and medical education

Nationally and internationally, medicine today is highly organised through professional structures that grant the profession considerable autonomy under state protection, while also purportedly protecting the public from malpractice and quackery. These ideals and structures are not timeless; nor can they be accepted at face value. Recognisably modern professional structures emerged in the nineteenth century. Before then, medicine was differently organised, or, in some cases, hardly organised at all – there was still a profusion of healers, with different skills and credit.

Medicine's organisation differed from nation to nation. In all the great kingdoms, medical professionals had succeeded from late medieval times in achieving some self-regulation and corporate identity. For the lesser ranks – country and small-town practitioners, apothecaries, surgeons – this involved apprenticeship to a master, for five or seven years, to be followed by entry to a guild conferring a licence to practice. The most prestigious practitioners, notably physicians serving as attendants upon the titled, tended to be dignified by a university training that culminated in an academic degree, followed by admission to a faculty and a college or court appointment. All such arrangements were authorised by royal or city government. Formal status conferred prestige and quasi-monopolistic privileges to practise specified arts within a defined region and also to prosecute interlopers. As was discovered, however, by many a German town physician, a price had to be paid for such rights. Official prerogatives presupposed official duties and supervision from above; and, for the aspirant junior practitioner, the formal regulation of the medical profession often meant that gaining initial entry and then climbing the ladder of promotion entailed long, arduous and expensive drudgery.

FRANCE

In *ancien-régime* France, medical regulation was chiefly in the hands of faculties attached to the main universities – Paris, Montpellier, Rheims, Toulouse, Tours and so forth. Candidates fulfilling prescribed conditions, passing examinations and paying fees, were licensed to practice within the local jurisdiction. Entry into such corporations was restricted, to cap numbers, reduce competition and swell rewards. Licensing a restricted pool of privileged practitioners, the French medical profession had a conspicuously corporate appearance, laying itself open in the Revolution to devastating attack, for, condemning professions as elite monopolies, the Jacobins dismantled all the traditional medical faculties. Chaos ensued. The Napoleonic regime restored order, replacing, through the Law of 1805, the old particular-ist, localist faculties with a unitary, Paris-based system of professional licensing under centralised government. The organisation of physicians changed from the corporate self-government typical of the *ancien régime* to uniform state regulation. To enlarge what was still rather an elite medical corps, a lower stratum of healers was created for the lower classes, the *officiers de santé*, the French equivalent of the paramedics or medical orderlies called *feldshers* in Russia and *sekundäre Ärzte* in Germany.

THE GERMAN-SPEAKING TERRITORIES

Medicine was regulated in the German-speaking principalities and the Austrian Empire through a system emphasising qualification via uni-versity qualifications. In states like Prussia where princes recruited a service aristocracy and cultivated the ideal of professional government service conducted by obedient functionaries (the *Beamtenstaat*), physi-cians tended, not surprisingly, to pride themselves upon operating as civil servants, fulfilling administrative ends in a rationally-organised, hierarchical bureaucracy. Top physicians and medical professors typi-cally belonged to a medical college (*collegium medicum*) attached to the royal court. Formal qualifications counted for much. In Prussia, for example, candidates for the *magister medicinae* (MD) were required to take anatomy and to discuss a clinical case (*casus medicopracticus*) before the Collegium Medicum and the Medicochirurgicum (state board of health). Similar requirements applied in the Austrian Empire, where licenses to practice were conferred by the universities of Vienna and Prague. In 1749, a state executive was designated in the Habsburg domains to superintend the curriculum and medical examinations.

In the German principalities, chains of command and responsibility descended from the collegium medicum through city councils to indi-vidual town and village physicians, whose local status was dignified by bureaucratic offices and bundles of parchment diplomas. In theory, offi-cial title conferred upon the licensed practitioner the exclusive right to local practice. In actuality, it standardly involved stacks of trivial and irksome supervisory chores, book-keeping and administrative obliga-tions – attending law courts, sanctioning military exemptions, regulat-ing poisons, making examinations of lunacy, pregnancy or paternity, inspecting the poor for venereal disease, documenting epidemic out-breaks, and serving as a public witness – and all for meagre pecuniary reward. In any case, in the face of itinerants and amateur healers, exclusive rights to practice proved impossible to enforce.

In England, the formal regulation of the medical profession instigated in the sixteenth century was threatened by rapid social change – while in the newly-independent United States, Congress had virtually no part in controlling or directing medicine's growth. The Royal College of Physicians of London, which under the Stuarts had aspired to extend its jurisdiction, dwindled into a gentleman's club, reserved for the fashionable elite. The College's statutes restricted its fellowship to graduates of Oxford and Cambridge and members of the Church of England. It resisted reformist pressures to open its fellowship to London physicians at large – despite the fact that by 1750, the finest physicians were Dissenters by religion, trained either at Leiden or at Edinburgh. Such eminences as William Hunter, John Fothergill, and John Coakley Lettsom resented being consigned to the status of mere 'licentiates' – non-voting members or second-class citizens. Their campaigns to democratise the College met successful opposition.

Yet if the College did little to promote medicine, it also did little to restrict its practice. Its jurisdiction extended only to a seven-mile radius of the capital; and it barely exercised its authority to debar interlopers. And when it acted, the College suffered reverses. Following the House of Lords' judgment in the Rose Case (1704), the College lost its monopoly of prescribing medicines; henceforth apothecaries might also prescribe and act as doctors.

London's Company (later College) of Surgeons failed to ripen into a teaching and examining body worthy of the modern world. The Surgeons' Company formally separated in 1745 from the Barbers, thus signalling that surgery was a craft in its own right; but one untoward consequence of the divorce was that the new hall occupied by the Surgeons long lacked that basic requisite, a dissecting theatre! The Society of Apothecaries officially regulated pharmacy in London, but dozens of unregulated chemists and druggists arose, provoking noisy but impotent protests from the Apothecaries. The consequence of this general atrophy among the regulating bodies was that quacks and fringe practitioners freely plied their trade in the metropolis.

Beyond London, there was a broad liberty to practise. In all but a few corporate cities, little medical regulation applied and a free-for-all ensued, in which assorted healers set up shop wherever they thought prospects were good. 'Without going a hundred miles from Clifton, Bristol, and Bath', lamented the hammer of the quacks, Thomas Beddoes, around 1800,

> you may meet with practitioners, whose genius has transported them at a single bound from the side of the mortar to the bedside ... As to consumption-doctresses, cancer-curers, mechanics professing to treat divers disorders, and particularly those of the female sex, there have arisen within my short memory, several, on whose behalf to speak with the cricket players, one might safely challenge all England.

In Britain, there was not even the pretence of a uniform system of medical education and qualification to channel entry onto and promotion up the professional ladder. Some doctors had degrees from English universities (though the output of medical graduates from Oxford and Cambridge dwindled almost to vanishing point, and all Oxbridge medical professors were nonentities). Many possessed degrees from Leiden, or a French or Italian university, and a swelling number had gained an education in Scotland, predominately Edinburgh, though by no means all had a degree (or a diploma issued by the Royal Corporation of Surgeons of Edinburgh). And many practised in England without any formal qualifications at all. There was no nationally or regionally enforced system of medical licensing; nor were there, as in France, provincial medical faculties. Prosecution for unauthorized healing was unusual and malpractice suits were rare. It was the market place rather than government or the judiciary that regulated practice in Britain. Yet the calibre of medical men was improving, not least because medical students commonly walked the wards of the new hospitals springing up in London and the provinces.

As Britain became a burgeoning free-market economy, medicine tacitly espoused the principles of Adam Smith, a sort of competitive individualism. In town and country alike, medical professionals were essentially on their own. Success depended upon a capacity to satisfy public demand, to be inexpensive, sycophantic, or cut a dash. Medicine in Georgian England was thus demand-led and beholden to its clients. Aspiring physicians had to bow to the behests of the fashionable, and common-or-garden practitioners tailored their services to market forces.

Criticism abounded. Proverbs expressed distrust: 'one doctor makes work for another' was heard alongside the Biblical 'physician, heal thyself'. Following Molière's barbs, physicians were pilloried in novels as 'Dr Slop', 'Dr Smelfungus', or collectively, in Hogarth's (1697–1764) engraving, as the 'Company of Undertakers'. Yet many practitioners proved highly successful, getting on and getting rich. For top physicians, incomes soared. William Cheselden reputedly charged £500 for a lithotomy operation (a stunningly good 'piece' rate, since his forte lay in extracting a bladder-stone in a few minutes – £500 was the annual income of many a country squire). London physicians like Lettsom topped £10,000 a year, while a provincial physician like Erasmus Darwin could make over £1000 a year. Whereas their predecessors had gone by foot or on horseback, by 1800 the cream of the provincial practitioners were gadding around in carriages – though doubtless they worked hard for their rewards, Darwin calculating he travelled 10,000 miles a year on his rounds. In his pioneering *Medical Ethics* (1803), Thomas Percival warned of a lack of professional *esprit de corps*, and insisted that the medical profession could not be upheld 'except as a lucrative one'.

MEDICINE IN THE COMMERCIAL SOCIETY

Doctors flourished because demand for medical services was rising. Much of Europe and the North American colonies was enjoying greater prosperity. In thriving consumer economies, the expanding middling ranks of tradesmen, shopkeepers, clerks and farmers had money to spare for services, of which medicine was one. And profitable sidelines were in the offing. English country practitioners increased their income by engaging in parish Poor Law practice. The 'trade in lunacy', based upon the private madhouse, proved profitable for others.

The first English medical registers, published in 1779 and 1783, list about 3000 practitioners (the total must have been higher). Thousands more made a living, or topped up their income, from healing. Grocers and pedlars sold drugs, blacksmiths and farriers drew teeth and set bones, doubling in human and horse medicine. In England at least, doctors seized the opportunities that booming consumer capitalism was offering. Yet the resultant 'sick trade' naturally attracted critics, who avowed that physicians pursued wealth more than health. The nineteenth century opened to a dawn chorus of critics demanding that medicine must elevate itself above mere trade. The new century was to prove an age of reform, dedicated to ending privilege and nepotism, opening up careers to talent, and enhancing professional dignity.

451

Developments in America resembled those in England. Medicine emerged without guild or university guidelines. Professional medical bodies arose fitfully from the 1730s, and regulatory legislation more slowly still. In 1765 the first American medical school was founded, at what later became the University of Pennsylvania. Its founder, the British-trained John Morgan (1735–89), in due course tried to promote qualifying examinations so as to ensure minimum standards of performance for military medicine during the War of Independence. Yet, after 1783, neither Congress nor state legislatures were anxious to reinstate old world monopolies; medical sects proliferated, and individualism remained dominant over *esprit de corps*. Only slowly did some semblance of licensing emerge. The Harvard medical school was established in 1783, and 20 years later it was agreed that either a Harvard diploma or a qualifying examination would serve as a Massachusetts license; in 1810 similar rules were formulated in Connecticut; South Carolina followed suit in 1817.

Overall, with its acceptance of a medical market place, the Anglo-Saxon world diverged notably from the Continental. Formal regulation under an absolutist administrative state set the mould for continental medical organisation, where the state assumed some responsibility for the health of subjects and the regulation of professions, and doctors became quasi-civil servants. In Britain, health became essentially an individual and family matter, and doctors served their clients on a private, contractual basis. But nakedly commercial medicine was a set-up that could not last. Rapid change and startling demographical growth meant that every nation became obliged in the nineteenth century energetically to interfere in matters of health and professional regulation. Questions of medical education also played their part in the turn of events.

It is unnecessary to explore medical education here in great detail, since eighteenth-century arrangements broadly perpetuated the sixteenth- and seventeenth-century patterns already discussed in Chapter 6. The rank-and-file learnt on the job by apprenticeship; the officer class enjoyed an academic training, with lecture courses, typically in Latin, leading to examinations, dissertations, and degrees. The yoking of academic teaching with the practice of anatomical dissection had confirmed the central place of the university, first and foremost Padua and Bologna.

MEDICAL TRAINING AND THE UNIVERSITIES

The eighteenth century saw other universities blossom. Developments in Paris have already been discussed in context of surgery. Leiden assumed towering prominence thanks to Boerhaave, a man who, if no great original genius, became the medical instructor of Europe for a generation. He began teaching anatomy at Leiden in 1701; in 1709 he became professor of botany and medicine, and by 1718 he was professor of chemistry – all the time keeping up an extensive private practice. His *Institutiones medicae* (*Medical Institutes*; 1708) and *Elementa Chemiae* (*Elements of Chemistry*; 1731) were popular teaching texts, and his strong personality inspired thousands of students. Like Cullen after him, Boerhaave endeavoured to create good clinicians. His inaugural lecture was significantly a call for a return to the study of Hippocrates. Boerhaave admired Sydenham's work, and might be said to have synthesised Sydenham for university use. Students flocked to his classes from all over Europe, and his influence grew especially powerful at the universities of Vienna and Edinburgh.

Leiden's success shows the importance of professors with a strong appeal. Personal factors were also crucial in launching modern education in America, where the great promoter was John Morgan (1735–89), a Philadelphian who learnt his medicine in Edinburgh from the Monros, Cullen, and Whytt. Returning in 1765, he published a *Discourse upon the Institution of Medical Schools in America*, founding in 1765 the medical department of the University of Pennsylvania, where he held the chair of practice of medicine. Another Philadelphia-born Edinburgh graduate, William Shippen, Jr (1736–1808), worked alongside Morgan, becoming professor of anatomy and surgery. In 1769 Benjamin Rush was elected professor of chemistry in the University of Philadelphia. Rush succeeded Morgan as professor of practice in 1789, assuming the chair of institutes of medicine in 1791. He was also physician to the Pennsylvania Hospital (1783–1813) and founder of the Philadelphia Dispensary.

Edinburgh's eminence, by contrast, derived from collective circumstances, in particular the handiness of Scotland as a tuition centre for English-speaking students. As Leiden's star waned, Edinburgh's rose. The Edinburgh University medical school dates from the appointment in 1726 of the Leiden-trained Alexander Monro (primus) (1697–1767) as professor of anatomy. By any standards, Edinburgh medicine in the following century affords a stunning success story. This was partly because of its galaxy of talent: the Monro family in anatomy (three, all Alexanders, were professors in succession Monro II (1733–1817) succeeded his father in 1758, and Monro III (1773–1859) followed his father in 1798; he stayed till 1846, the three Monros holding the post some 120 years); Black in chemistry; Cullen and John Gregory (1724–73) in theoretical and practical medicine, and other lesser lights besides. But Edinburgh's eminence was largely due to its collective identity and its operation in a university environment that was uncommonly user-friendly and responsive to demand. By the 1780s, when medicine was moribund at Oxbridge, Edinburgh University was attracting, from all corners of the English-speaking world, around 200 medical students a year – a tally that had doubled by the 1820s; a staggering 17,000 medical students studied in the first century of the School and there were additionally apprentices studying surgery at what was known from 1778 as the Royal College of Surgeons of Edinburgh.

Edinburgh had unsurpassed attractions for a student. It was cheap, there were no religious tests, and the lectures were in English. True, graduation examinations were held in dog-Latin, but there was no obligation to graduate, or even matriculate, and many students felt no need so to do. Above all, Edinburgh's appeal lay in the fact that it operated on a supermarket system: students attended only the lecture courses they desired, and paid for those alone. This student-power, payment-by-results regime kept the professors on their toes. If pupils occasionally griped that Cullen and his cronies droned from old notes, the remarkable thing about the Edinburgh professoriate, in an era when Oxbridge dons routinely forgot their duties while pocketing their fees, is that a cohort of Europe's pre-eminent medical men performed so conscientiously, sometimes twice a day, six days a week. Edinburgh, judged Thomas Beddoes, who knew it first-hand, was 'almost the only place in the three kingdoms, where at once degrees were conferred and lectures systematically read'.

What did the student want, or get, out of Edinburgh? Not an intensive bedside training. Though Edinburgh pioneered infirmary-based teaching, only around a third of the students signed up for clinical lectures. Nor did they want, it seems – and they certainly did not get – prolonged personal practice with the dissecting knife. Edinburgh's Burke-and-Hare image did not apply to the eighteenth century – students typically had to take the high-road south to London to get their knives into cadavers. The strength of an Edinburgh education, rather, lay in inculcating the elements of anatomy, surgery, chemistry, medical theory, and practice, with system and clarity. After just three years of learning medicine by the book, an Edinburgh man was ready to go out into the world and make his fortune as a medical practitioner, trained in both medicine and surgery, and hence fit to practice the new trade of 'general practitioner' or family doctor; and his patients would feel tolerably confident he would heal not harm. Someone falling sick in 1810 in Newcastle, Newfoundland, or New South Wales would almost certainly have been examined by an Edinburgh man.

Britain developed two other modes of medical instruction that served the needs of paying students, eager to acquire, rapidly and cheaply, a practical medical training. One was the private anatomy school. Private medical lecturing was a key feature of the English commercial approach to learning. From the 1720s, primarily in London, medical lecture courses mushroomed, delivered by first-rank instructors and open to anyone caring to pay class fees. At least 26 medical lecturers had performed in the metropolis before William Hunter started in the mid-1740s; by the 1780s, over 20 classes were running during the course of a single year. The core subject was anatomy, but practical physic, materia medica, chemistry, and specialisms like obstetrics were also taught. Courses typically extended to 30 or 40 sessions, but some were more elaborate. William Hunter's series ran to 112 meetings, held six days a week for three and a half months, ensuring comprehensive coverage of anatomy, practical surgery, and midwifery.

PRIVATE LECTURES AND ANATOMY SCHOOLS

Offering thorough and inexpensive vocational instruction for students, such lectures were delivered by the cream of the profession, men such as William Cheselden, the leading early eighteenth-century surgeon; by the chemist, George Fordyce (1736–1802), who lectured six days a week, from 7 to 10 a.m. throughout a teaching career spanning 30 years; and, above all, by the Hunter brothers, unmatched for anatomical, physiological, and obstetrical expertise. In 1768 William Hunter set up in Great Windmill Street, Piccadilly, what became the capital's leading anatomy and obstetrics school, where he trained leading British anatomists and surgeons, including his brother, John, William Hewson (1739–74), William Cruikshank (1745–1800), and Matthew Baillie. Hunter prized his position as a 'breeder of anatomists'.

Such courses had many attractions. Some imparted discoveries unavailable elsewhere. William Hunter's auditors heard of his researches on aneurysm, the placental circulation, the lymphatic system, and the gravid uterus, nowhere available in print. Hunter never distilled his findings into a textbook, knowing, as a canny Scot, that his livelihood came through the spoken word. Another attraction lay in the high-grade specimens, preparations, models, and demonstrations devised as teaching aids by such instructors as the Hunters and Joshua Brookes (1761–1833), who developed vast private museums of specimens available to students. Pupils of the top midwifery lecturer, William Smellie, could practice delivery techniques on his life-size dolls. At William Hunter's school, they had the benefit of the teaching and specimen collections of William Hewson, who had gone into partnership with William Hunter. Hewson was an experimental physiologist of note. His *Experimental Inquiry into the Properties of the Blood* (1771) explained the coagulation of the blood, showing it was due, not to mere cooling or exposure but to a coagulable plasma. Between 1768 and 1771 Hewson made more than 200 preparations, dry and wet; many were injected with highly-coloured substances rendering them striking for teaching purposes. Another important teacher was William Cruikshank, a Scot who succeeded Hewson as William Hunter's assistant, becoming a partner in the Great Windmill Street School, and, on Hunter's death, joint proprietor with Matthew Baillie. Cruikshank investigated the regeneration of divided nerves, the passage of the impregnated ovum through the Fallopian tube, and, in his *Anatomy of the Absorbing Vessels of the Human Body* (1786), the physiology of absorption. In his *Experiments Upon the Insensible Perspiration of the Human Body* (1778) Cruikshank demonstrated that the skin, not just the lungs, gives off carbon dioxide.

Private lecture schools, in short, could be centres of research excellence. They also proved popular with students because of the superb opportunities they offered – unlike the universities – for practical anatomy. 'The young Surgeon', noted Robert Campbell's *The London Tradesman* (1747), 'must be an accurate Anatomist, not only as a speculative but practical Anatomist; without which he must turn out a mere Bungler. It is not sufficient for him to attend Anatomical Lectures, and see two or three Subjects cursorily dissected; but he must put his Hand to it himself, and be able to dissect every part, with the same Accuracy that the Professor performs'. Yet this was easier said than done. For the law and popular antipathy to dissection restricted legal supply of cadavers. From 1752, the Company of Surgeons was granted the corpses of all executed felons but Surgeons' Hall dissections were formal exercises, students being mere spectators. By contrast, the best private anatomy instructors won customer loyalty by ensuring that students had personal access to bodies. George Fordyce, while one of 'Hunter's men', dissected three corpses. To achieve such a supply, operators like William Hunter needed to be in cahoots with shady body-snatchers. Their willingness to turn a blind eye to legal niceties ensured private lecturers student devotion and meant they could offer unmatched hands-on anatomical experience. Hunter had studied at Paris, supposedly the finest anatomy school in Europe; 'there I learned a good deal by my ears', he recalled, 'but almost nothing by my eyes; and therefore hardly anything to the purpose. ... The professor was obliged to demonstrate all the parts of the body ... upon one dead body'. Even at Edinburgh, corpses for dissection were notoriously scarce, and the Monros taught mainly from models. Things were different in London.

The half-century after 1760 was the great age of the private anatomy school. Alongside William Hunter's, Joshua Brookes' Great Marlborough Street school began in 1787, Brookes supposedly taught 5000 students, and at its peak, his museum was reckoned to be worth £30,000. Academies outlived their founders. On Hunter's death in 1783, Matthew Baillie and William Cruikshank inherited it; later James Wilson (1765–1821) took it over; subsequently Charles Bell (1774–1842), Herbert Mayo (1796–1852) and Caesar Hawkins (1798–1884) ran it till its demise around 1831, by which time the state, the hospitals, and London University were insisting, in the name of professional regulation, on a more structured and less demand-led mode of medical education.

THE TEACHING HOSPITAL

The other new site for medical teaching was the hospital. The life of the infirmary will be examined below. Here the point must be made that hospitals increasingly opened themselves to students as places to learn, and teachers used instructive cases on their doorstep as training material. In Vienna, for example, the hospital reforms carried through in the 1770s by Anton Stoerck (1731–1803) led to clinical instruction on the wards. 'This great man, born for the good of science, his country and those who govern it', remarked Maximilian Stoll (1742–87), has undertaken a great number of improvements facilitating clinical study... The students have ... the advantage that when they have learned enough from the restricted number of patients contained in the hospital clinic they can be presented with a much larger field in which to perfect their practice. They may then be let into the large wards which daily contain all species of disease... and by practising at their own expense, they form a certain practical judgement and obtain a singular faculty of discernment, indispensable qualities for whoever wishes to practise medicine with success and which reading alone will never give.

The Edinburgh medical school's success owed much to its links with the town infirmary. Professor John Rutherford (1695–1779) inaugurated clinical lecturing there in the 1740s, and from 1750 a special clinical ward was set up, whose patients served as teaching material for professorial clinical lectures. 'A number of such cases as are likely to prove instructive', noted the medical student, John Aikin (1747–1822), in the 1770s,

> are selected and disposed in separate rooms in the Infirmary, and attended by one of the college professors. The students go round with him every day, and mark down the state of each patient and the medicines prescribed. At certain times lectures are read upon these cases, in which all the progressive changes in the disease are traced and explained and the method of practice is accounted for.

Students were expected to visit patients' bedsides for themselves, studying the professors' reports. This practice became normal throughout Europe.

Similar developments occurred south of the Border. Hospital facilities mushroomed in Georgian England and developed in them on-site lecturing. Cheselden started private surgical lectures in 1711. From 1718, he moved his lectures to St. Thomas's, delivering four courses a year. The practice spread. It offered an excellent way of learning. The Philadelphian William Shippen (1736–1808) attended London's hospitals in 1759. '4 August', he recorded,

> saw Mr. Way surgeon to Guy's hospital amputate a leg above the knee very dexterously 8 ligatures...(23 August) attended Dr Akenside in taking in patient and prescribing for them, 58 taken in...(5 September) examined particulars in hospital several smallpox 3 out of 4 die, saw Mr. Baker perform 3 operations, a leg, breast and tumor from a girl's lower jaw inside, very well operated. ...(7 November) went to Bartholomew's Hospital and saw the neatest operation of bubonocele that I ever saw by Mr. Pott a very clever neat surgeon.

And so forth. In his poem, *The Hospital* (1809), the actor, Joseph Wilde, laid up in the Exeter Hospital with a gammy leg, noted the house surgeon and the physician were routinely attended by their pupils, 'sprightly harbingers of their grave principal', a 'train/ Of youths, observant of his every motion'. Pupils became common in provincial hospitals. Student training likewise was essential to specialist institutions like maternity hospitals. One such, London's General Lying-In Hospital, admitted student man-midwives as pupils to the attending accoucheurs. By 1800 London was, according to Thomas Beddoes, 'the best spot in Great Britain, and probably in the whole world where medicine may be taught as well as cultivated to most advantage'.

These developments highlight the wider question of the organisation of medicine. In Enlightenment Britain, high-quality student-centred, demand-led medical education emerged precisely because medicine was thrown back upon its own resources, having to tailor itself to market needs in an age in which the state and the universities kept what might euphemistically be called a low profile. In Britain, doctor training and the practice of medicine had remarkably little interplay with government. Medicine became detached from academe and the state. Nineteenth-century Britain was to witness a double transformation, two interconnected movements; the reconstitution of organised medicine under the state, and the consequent centralisation and systematisation of medical education. These processes of professionalisation must be read not as 'progress' but as realignments of priorities to meet new needs.

Quackery

The eighteenth century has been dubbed the golden age of quackery. Where state and professional control are weak, quackery (that is, market-oriented healing) flourishes. With growing central and professional regulation after 1800, quackery was squeezed and 'alternative medicine' blossomed – or, so to speak, quackery dignified itself into a matter of principle.

As demand for regular medicine grew, so too did the call for irregular medicine. After all, regular medicine had no monopoly on effectiveness. From the 1780s, the French state attempted to limit quack medicines through the policing powers of the Société Royale de Médecine, a body whose prerogatives included the right to assay and certify proprietary preparations. English common law, by contrast, presumed the free-market maxim of *caveat emptor* ('let the buyer beware'). In English conditions, irregulars, quacks and nostrum-mongers seized the opportunities a hungry market offered.

To speak of quackery is not automatically to impeach the motives of empirics (i.e., unqualified practitioners), nor is it to pass negative judgment upon their cures. Many of the most notorious Georgian quacks – such as James Graham (1745–94), advocate of mud-bathing, vegetarianism, and sexual rejuvenation – were not deliberate charlatans but fanatical believers in their personal gifts. Many proprietary remedies were look-alikes to those prescribed by physicians, sharing the same active ingredients like opium and antimony (which induced sweating to reduce fever). It could make good sense to buy ready-made nostrums, because they were commonly cheaper.

Quackery formed medicine's entrepreneurial sector. Empirics touted their wares in the market rather than relying on the slower business of cultivating a practice by patronage and word-of-mouth recommendation. They made their profits out of selling commodities rather than from receiving fees for advice, expertise and bedside attendance. They excelled in the arts of publicity. Rose's Balsamic Elixir, its vendors claimed, would cure 'the English Frenchify'd' (i.e. venereal patients) beyond all other medicines: 'it removes all pains in 3 or 4 doses and makes any man, tho' rotten as a Pear, to be sound as a sucking lamb'. In short, that elixir, like so many others, worked like magic. The traditional Italian-style charlatan, gaudily dressed and flanked by a stooge and a monkey, erecting his stage on the street corner, drawing first a crowd and then a few teeth, both to the accompaniment of loud drumming, giving out bottles of julep free, selling a few dozen more, and riding out of town – such a figure was by no means extinct in Georgian England or the Dutch Republic (that other densely urbanised and politically liberal nation was another happy-hunting ground for quacks). Such figures could still cut a dash and make a fortune.

Most mountebanks were small-timers, like the man with a circuit in mid-century rural Sussex, about whom the local grocer, Thomas Turner (d. 1793), noted that he had seen through the fellow, though his wife was taken in. But some irregulars made big money. Joanna Stephens (d. 1774) hawked a remedy that promised to dissolve painful bladder-stones without the need for surgery. Parliament raised a £5000 subscription to buy the recipe from her. Joshua Ward (1685–1761) made a fortune out of his 'pill and drop' panacea. In many cases, the knack was to claim to satisfy needs that regular doctors failed to supply. Thus patent medicines promised to cure tuberculosis and cancer, to restore lost youth and vigour, or to alleviate conditions like venereal disease about which patients might be embarrassed to consult their family physician.

From Stoughton's Great Cordial Elixir to Della Lena's Powder of Mars, myriad proprietary medicines were advertised in newspapers. The Duke of Portland's Powder was widely recommended as a gout cure (then as now, great names sold products). Another gout nostrum, Husson's Eau médicinale contained colchicum, which made it the most effective remedy available. Most famous of all in England were the antimonial fever powders and analeptic pills of Dr Robert James (1705–76), an Oxford MD, author of a learned *Medicinal Dictionary* (1743), and a friend of Samuel Johnson.

Quackery also promoted certain 'technological' inventions, like the metallic or magnetic tractors patented in 1798 by Elisha Perkins of Connecticut (1741–99). This contrivance, resembling a tuning fork, with its prongs of unequal lengths and made of different metals, worked by stroking, by analogy with galvanism or the animal magnetism then being promoted by Franz Anton Mesmer (1734–1815), the Viennese physician who, despite his own impeccable credentials, developed hypnotherapy, the basis of much subsequent charlatanry. The sublime powers of electricity and animal magnetism were used for sex therapy by James Graham (1745–94) of Edinburgh, whose 'celestial bed' promised to rejuvenate the impotent at a stroke. Opened in London in 1780, Graham's Temple of Health combined medical lectures, medicine-vending, and a multi-media entertainment centre, including alluring, soft music and near-naked nymphs – supposedly one was the later Emma Hamilton (1761–1815), posing as a Goddess of Health.

Leading captains of industry, like the potter Josiah Wedgwood (1730–95), developed consumer psychology and advertising. Similar arts were perfected by the luminaries of irregular medicine. Large promises, attractive packaging, seductive names, free gifts, special offers, and money-back-if-not satisfied guarantees were the common coin of these trailblazers of the pharmaceutical industry. Supreme showmen included such men as John ('Chevalier') Taylor (1703–72), the itinerant eye specialist whose patter was a spellbinding, or preposterous, mix of Latin and Johnsonian English, and Gustavus Katterfelto (d. 1799), the flu-remedy peddlar accompanied by a bevy of talking black cats whose

461

advertisements ran 'WONDERS! WONDERS! WONDERS!' – those were names to conjure with. If some quacks kept magic alive, they were also go-ahead business men who pioneered the saturation advertising that became ubiquitous in Georgian life. Newspaper agents also undertook to distribute drugs, so that country readers might find readier access to 'mail order' patent medicines than to regular doctors. In these ways, medical opportunists cashed in on the self-diagnosing, self-help medical traditions ingrained among the laity, while pandering to consumers' desires for miracle cures and something new.

Nostrums and patent medicine did not amount to a medical 'fringe', if by that we mean unorthodox medicine advanced by adversaries of the dominant elite. Indeed, the top quacks of the Netherlands and Georgian England are more noteworthy for their itch for acceptance in fashionable society than for championing the people against the Establishment. Some quacks had official approval. In Britain, mounte-banks from the Continent could purchase royal privileges to practise, just as 'empirics' (practitioners without formal training) could patent their proprietary medicines. Ever pinched for revenue, Stuart monarchs had been glad of the income derived from selling these rights, although the medical elite found it a scandal. Quack medicines made money for the government through the stamp duty they paid. After 1800, things began to change. The age of fringe medicine, hitched to radical religion and popular politics, was dawning.

In this blossoming of market-place quackery, Britain presents a con-trast to most of the Continent. In France, Spain, Prussia, and Russia, quackery was not allowed the freedom it possessed in Britain and so did not become big business. The case of Franz Anton Mesmer (1734–1815) is instructive. Mesmer developed his unorthodox healing methods – first using the power of magnets, and then the eye, to remove 'obstructions' in hysterical and nervous cases – in Vienna in the 1760s. Though a qualified physician, friendly with the Mozarts, he was drummed out of the City by faculty opposition. He migrated to Paris, winning celebrity for his fashionable séances, curing nervously-afflicted ladies through animal magnetism. A Royal Commission estab-lished by Louis XVI (1754–93) found him guilty of charlatanry (his cures might work, it was found, but they were scientifically bogus and therefore unacceptable), and he was obliged to leave Paris. By contrast, Mesmerists were able to perform in London with no obstructions what-soever.

Medicine and the state

The organisation of medical training and practice, as already suggested, differed from nation to nation, depending upon the force-fields of society, economy, and the state. The same applies to the public endowment of health and healing. In Northwest Europe in particular, the eighteenth century saw rapid socio-economic change, steep population rise, urbanisation and the take-off into industrialisation. *Ancien régime* Europe was also marked by distinctive political formations, notably the triumph of absolutist princes whose power was legitimated not through crude military dynasticism but through ideologies of public welfare (mercantilism, cameralism, physiocracy). This section examines medicine's official role in different policies.

As shown earlier in this volume, in many European regimes there had long been posts for doctors as public functionaries. The city states of Renaissance Italy had appointed town physicians and health boards to enforce often draconian anti-plague ordinances, and health bureaucracies were in place by 1700 in various German principalities. Even in England, where official responses to the plague were tardy, writers like John Graunt (1620–74) and William Petty (1623–87) had emphasised the need to digest knowledge of population, health, and wealth within a new science of the state. On the basis of the Bills of Mortality (weekly burial figures), they called for the gathering of official statistics. The 'life table' was devised in 1693 for actuarial purposes by the Newtonian natural philosopher, Edmond Halley (c.1656–1743).

THE POOR

England lacked the health bureaucracies common on the Continent, the Poor Law, inaugurated under Elizabeth I (1533–1603) and updated in 1660, gave extensive welfare rights to all subjects in their own parish, and led, over successive generations, to expanding parochial provision of medical care for the needy. Within the Poor Law framework, parish paternalism frequently involved outlay of ratepayers' money on the sick, disabled, or infirm, spurred by a mix of genuine neighbourliness with enlightened self-interest. The sick were commonly committed to the care of other parishioners paid to nurse them. Medicines, foods, and funerals might be provided, and surgeons' fees reimbursed for treating the destitute. It became common for a parish to contract a general practitioner to treat its paupers for an annual sum.

The amounts laid out on individuals sometimes appear surprisingly generous. It was not unknown to pay to send a sick person to a spa or to London for treatment, in the expectation that such outlays would in the long run prove cheaper than the burden of permanent parish relief.

In England, pauper hospitals were a rarity (Bristol set one up in 1695); but before the rise of the friendly societies and other self-help benefit associations, charity and Poor Law relief combined to offer at least some medical attention to the lower orders. Pauper hospitals were, however, common on the Continent. The great cities of northern Italy possessed flourishing and well-endowed institutions for the sick poor, orphans, and widows. These institutions, funded by donations, bequests, and public charity, tended to operate a flexible regime combining both indoor and outdoor relief.

Facilities for health care and destitution relief provided opportunities for medical men to enter state service. For status reasons, this they were pleased to do, though it was frequently onerous and ill-paid. Outpatient care for the needy was provided in some cases by volunteer doctors or by low-paid practitioners working for municipal government or philanthropic agencies. Enlightenment philosophy – serviceable to absolutism as well as to liberal regimes – also deemed it a government duty to deploy medico-scientific knowledge and resources for public benefit, that is, for the good simultaneously of the state, the sovereign and the populace at large. Enlightenment demands for reform and improvement took various forms, including *Cameralwissenschaft* (rational administration) and utilitarianism (pursuit of the greatest happiness of the greatest number); but everywhere promotion of thriving populations and amelioration of state institutions were central to reformers' campaigns. Alongside military success and economic prosperity, a rising birth rate and a healthy citizenry became, for enlightened statesmen, touchstones of good government.

STATISTICS

States began collecting population data. The westernising Czar, Peter the Great (1682–1725), initiated a nationwide Russian census, characteristically for taxation purposes. From 1748, Sweden established a centralised system for compiling statistics, enabling Pehr Wargentin (1717–83) to publish in 1766 the first mortality table for an entire country. The United Kingdom established a national census from 1801 – earlier proposals had been frustrated by a scare rhetoric of 'liberty in danger'.

The culmination of Enlightenment calls for action to promote public health came in post-1789 France. Revolutionary France began collection of detailed social statistics, and *philosophes* and physicians like the Marquis de Laplace (1749–1827), the Marquis de Condorcet (1743–94), and Philippe Pinel (1745–1826) strove to apply vital statistics to public health questions. The Revolution also advanced a bold programme of social medicine and hygiene formulated in terms of the idea of the 'citizen patient', which acknowledged the state's duty to minister to the health needs of its population and the individual's reciprocal obligation to tend his well-being as citoyen. Between 1790 and 1794, comprehensive programmes for a national system of health were brought before the revolutionary assemblies. In 1791, the Legislative Assembly advanced a combined health and public assistance package in a single commission under Rochefoucauld-Liancourt (1747–1827). A scheme was approved covering health inspectorates, child care, a national inoculation campaign, and medical services for the young and the poor. Under pressure of war and the Terror, however, little was achieved.

Promotion of the people's health lay partly in the desire of Catholic rulers to supplant the Roman Church as the primary agency of aid, or, in other words, to transform charity from pious offerings into regular schemes of public benefits. The motives were varied, ranging from naked expropriation of religious charities to a principled desire to see to more efficient and equitable benefits distribution. In Austria, Joseph II (1741–90) closed the monasteries to redirect charity to socially more useful objectives, and reformed Vienna's hospitals. Revolutionary France transformed philanthropy more drastically. As part of a wholesale attack on the Church, religious nursing communities were abolished and charities nationalised. Revolutionaries confiscated the coffers of religious foundations to divert them to public use to relieve distress. In the event, however, political corruption and rampant inflation led to a spectacular reduction in the welfare and hospital services provided for the penurious. By choice and necessity, Napoleon largely reverted to the status quo ante, with hospitals being financed by pious donations and staffed by religious orders, above all the Daughters of Charity, who flourished in the nineteenth century.

MEDICAL POLICE

Enlightened rulers like Frederick the Great of Prussia prized rational administration (often nowadays called mercantilism and cameralism).

Medicine and law were seen as sister professions serving the ruler. Forensic medicine was codified in works like Friedrich Hoffmann's (1660–1742) *Medicus politicus* (The *State Doctor*; 1738) and Johann Wilhelm Baumer's (1719–88) *Fundamenta politica medica* (*Foundations of State Medicine*; 1777), which defined the role of medicine within legal procedures. Enlightened absolutists paid increasing attention to medical and hygiene issues, developing for instance, centrally-administered schemes for epidemic control, administered by a corps of functionaries acting under public licensure. Influential thinkers publicised welfare questions, developing the notion of statistics (*Staatistik*, derived from *Staat*, state), in which health data would be included in civil information on such topics as population, topography, climate, natural resources, trade, manufactures, military strength, education, and religion. The Prussian army chaplain, Johann Peter Süssmilch (1707–77), was a pioneer of vital and medical statistics, assembling extensive data relating to public hygiene, life insurance, and epidemics. Of top significance, however, was the concept of medical police, a doctrine exhaustively expounded in works published by Johann Peter Frank (1745–1821).

Hailing from Rotalben in the Palatinate, Frank became a physician to the Habsburg Court and director of the General Hospital in Vienna. In his *System einer vollständigen medizinischen Polizey* (*Complete System of Medical Police*; 1779–1819), he outlined procedures for state regulation of personal and community behaviour liable to spread ill health – pregnancy, marriage, personal hygiene, child welfare, school hygiene, sexual conduct – and proposed public hygiene measures – hospital reform, pure water supply, street cleaning, drainage, marriage regulation, vice control, and measures against urban overcrowding. Frank's system built on traditional Habsburg public administration and maintained that a thriving, healthy population should be the basis of imperial strength. Through *Polizey*, the well-disciplined body of the subject was to become the productive property of the state.

MILITARY MEDICINE

Statecraft required attention to health in many other fields, not least military hygiene. For centuries, every army had lost far more soldiers in camp through appalling sanitary conditions than on the battlefield. Strenuous efforts were made to change this. Outstanding was the work of Sir John Pringle (1707–82), a Leiden-trained Scotsman who was physician general of the English army from 1742 to 1758. Pringle is memorable for developing the idea of the neutrality of the military hospital. At the battle of Dettingen (1743), he proposed to the French commanding officer that the hospitals on each side should be immune from attack. The idea caught on. More importantly Pringle gave his attention to gaol fever, noting the parallels between military and civilian diseases of dirt and overcrowding. In *Observations on the Diseases of the Army* (1752), he advocated barrack-room ventilation, good latrines and sanitation. Pringle was a promoter of the notion of antisepsis – the struggle against 'putrescence' – which became so prominent in the hygiene movement for the cleansing of ships, camps, and gaols.

The health of sailors also received great attention, not least after scurvy ravaged the crew of Lord Anson's (1697–1762) round-the-world expedition of 1740: 75 per cent of Anson's men were stricken. As noted in Chapter 6 (pp. 227–30), scurvy was investigated in a scientific manner from the mid-eighteenth century. Since hindsight teaches that scurvy is a deficiency disease caused by lack of vitamin C, historians have praised Lind for his advocacy of citrus fruits. In truth, Lind and his followers, including James Cook (1728–79), Thomas Trotter (1760–1832), and Sir Gilbert Blane (1749–1834), recommended an integrated regime, emphasising proper diet, cleanliness, ventilation aboard ship, discipline, and good morale. On Cook's first circumnavigation in 1770, good management meant that there was very little illness and only one death among his seamen. Alongside fresh lemons, limes, and oranges, Cook extolled the antiscorbutic virtues of onions, cabbage, sauerkraut, and malt. Through the political skills of Blane, an admiralty order enjoining the use of lemon juice was issued in 1795, leading to dramatic reduction of scurvy – it has been suggested that lemons did as much as Nelson (1758–1805) to defeat Napoleon (1769–1821).

But the wider significance of experiments like Lind's lay in tackling the broad hygiene problems created by crowded populations, and appreciating the analogues between civilian and military sickness. Lind's efforts parallel those of the Dissenting philanthropist, John Howard, who conducted pioneering investigations into prisons, bridewells, and lazarettos. On the basis of extensive gaol and hospital visiting in Britain and on the Continent in the 1770s and 1780s, Howard concluded that their filth and close, contaminated atmospheres were responsible for endemic conditions like gaol fever (typhus).

PUBLIC HEALTH

Some attention was also being paid to occupational disorders, thanks to the inquiries of Bernardino Ramazzini (1633–1714). Ramazzini called attention to such conditions as stonemason's and miner's phthisis (pneumoconiosis) and the eye troubles of gilders and printers. Little in truth was done to counter occupational diseases – even enlightened absolutists saw scant reason to interfere with the laws of trade. But attempts were made to improve urban hygiene, through measures including waste disposal, drainage of surface water, improved street ventilation, slum clearance, and so forth. John Bellers (1654–1725), a Quaker cloth merchant living in London, wrote perceptively on the health of towns, highlighting the role of overcrowding in propagating disease. He urged municipal street cleaning, refuse collection, regulation of dairies, abattoirs and noxious trades, and other measures that, initially visionary and impossible, found their way onto the statute book over the next two centuries. Equating dirt with danger, John Haygarth (1740–1827) argued that the contagiousness of typhus fever was responsible for its prevalence amongst the urban slum-dwelling poor. Like Pringle, he placed great faith in better ventilation. Commissioned in 1750 to purify the noxious air of Newgate prison, Pringle and Stephen Hales recommended the introduction of ventilators. Having advocated hand-operated bellows for ventilating ships, Hales invented a 'windmill' device to be placed on roofs, to ensure free air circulation.

THE HOSPITAL

Central to public health provision was the hospital; but it was also the heart of the problem. Nominally a site of recuperation, the traditional hospital was all too often a place of disease and death, spreading the maladies it was meant to relieve. Hospitals took many forms and served many functions. In France, the *hôpital général* (an institution similar to the English poorhouse) sheltered beggars, orphans, vagabonds, prostitutes, and thieves alongside the sick and mad. The Hôtel Dieu in Paris was more specifically designed as a healing institution, but this was administered by religious orders, with the medical staff merely making occasional visits. The medical profession sought hospital reform, in particular the medicalisation of the hospital. When Louis XVI invited the Académie des Sciences to explore hospital reform, Jacques Tenon (1724–1816) was sent to visit England. Impressed with the Royal

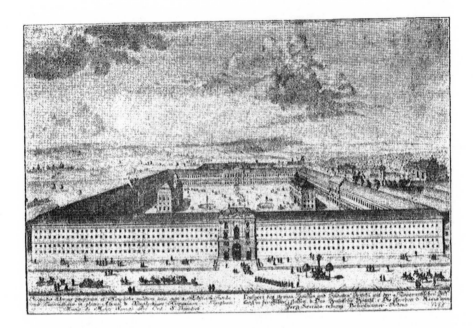

Fig. 61. Allgemeines Krankenhaus, Vienna. This print gives some idea of the scale of the new eighteenth-century medical institutions. (The Wellcome Institute Library, London. M8519.)

Naval Hospital in Plymouth, and the through-ventilation permitted by its pavilion style, he returned to Paris with noble plans of new buildings. But the Revolution distrusted hospitals, seeing them as agents of religious indoctrination, and no serious hospital programme was begun in France until after 1815. Innovations occurred elsewhere.

The most notable continental hospital was Vienna's Allgemeines Krankenhaus (general hospital), rebuilt by Joseph II in 1784, a perfect expression of the Enlightenment absolutists' drive towards administrative centralisation. In traditional manner, the Vienna hospital sheltered the poor as well as providing medical facilities for the sick. Planned for 1600 patients, it was divided into six medical, four surgical, and four clinical sections, and 86 clinical beds met teaching needs. Serving Joseph II's grand design, provincial hospitals were also built in Prague (1789), Olmütz (1787), and Linz (1788). Comparable institutions were set up in other German states, including the Juliusspital at Würzburg (1789), which had a well-planned operating theatre. Berlin's Charité Hospital was built in 1768, and in St. Petersburg Catherine the Great (1762–96) erected the huge Obuchov Hospital.

Georgian England witnessed a rapid expansion of hospital building. In London only St Thomas's Hospital, St. Bartholomew's Hospital and Bethlem Hospital (popularly called Bedlam – for long England's only madhouse) had survived the Reformation. By European standards, England in 1700 was exceptionally ill-endowed with hospitals or plague-houses, or with sister institutions like orphanages. Enlightened philanthropy, both secular and religious, raised new foundations. English provincial hospitals were typically meant for the poor (though not for Poor Law paupers), who would receive care without charge, thus, it was hoped, confirming ties of deference, paternalism, and gratitude. London benefited earliest. To the metropolis' two ancient hospitals, a further five were added between 1720 and 1750 – the Westminster (1720), Guy's (1724), St. George's (1733), the London (1740) and the Middlesex (1745). These were all general hospitals. They spurred similar institutions in the provinces, where no genuinely medical hospitals had previously existed at all. The Edinburgh Royal Infirmary was set up in 1729, followed by Winchester and Bristol (1737), York (1740), Exeter (1741), Bath (1742), Northampton (1743) and some 20 others. By 1800 all sizeable English towns had a hospital.

Augmenting these general foundations, Georgian philanthropy also pumped money into specialist institutions for the sick. St Luke's Hospital was opened in London in 1751, the only big public lunatic asylum in the kingdom apart from Bethlem. Unlike Bethlem, extensively criticised for its barbarity, St. Luke's was launched to an optimistic fanfare, its physician, William Battie (1703–76), asserting that, if treated with humanity, lunacy was no less curable than any other disease. By 1800, other great towns like Manchester, Liverpool, and York had public lunatic asylums, philanthropically supported. As well as lunatics, sufferers from venereal disease also became objects for charity, indicating the replacement of the religious judgment that such diseases were salutary punishment for vice by the Enlightenment view that humanity demanded relief of suffering. London's Lock Hospital for venereal cases opened in 1746. It was paralleled by another new charitable foundation, the Magdalene Hospital for Penitent Prostitutes (1759) – less a medical hospital than a refuge where prostitutes wishing to 'go straight' could learn a trade.

Another new institution was the lying-in hospital. In London, the earliest of these maternity hospitals were the British (1749), the City

(1750), the General (1752), and the Westminster (1765). Maternity hospitals met major needs, not least guaranteeing a few days' bed-rest to poor women. They also enabled unmarried mothers, mainly servant girls, to deliver their bastards with no questions asked. Many of these babies then ended up in the Foundling Hospital, opened in 1741 as London's first orphanage. Unwanted children could be deposited there anonymously; they would be educated and taught a trade. The benevolent designs of lying-in hospitals were thwarted by the appalling maternal death-rates from puerperal fever.

Hospitals provided treatment, food, bed-rest, and convalescence. By 1800, London's hospitals alone were handling over 20,000 patients a year. But they restricted themselves to minor complaints that would respond to treatment, excluded infectious cases (no one wanted fevers raging uncontrollably through the hospital), and in any case, could treat only a fraction of the sick. Hence it became important to augment hospital facilities. One device was the fever hospital, designed only for infectious cases. London's fever hospital (tactfully known as the House of Recovery) was opened in 1801. Another new instrument of healing was the outpatient department.

Similar developments occurred in the North American colonies. The first general hospital was founded in Philadelphia in 1751. The Pennsylvania General Hospital received a grant of £2000 from the Pennsylvania Assembly to match private subscriptions. The New York Hospital was established some 20 years later; the Massachusetts General Hospital was founded in 1811. All such hospitals catered for the sick poor.

Alongside hospitals, other medical institutions were opened. The first London dispensary was set up in 1773. By 1800, sixteen dispensaries existed, treating up to 50,000 cases a year, and many in the provinces besides. Dispensaries provided outpatient services, supplying advice and free medicine to the sick poor whose complaints were unsuitable for hospitalisation. The dispensary system involved domiciliary visits by physicians into the homes of the poor. This firsthand experience of how the other half lived fired the reforming zeal of progressive doctors for improved housing, better sanitation, and popular health education.

Also in England, the Humane Society (1773) aimed to heighten awareness of industrial hazards through teaching life-saving techniques. With ports, rivers, and canals central to economic expansion, many fell victim to the hazards of water (the proverbially suicidal English were said to make a habit of throwing themselves off bridges). Other societies were set up to provide free surgical appliances to labourers suffering from hernia. Initiatives like these changed the British medical landscape. The voluntary hospital movement did not amount to the comprehensive, state-funded medical system that far-sighted seventeenth-century Puritans had envisaged (that had to wait until 1948). Neither did it spark any major breakthroughs in medical science or therapeutic powers. Such foundations did, however, signal a new recognition that the people's health was the concern of society and even the state.

They also testify to the complex relations between laity and medical profession regarding medical provision. Piety and humanity demanded compassion for the sick; utility taught that neglect of disease ran counter to enlightened self-interest, for epidemics spread from the indigent to the affluent, and sick and disabled labourers made inefficient employees. Hence it is not surprising that initiatives generally sprang from people other than physicians. Thomas Guy (1645–1724), whose wealth set up Guy's hospital, was a London printer; Thomas Coram (1668–1751), inspirer of the foundling hospital, was an old sea-dog; Alured Clarke (1696–1742), who laid the blueprints for many provincial voluntary hospitals, was a cleric. Subscriptions generally came from nobles, gentlemen, and civic worthies; and the management of these hospitals largely remained in lay hands with physicians taking a back seat.

Of course, the hospital movement greatly benefited the medical profession. Every hospital had honorary appointments for physicians and surgeons, who would give their services free as an act of public liberality. The honour accruing from hospital appointments proved career 'leg-ups' for aspiring practitioners, who could expect to hobnob with the governors, gaining powerful patrons and prosperous patients. Hospital appointments, especially in London, could prove more directly lucrative – hospital staff, especially surgeons, took apprentices who would walk the wards and learn the craft while acting as an assistant. Thus hospital expansion gave rise to hospital teaching, and institutions largely set up by the laity gradually served to advance the medical profession.

Conclusion: disease, medicine, and society

By 1800, Europe and its overseas colonies were on the brink of momentous change – industrialisation. Already, population was beginning its inexorable rise, especially on the Atlantic seaboards. And, first in Britain but soon in France, the Low Countries, and the Atlantic states of America, urban growth, commercial expansion, technological innovation, and vast growth in manufactures were to transform civilization. There is no change that medicine had wrought that indubitably helped launch industrial society or eased its birth-pangs. The rapid rise in population indispensable to urbanisation and industrialisation was nowhere due to any significant decline in the death rate, but rather rising birth rates. And most historical demographers believe that rising birth rates were chiefly the result of social changes like earlier marriage, a more permissive sexual climate, and the greater economic earnings-power of children, and owed little to medical factors, however broadly construed. It is far from clear that population rise even went with improved standards of nutrition. Research on Central Europe suggest that industrialisation was attended with worsening standards of living, nutrition, and health, though studies of working class height (a fairly reliable proxy for health) suggests things may slowly have improved in Britain between 1750 and 1840.

The health profile of the West around 1800 defies easy generalisation. A few unambiguous changes had occurred. For instance, after four centuries of terror, bubonic plague had finally receded from Western Europe. But the picture generally remains complex and opaque. Large questions loom regarding social change, the empire of disease and medicine's capacity to resist death and relieve sickness – questions easier to pose than resolve. At least till 1760, epidemic and crisis mortality remained high on the continent of Europe, associated with severe winter famines. Health and medical measures were having no more than marginal effects in tipping the demographic balance. Administrative measures can take a certain credit for the elimination of plague. On the other hand, unregulated urban growth, particularly the rise of industrial pollution, slums and overcrowding, and swifter communications and trade-links spread air- and water-borne filth diseases like typhoid, and urban maladies like tuberculosis and rickets. These were later to grow into appalling urban threats, in turn requiring public health responses on a hitherto unparalleled scale in the nineteenth century.

The Enlightenment brought transformations in perceptions of population and hence of healthiness. It opened with mercantilist fears of depopulation – it was the job of the monarch to take political and public health measures to boost populousness. Such views were widely

473

reiterated. The century ended, however, at least in Britain, with this picture being reversed. In his *Essay on ... Population* (1798), Thomas Malthus (1766–1834) prophesied runaway population growth leading to wars, plague, famine, vice, and social catastrophe. Malthus was right, in part at least. By 1800, Europe was beginning a population explosion. Malthus was also right to attribute this demographic new regime to rises in the birth rate not the death rate. With the possible exception of smallpox inoculation, Enlightenment medicine did little to keep people alive that would have weighed heavily in the demographic balance. Newly-rampant disorders like tuberculosis, rickets, diphtheria, and the 'filth diseases' counterbalanced the benefits of the disappearance of plague and the containment of smallpox. Though the eighteenth century campaigned against disease, such crusades had small aggregate results, though fortunate individuals and families benefited.

Globally, the eighteenth century was an unmitigated health disaster. For the accelerating pace of overseas exploration and discovery, and the internationalisation of capitalism and warfare turned localised diseases into universal ones. The slave trade spread Old World diseases to the New World, while tropical diseases like yellow fever were transported across oceans. The opening up of the North American heartland and the infiltration of the Pacific resulted in European diseases like smallpox, measles, and syphilis decimating populations that had no experience of, and hence no resistance to, such disorders. The effects were cruel and cataclysmic – germs did more than guns to spread European imperialism. Soon cholera, for thousands of years confined to Asia, would be exported throughout the globe.

Within Europe, disease left existence precarious. Medical interventions had some effect in individual cases, though unpredictably. Aged 50, the wealthy and worldly-wise Edward Gibbon complacently looked forward to a further 20 years of life, but he was dead within four of a hydrocele (a swollen testicle) – or, more probably, as a result of sepsis following surgery. His contemporary, the quack James Graham, claimed to be able to prolong life to 150 years. He died at 49. Medicine did little to improve longevity.

Medicine perhaps contributed to a new confidence in an individuals's capacity to master the environment, society, and his own circumstances. Medicine was increasingly complementing religion as the source of meanings of existence. More people were being born in the presence of a medical attendant, the new man-midwife. More were dying with the ministrations of a physician rather than a priest, gliding perhaps into a peaceful death thanks to opiate cocktails. Commentators like Ivan Illich (b. 1926) have criticised the Enlightenment for speeding the 'medicalisation of life' and the 'medicalisation of death'. Though endlessly satirised, medicine was gaining cultural presence. Medicine was well represented in continental and American academies, for example, the American Philosophical Society, the Berlin Academy of Science, the Academy of Sciences in Paris, the Royal Society of Göttingen, or academies in such places as St. Petersburg, Madrid, Uppsala, Bordeaux, and Haarlem. Doctors were also important in intellectual gatherings like the Lunar Society of Birmingham and the Manchester Literary and Philosophical Society.

Enlightenment thinkers, seeking to understand and change society, looked to science for their model. Science was seen as a matchless engine of analysis – objective, critical, progressive. Natural order promised models of social order, in particular (for many philosophes) a vision of free individual activity in systems governed by natural law. If humanists were looking to science, medical men were, as it were, returning the gaze, and looking out at society. The scientific spirit encouraged medicine beyond individual cases in search of the laws of health and sickness in wider contexts, examining climate, environment, and epidemic rhythm over the centuries. The Enlightenment was marked by energetic medical environmentalism. Certain eighteenth-century physicians developed an enlarged social awareness, confronting the interplay of sickness, medicine, and society. What determined the patterns and pathways of community illness? Why did sickness vary from society to society, from region to region, from group to group? Confronting such wider variables, many physicians felt driven to be more than bedside healers – they had to become anatomists and doctors of society itself. These questions were asked more insistently in the Enlightenment than ever before. The eighteenth century witnessed certain advances in medicine, but it also transformed perceptions of medicine's place in society.

8   Conclusion

MICHAEL NEVE

No idea of tradition, let alone an idea of the 'Western medical tradition' can be coherent without making certain assumptions. One of them is that this proposed tradition is visible, or comprehensible, through the examination of the historical record, and through other texts that guide the reader through that record – these other texts being the work of historians. As with certain ideas of literary tradition, the use of the concept of greatness may, in some versions of the tradition in question, be invoked. Indeed, as suggested in the introduction, current writers of medical papers often appeal to this idea of greatness, thereby misconstruing the historical record and producing a series of historical icons instead of a historical context. The appeal is made to what currently passes for orthodoxy, marginalising other parts of the historical story.

Another similar assumption may be present (indeed almost always is) that is equally important. This is, that the tradition in question has a kind of a backbone, a backbone that is the product of evolution and a backbone that is the mark of progress. One way of thinking of what this backbone may look like is to trace the history of influence, the influence of ancestors for example, in the historical record. These ancestors can be imagined as founding fathers whose work still counts, or as past masters whose work has been acknowledged as great and then improved on, even overthrown. But especially in the history of medicine, conceived as an account of mankind's struggle with disease and with death, the possibility that the historical record is not just a story of progress is hard to accept. And the related possibility, that there has been a successful struggle within human history against disease and death, but that medicine's part in that struggle has been marginal, may be equally hard to come to terms with. The historian's task, once these possibilities have been included, becomes complicated; the idea of progress can seem more a fantasy than reality, and the backbone of tradition begins to disappear. 'Progress' begins to look too simple a story, attractive for that reason but needing to be examined with scepticism, with a sense of historical flexibility rather than iron law.

The Western medical tradition, as an idea, speaks not only of the history of learning, of the history of natural enquiry and more recently, the advances of a medicine that employs scientific procedures. It also assumes a comprehensible story about the *making* of that tradition, the long journey from fake remedies to technical understanding, from magic and superstition to rationality and practical defeats of disease. At its most ambitious, the Western medical tradition turns out to be an account of how a certain trained body of activists, called doctors, or healers, gradually pushed back the frontiers of ignorance in the hope that (at the culmination of the tradition as it were) they would conquer death itself. Few histories, in the human story, involve such urgent issues as those that surround the history of medicine. To call into question a simple idea of progress, to attempt a different history, can sometimes be seen as doubting the purposes and longings of medicine itself, out of an unhappy combination of ignorance and spite.

One way to begin to grasp the nature of Western medicine and the history that it is made from is to remember just how different the world of modern medicine, with its organised profession, its hospitals, its technical know-how, indeed its sheer size, is from any conceivable earlier world, from the classical era to the end of the Enlightenment. It is this pre-modern world, its municipal organisations, its hospitals, its charities, its monasteries, its universities, and its many varieties of medical practitioner that have been covered in this volume. All kinds of assumptions, about who practised medicine, and where; about the qualifications required; about the number of human individuals who would automatically assume that their health was something a doctor should be consulted over; all these assumptions have to be put to one side. To enter the historical arena is to enter a world where we see what we assume has always been present actually being manufactured, being created in political circumstances, in educational contexts, even in the marketplace, where we may think doctors, in the modern sense, are out of place. The importance of this part of the story is that it allows the reader to imagine that the history of the Western medical tradition is in fact an account of the doctor's rise to social power and social prominence in ways that are not simply explained by the successful therapeutic outcomes of a doctor's knowledge. Medicine, to put it simply, is not necessarily the historical possession of the doctor. The story of the Western tradition may indeed be the story of how this came to be achieved, how this argument was won and, in that sense, it may be partly the story of the subordination of the lay community and the marginalisation of the patient.

In not a few previous histories of the Western medical tradition, that is indeed the forgotten part of the story. We travel, thankfully as it were, from the suspect world of folk-mythology, numerology, priests, shamans, and the 'evil eye', to the world of learning, of honesty, and of heroic, and often unpaid, labour. Furthermore, this merciful release from the fake past is achieved because doctors come to understand, not just funny talk about herbal remedies from village ladies, but the independent existence of diseases themselves. The doctor will be different, in the Western tradition, because he will be looking *through* the ill person to the disease that is causing the illness. The trained doctor will have a form of contact, not with individuals, but with the diseases that use these individuals as media. The celebrated medical historian Owsei Temkin has written on the tradition of medical science which emphasises the independence of diseases as an 'ontological' one. The alternative, where the individual's own circumstances are as important, for example in the work of Hippocrates and his followers, Temkin calls the 'physiological' tradition. It would not be fruitless to see the advantages and disadvantages of these two ways of thinking about disease as appearing and reappearing throughout the history of Western medical practice. Physicians attempt to relate individuals to independent disease entities, while at different times, ontological thinking predominates in medical theory and practice, especially in the era of modern clinical medical work, starting in the Enlightenment. This contradiction is an important one in the development of Western medicine.

It may follow from this that one aspect of the doctor's education is to propose that, should the patient have particular views on the nature of his or her illness, such views in fact constitute a feature of the patient's disease. Part of the progressive ambition of the history of Western medicine, some of its backbone, will be the attempt to see off various 'backward' forms of thinking, recasting them as the language of a pre-scientific world of magic and superstition. This will be as true in Christian Europe, with its apparent privileging of the ill person, as in classical or secular Europe.

Anthropological writers have provided the evidence that suggests that all human cultures, Western and non-Western, ancient and modern, display certain beliefs about bodies, food, and the environment, that pre-date the successful development in Western medicine of the so-called biomedical model, the model that proposes that explanations of disease and of illness can be explained by materialist biology as the true order of reality, the reality that underlies everything else. Before the rise to power of this model, in the period from roughly 1700, the cultures of the world, including the West, display what might be rather grandly called 'transactional' medical systems of belief. Bodies, for example, are healthy if they balance the elements at work within them, if they can inhabit the right harmony between diet, environment and supernatural agency and the internal influences, for example, humours, at work within bodies. The external and the internal, if balanced, produce health. Disease is imbalance, and needs to be harmonised out of existence by the removal of excess (by bleeding or purging, say) or by the replacing of a deficiency (by special diets). At the origins of the Western medical tradition, in the work of the Hippocratics, humoral theory played as central a part as it did in the medicine of ancient China and India, based on the idea that health was a balance between the internal humours and the external environment, not least as it changed through the seasons. The emphasis on diet was especially stressed, with divisions between food and non-food, or some foods that were sacred, others profane, being culturally widespread. In discussions of mental illness, the power of supernatural forces, the actions of the gods, or the activities of witches and of witchcraft were widely agreed to be causal agents. But the essential point is that interactionist, processional ebbs and flows constitute the pre-biomedical idea, and that part of the history of Western medicine is the journey away from this world, one that earlier had been shared with non-European cultures.

It would be quite wrong and even insulting however to assume that the history of, say, Arabic medicine, and the history of medicine under Islam, were merely footnotes to a mainstream Western tradition that had its mythical roots in Hippocrates and Galen. As with the rise of Islamic science from the middle of the eighth century, the growth of Arabic medicine derives from a rich and varied heritage which it would be a caricature to incorporate into an idea of the Western medical tradition as if it were a footnote to Western ideas of medical classicism. This fact also makes it difficult to portray the rise of Islam as simply part of an inexorable move from interactional models of sickness to scientific understanding of actual disease entities. The rise of Islam does see the policing of certain animistic beliefs, but not the banning of practical therapies, some of which may have had their historical roots within such earlier belief systems. Throughout the centuries, as discussed in the preceding chapters, religion and medicine display complicated relationships, sometimes appearing inseparable, sometimes coexisting in their separate spheres. The rise of Christianity, as we have seen, does not lead to the overthrow of Galenism. Indeed, an emphasis on the divine creator helped to strengthen Galenism against alternatives. In the middle of the eighteenth-century Enlightenment and its secular hopes, ordinary sufferers might well go on believing in witchcraft and folk remedies. The medicalisation of life, as an Enlightenment task, was as much an agenda as an actuality, meeting resistance in ordinary life. Despite these external facts, the particular goals made within the profession of medicine in the West, from Galen onwards, can still be usefully seen as the task of replacing individual stories with a scientifically understood, physico-chemical, and properly classified diseased world. Medicine's past can be characterised as an age when such a diseased world was not understood or properly mapped.

All social systems of healing may thus share certain characteristics – categories for diagnosing illness, or socially derived metaphors that improve the modelling of pathological states, or various competing groups of healers from the folk, or popular, or professional sectors. What makes the Western medical tradition different is the prolonged move away from an explanatory world that was also shared with other social systems to one that attempted to do away with such religious or folk dimensions. But as we have seen, this story took up centuries of time, and may not even have been achieved by the end of the eighteenth century. But a commitment to explaining illness by invoking diseases that have an independent natural existence is a hallmark of the idea of medical progress.

Other areas of 'reality' (the psychological, the social, and the moral) become cover stories, that hide the bedrock of natural truth. The medical practitioner, freed from the need for an individual patient's version of their story to be seen as part of their history, looks through the patient to the disease. Illness as an experience becomes replaced, or pushed to one side, as the trained doctor tracks the authentic but hidden world of disease as biological pathology. The disease entity, the object of attention, splits from the experience of suffering with which it had once been linked, not least in humoral theory. Importantly, this

split may be accompanied by a marked increase in professional responsibility, at least theoretically, with a move away from the charismatic
emphases in folk medicine and a corresponding de-mystification of the
previous languages of what will now be called superstition.

Medicine and its claims to see through to the disease embody the
progressive ideal of the Western medical tradition. Forms of non-
Western medicine – acupuncture, or herbal remedies – become relegated as do Western medical practices that do not fully enjoy the
organic, therapeutic interventions of mainstream medicine – psychiatry, chiropraxy, sexual therapy. Medicine has, in that sense, departed
from the population and community-based public health orientations
that constituted the explanatory systems of early man. The backbone of
progress that makes up one version of the Western medical tradition is
formed out of the possibility of the successful application of biomedicine
and its technology.

As the chapters in this book show, and show quite often with that
important historical aid a sense of humour, the idea of a backbone of
progress must not be allowed to oversimplify the historical story.
Tracing the long journey from the Greeks to the late Middle Ages for
example, the reader's attention is drawn to a number of historical
lessons. Firstly, that part of the Western medical tradition may itself be
the invention of doctors evoking other doctors. Greek-born but active in
Rome in the second century AD, the physician Galen may among other
things be thought of as the inventor of the historical figure we think of
as Hippocrates. Famously prolix, self-aggrandising, dismissive of quacks
and even partners, and emphasising the ability to make a prognosis as
the true sign of the able doctor, Galen was also a historian, bringing
Hippocrates to life, partly to enable himself to be seen as his legitimate
successor. Uncovering some of Galen's medical politics does not detract
from his philosophical and practical genius, nor does it disfigure the
nature of his enormous historical influence. The history of medicine
can easily accommodate both aspects.

Such a medical history illustrates how traditions are made up, in this
case with the doctor acting as a historian of himself. It also indicates, as
historians of science have recently done, that certain stresses on conflict or disagreement in medicine can be historical exaggerations. That
disease is spread by *either* contagion or miasma would not have been
the choice for a medieval Galenist. The two explanations were often not
separated. The same holds in searching for explanations of illness that

might be religious or natural. Once again the two would mix. Even with the arrival of Christianity, the historical notion that this would see the disappearance of partly natural explanations of disease is false. Sometimes the humours were responsible, sometimes sin. As we have seen, the sixteenth century in Europe saw bitter contests between Galenists and Paracelsians, contests that were certainly about agencies of disease and about therapies. Even more importantly however they were quarrels about social authority, about medical elitism, about institutions and their relevance. The importance of institutional life and circumstances, as directly affecting developments in medical practice and medical theory, has been stressed throughout this volume. These would include armies, monasteries, universities and just as important, the appearance in thirteenth-century Northern Italy of doctors working on behalf of magistrates and civic authorities. The politics of the profession of medicine is historically linked to the presence (or indeed absence) of governing institutions. The commitment to Galenism in the late medieval period received an institutional setting in universities and hospitals, which in turn permitted the historical creation of a new figure, the graduate physician. By providing an institutional context and a social history, historians can for example examine plague in Europe in 1348 and speak properly of the power of sheer terror as reaction to such an event, and insist nonetheless on historical differences between plague and modern epidemics such as AIDS. The historian comes to stress the local history of actions taken, in individual cities and towns in the attempt to deal with plague. Even something as apparently simple and fatal as the Black Death has a complex social history.

Another danger of an over-simplified model of progress in the Western tradition would be to ascribe revolutionary breakthroughs to historical figures who might actually have regarded their actions as homages to past authority. The most famous case in the period covered by this book is perhaps William Harvey, publishing on the circulation of the blood in 1628. Placing this achievement in a much broader historical context, a strong case is made for Harvey's practical skills (that one can actually see for oneself, and draw real conclusions) and for his completing a task, not as a revolutionary in anything like the modern sense, but as a firm follower of Aristotle, whose remarkable influence in the medieval and post-medieval periods has been traced with care. In a historical story full of endless divisions between medical theory and practice, where diagnoses based on reports or specimens from unvisited individuals were common, this account of Harvey combines the theoretical and the practical, while reminding the reader that what later generations see as innovatory, contemporaries may have seen as confirming the authority of the distant past.

The making of a tradition then, and the slow growth of biomedical explanations of disease and sickness, is not to be oversimplified. The history of midwifery for example, or the relationship between religious beliefs and medical explanations help us to see this.

Disease and the environment

The question that nonetheless has to be asked is: what is the evidence for the *progressive* history of the biomedical model? Have the historians of medicine been persuaded by the progressive history which argues that the history of medical relief has gone from a time that saw most human beings believe that illness was caused by things, or other people, or, sometimes, spirits or departed souls, to a time when the beliefs of such human beings were circumvented by the medical practitioner? Does the practitioner see through all such subjective beliefs, to an esoteric knowledge about natural causes? Does the orthodox history of medicine play no part in questioning the progressive account that medicine then chooses to give to itself?

One famous and well-documented history has proposed that when examined from a demographic point of view, and from a historical perspective that examines the geography of diseases and their periodicities, medicine's part in the prolongation of human life is slight. In this work, the idea of diseases as objects of scientific understanding is left to one side. Instead, human cultural evolution is examined alongside the main parameters of such an evolution: social structure, food supplies, economic organisation, and patterns of social hierarchy. Placing particular emphasis on the importance of nutrition, and the effects of nutrition on human health, this demographic analysis attempts to keep alive an influential tradition in the history of medical history, one that accepts the connection, not between medicine and health, but between social status, social position, social experience, and health. Medical demography, partly by employing the medical statistics that were developed from the eighteenth century onwards, stresses the causal connection between health and class, and between health, water and food. Much of the controversy in medical historiography in the West, during the twentieth century, has been to do with the political claims, made in a decidedly socialist, often Marxist, historiography, of the causal connection between health and poverty. For some observers, the absence of such a committed historiography helps to explain the absence of a persuasive, or accurate, social history of medicine.

Employing rather ambitious models of social evolution – from hunter-gatherer cultures through to industrialisation – a history of medicine based on demographic evidence, rather than one persuaded by the progressive claims of biomedicine described earlier, has proposed the following. Disease is not a fact of life, nor is it a group of conditions that are easily brought under control by the activities of doctors. Instead, patterns of human cultural practice – forms of economic activity, migration, warfare, and not least ideas on what constitutes a proper trade with other countries – all help to provide what might be called a natural history of disease, a history that deliberately chooses not to concentrate on the claims of the progressive record. In this historical work, removed from the heroic ideas and images of other medical histories, public health is the issue; public health conceived as a relationship between human beings and their social environment, rather than a relationship between human beings and their doctors.

The story might go something like this. Hunter-gatherer societies had small populations, mobile, and without experts, especially 'medical' experts. Concern over health, in these groups, would play a relatively small role, in the face of other concerns, and the general shortness of life would be due to food deficiency. Early human groups did not suffer from smallpox, yellow fever, typhoid, measles, polio, let alone hypertension, obesity, or coronary heart disease. With the arrival of settled, agricultural society, the historical record suggests an increase in the size of the general population, with competing social groups, and an increase as well in the sedentary nature of much economic activity. An increase in trade between these settled groups led to an increase in epidemics partly due to the growth of irrigation and an increase in the prevalence of faecal–oral transmission. So, at the agricultural stage, as it were, infectious diseases become the predominant causes of sickness and death, both *within* agricultural societies and between them. In no serious sense does the existence of a medical corps of practitioners effect these social fundamentals. In terms of the overall incidence of mortality, not least in early life, the medical presence counts for little in the face of social forces and economic practice, with their accompanying disease outcomes.

In a third stage of social evolution (or historical change), urbanisation and then industrialisation, historical demography has proposed that human beings create conditions of life far removed from those in which they initially evolved, and that this stage sees an increase in the destructive effects, not of infectious diseases (although these by no means disappear) but of non-communicable disease, sometimes called diseases of civilisation. Cardiovascular disease, cancer, diseases of degeneration, become, within industrialised societies, more prevalent than in the agricultural stage. The increase, at the same time, of the industry of medicine, and medical research (not least for possible cures for cancer) does not, in this version of the story, make a huge difference. Rather, as an irony, an infectious disease, such as smallpox, is conquered at the very time that non-communicable diseases defy scientific medicine, and become matters of public health in the old-fashioned sense. The plagues of earlier periods disappear, not for medical but for socio-historical reasons. This irony is overseen, as it were, in the industrial world, by a now highly organised medical profession, facing the incidence of non-communicable disease.

The usefulness of the demographic perspective in the history of medicine and its Western tradition is nowhere better served than in discussions of Western imperialism and its ecological outcome; that is to say, the diseases that Europeans exported to ecological worlds that were not unlike Europe but which had known little of European disease. The historian A.W. Crosby has shown in his book *Ecological Imperialism* (1986) that in most temperate zones of the world (what he calls 'neo-Europes') the bulk of the population in the modern age are people of European descent. In migrating to these ecologically attractive places, the Europeans took with them not just firearms, but their common diseases – smallpox, whooping cough, measles, TB, mumps, gonorrhoea – and these granted the Europeans a way of visiting death on the indigenous inhabitants of the Americas and Australasia. Without any prior immunity (as might also be said of their experience of alcohol), native populations were decimated. Diseases played an evolutionary part in the history of human migration, not simply because diseases themselves might be thought to evolve, but because medicine had not seen their elimination, and they went on to play their part in the occupation of appropriate ecological worlds at the expense of native populations. And the important point is that these sudden depopulations in areas of contact did not occur just through viral or bacterial assault. This assault was made manifest through social collapse, through an increase in infertility, through – once again – the social and political structure. The biological expansion of Europe therefore occurred at the same time as the biomedical model of disease, in the Western tradition, was most (theoretically) prominent. Once again, the demographic story, linked in this case with colonialism, suggests the limits to medicine's achievement, and the merits of the natural history/anthropological model in the discussion of the history and geography of diseases.

Doctors, patients and medical history

The wide-ranging character of the demographic and anthropological accounts of medicine and its history provide useful insights, from a very broad perspective. These insights are less obvious if the historian is anxious about the details of medical practice and the scientific developments within medicine itself. Many of the chapters in this book provide these details and the advances made in medicine up to 1800. But the anthropological perspective stresses that the increase in medical commitment to the biomedical model, with diseases as alien entities attacking the body from the outside, and then seen off by the trained doctor, fundamentally altered previous historical ideas of what illness was. From the Elizabethan age to the mid-nineteenth century, illness and suffering were events that occurred *within* the life of the sufferer, and gave reasons to suppose that the personal story (self and environment) or the personal relationship to Fate or to Providence, was badly arranged, and that the patient had to learn from this and not necessarily learn what it meant from a doctor. Your life in your hands. It is of considerable importance to remember that in many of life's *rites de passage* and duels, not least birth and death, physicians may have been rarely present until at least the end of the seventeenth century. The anthropological account of medical history reminds the student not merely of medicine's weakness in the face of infectious disease and a large number of surgical mishaps, but of the relative absence of doctors from what might now be seen as events in life that doctors have understood and made their own. Not merely does the history of medical advance seem less of a progressive surge, more of an ebb and flow. So too is the varying amount of medical interest in the experience of sufferers themselves. Under some extreme versions of the biomedical model of disease and illness – the extreme versions of the ontological approach mentioned earlier – the patient can bring no real news from the land of suffering, only haphazard misreporting that has to be decoded and explained away. It may be, again ironically, that patient power has been strongest when the commercial element in the doctor/patient relationship has also been strongest – a good example here is the English experience of the eighteenth century, an age when the patient answered back, or even ministered to himself or herself.

It is a notable feature of previous histories of medicine, designed for students and the lay public, that the bulk of the evidence for medicine's advances appears in three historical epochs. There is, initially, a foundation stone laid down in the classical era, with the Hippocratics receiving their reward from Galen (and maybe even being partly historically invented by him) and with high regard being placed on the philosophical and natural – the historical work of Aristotle. There then follow long periods of blankness, before the anatomical renaissance of the period 1500–1700, and various individual achievements in the description of bodily function (the circulation of the blood, the physiology of respiration and digestion and so on). From the late eighteenth century onwards, with the establishing of reformed medical education, the arrival of the germ theory of disease, of bacteriology, of radiology, and the rise of the clinical laboratory, the story becomes more heartening – the Western medical tradition alters its historical form, and becomes recognisable to the modern mind: scientific, technical, and professional. Much of the history of the preceding period can again be forgotten: it was as an age of agony, of quackery, of ignorance. Of course, there were heroes, fighting back against charlatans and against folly, but the nineteenth century sees medicine in the West (in this account) leaving behind another Dark Age.

The chapters in this book have examined the history of this 'pre-scientific' era. They suggest that in the period 1650–1800, it would not be necessary to hold a cynical view of the medical profession to propose that medicine's achievements were limited, and not just because of ignorance or malpractice. When the plague disappears in the late seventeenth century from Britain, it was probably to do with the political decisions made over quarantine. There can be little doubt that human populations developed immunity – to certain fevers for example – and not because medical breakthroughs had taken place. Remarkable achievements, notably vaccination against smallpox, stood out on their own, rather than being part of a general story. The history of medicine until modern times has been at least as much the story of knowing what cannot be done (not least in surgery) as of what can be done. The partial destruction of infectious diseases by antibiotics, first developed in the 1940s, leaving aside the difficulties of employing such drugs against destructive viruses rather than bacteria, should not require a heroic history of the past to heighten current achievements. The best histories of epidemics show this conclusively. Likewise, responsible histories of public health movements, or the hospital, or the history of fighting against cholera or tuberculosis, all have as strong a sense of defeat as of victory. Cholera and tuberculosis – and even bubonic plague – are as likely to reappear, perhaps even in strengthened forms in the late twentieth century, as to disappear. The late twentieth century is certainly witnessing the evolution of drug resistant bacteria, with obvious implications for bacteriology and health policy, not least because of the relationship between the spread of such bacteria and the scale and rapidity of international travel. The remarkable breakthroughs of the biomedicine of the twentieth century do not need histories that conceal the distresses, the failures, and the courage, of past doctors and past patients. The face of the medicine, and the suffering, of the Western past may well be the face of scepticism combined with knowledge, not the face of certainty combined with victory. Employing both demographic and anthropological models of Western medicine can assist in generating a more accurate account than the progressive clichés of some medical history.

One great advantage, from a historical point of view, in toning down medicine's language of (recent) triumph is that the shadowlands of fringe practice, or of medical techniques that elite physicians found improper but which continued to find a market, can be properly examined. Take quackery. Recent accounts of quackery, of how quackery was made into something it was not appropriate to endorse, have managed to rescue the subject from cliché by showing that in an age of commercial medicine and with all kinds of practitioners peddling their wares, quacks had their place. Indeed, quacks and formally qualified practitioners, in the early modern world were similar in the use of advertisement, in therapeutic methods, and, perhaps most surprisingly, in a shared sense of conservatism in public life. Not until the nineteenth century was this a conflict between professionals and disreputable outcasts – in the pre-Victorian world, medical men were entrepreneurs, and the public could pick and choose. It is in the historically specific context of Victorian medical specialisation and professionalisation that 'fringe medicine', be it homeopathy, hydropathy, or hypnotism, fights back, in an organised manner, against a profession now closing its doors partly through the involvement of the state and the ending of the outright *laissez-faire* beliefs of the previous century. And rewriting the history in this way does not, in any necessary sense, detract or make less persuasive the nineteenth-century denunciations of quacks and quack remedies. These attacks could be heartfelt, even accurate, but at last can be seen inside a historical context – the developing of the biomedical model as the true science of modern Western medicine. In such a story, the emergence of the hospital as the headquarters of the qualified practitioner is of great importance, quackery being excluded. Quackery has been rewritten, and its history opened to view, by relating the practice of medicine to the concrete social world where it resides. The story gives additional force to the already existing accounts of the revolution in 'scientific' medicine in the nineteenth and twentieth centuries. And this in turn connects the history of scientific medicine to the financial role of the state and the growth of a health industry on a huge scale, leading in its turn to the appearance of a dependent civilian population – dependent that is on the doctor and the hospital, and perhaps, the state – in ways that form a marked historical contrast with the commercial marketplace of the eighteenth century.

It is the nature of that market and the kinds of medicine that it generated that is one of the concerns of the chapter on Enlightenment medicine. Previous histories of medicine have tended to concentrate on disputes within what comes to be called 'the medical profession' (the most famous of these being debates between physicians and surgeons) without paying quite enough attention to the economic history underlying such disputes. Whether in societies based on slavery, or within feudalism, or monarchical courts, or the liberal commercialism of much eighteenth-century life, doctors had to take their place within the context of social life. In the eighteenth-century example, the commercial relationship between doctor and patient allowed the patient certain claims on the doctor that may not have existed previously. Furthermore, the patient's own ideas as to how to negotiate illness were often as important as the doctor's, and this examination of the historical record allows us glimpses into lay perceptions of illness that are particularly valuable. We can also see how non-medical individuals could involve themselves in the financing and administration of hospitals and medical charities.

The Enlightenment also saw an enormous increase in medical theories and in the aspiration towards an environmentalist and naturalistic medical science. And there were apparently heroic medical advances, for example in the war against smallpox. But the eighteenth century again tells an ironical tale, one that was understood as such by Enlightenment writers and doctors. Firstly and most simply, advances in medical theory did not always mean changes in medical practice. Indeed the scale of this paradox becomes itself a major issue in the medicine of the late Enlightenment. Just as the disappearance of plague and the control of smallpox could be cruelly counterbalanced, as discussed earlier, by Europeans exporting their diseases to North America and the Pacific, and then by the appearance in Europe of new diseases like venereal syphilis, so the medicalisation of the human sciences in the Enlightenment was by no means the same thing as the successful conquest of sickness and disease. For as we have seen, the final paradox in Enlightenment medical thinking was that commercial and urban society might itself turn out to be the chief cause of many forms of sickness, including a renewed emphasis on mental illness and diseases of the nerves. An organised commitment to biomedical and naturalistic models of human nature, the growth of sea bathing and of versions of popular Hippocratic medicine, did not make huge inroads, did not for example bring much change to the death rate in European populations. Enlightenment medical writings stand on the brink of what will come to be called the scientific medical revolution of the nineteenth century, when the pursuit of ontological, biomedical explanations of disease would be advanced in the clinic, the hospital, and the laboratory. But the Enlightenment paradox – where might nature be found in commercial society to allow its healing power to do its work? – set new terms for discussion. Neither a desert nor an oasis, the Enlightenment as discussed in Chapter 7 invented an extended idea of public health and its problems and suggested a social explanation for what might have been seen in some earlier writings as an individual problem.

The healing power of nature

No version of the possible historical claims made by the Western medical tradition can avoid being simplistic, and an explanation of the biomedical project in the terms laid out here is no exception. Other forms of medical project, forms that did not commit themselves to this disease model and to seeing the sufferer as simply a presenting vehicle, have played important roles in the West. The development of certain medical skills – the classical Greek emphasis on prognosis as the chief sign of medical acumen, for example, cannot be entirely explained by biomedical imperatives. Likewise, to seek a connection between biomedicine and its origins with, say, monotheism makes little historical sense in the pre-Christian context, or if crassly employed in the Arab-Islamic context, and is not a causal story that holds good for all periods of Western medicine. The one advantage of concentrating on the development of biomedical arguments is that it does help present one story of Western medicine's development that helps explain the *idea* of progress that has constituted that development. As the medicalisation of culture increased, and as doctors began to appear in places that they had not done so before, medicine can be seen to be approaching an understanding of natural facts, and natural explanations for illness. Even in Christian culture and the moral ideas on illness that Christianity teaches, the naturalistic model, inherited from the ancients, played its part, coming eventually to undermine certain Christian doctrines about disease causation. The powerful mixture of humoral theory, combined with the search for independent diseases that appeared and disappeared in human populations constitutes the historical origin of Western medicine.

This hunt for natural causes and for a natural history of disease is especially evident in the growth of that very recent medical speciality, psychiatry. The history of the agencies thought to be behind what comes to be called mental disease is a kind of miniature history of the Western medical tradition. From the gods, through to the humours, to social misfortune, to nerves and (in recent views) to the brain and to genes, the search for agencies has characterised the history of Western medical views on mental pathology. Yet at the same time, non-biomedical factors – the death of loved ones, or failure in business – have never been entirely removed as causal factors. Psychiatry has been literally divided between the supporters of the organic model and those who doubt that such a model can be found. In its most extreme version, the search for a biomedical psychiatry has been called a medical conspiracy, a professionalised medical research programme that has no chance of realising its goal, and an activity that could as easily be conducted by untrained laymen with moral commitments and moral understanding. Whatever the truths in this debate, the aspirations of psychiatry bring out the more general aspirations of the Western medical tradition. A psychiatry without a disease model based on natural agencies and presenting as mental illness would not appear scientific, or an activity peculiarly appropriate for professional doctors to organise and administer. The remarkable growth of clinical medicine, in the laboratory, the hospital, and the research clinic in the period from around 1850 made this priority for a scientific psychiatry of the greatest importance.

The chapters in this book have given details of the history of the practice of medicine, and the extraordinary number of individuals – from herb-gatherers to barber-surgeons – involved. One important story, treated in part here, is the place of women, apparently excluded at various points in the history of the medical West from any part in the idea of a profession of medicine. This historical discrimination has been of fundamental importance, accompanied by various kinds of rationale and explanation. But once again the story is both evidence of discrimination and yet not quite so simple.

Appearances have also been made by some of the most important actors in the medical drama whom it is easy to forget when concentrating on the human story – rats, fleas, lice, and mosquitoes.

At the heart (not, until fairly late on, its most revered organ), the Western medical tradition contains all kinds of contradictions. Doctors, who nowadays can seem to come from the future, have histories where they look like slaves, or wanderers, or craftsmen, or individuals who read some academic medicine and then go on to read something else – like divinity. From the classical age to the nineteenth century, Western medicine seeks out an enterprise that contained the idea of medicine's endless future, the future that will be the act of closing in on the hidden world of disease. In modern times, this has, in turn, produced its own contradiction – a vast health industry, without any guarantee that public health will improve, or that all citizens of an industrial society will have access to organised health care. This is especially true of the modern United States, and no doubt becoming true of the once totalitarian Soviet Union and its satellites, in whatever idea of the future they will occupy. Because of the scale of this contradiction, the question of medicine's relationship with true public health will never be easy to answer, despite the astonishing achievements in bacteriology and drug therapy.

Michael Neve

At the origins of the Western medical tradition, set out in the Hippocratic writings and endorsed by Galen (like many doctors, and not a few medical historians, a man inhabiting a foreign land) lay the belief in the healing power of nature. Nature, if properly comprehended, and seen as a balancing act between the external and the individualised internal, could heal. She had the power so to do. As the Western tradition comes into the era of modernity and even the world of the future, it still carries its great, and as these chapters hope to have shown, fundamental historical paradox: can the doctor, as the student of the healing power of nature, meet the patient who believes that this makes one responsible for oneself? In the professionally organised, scientific, and often state financed world of medicine from 1800, the oldest questions of the Western tradition will still remain. Can the technical ambition that describes much of the Western medical tradition meet patients who remember (with the mythical founders of that medical tradition) that the healing power of nature is available to all? Does modernity's commitment to scientific, technical and usually ontological disease models, and the means to combat them, indicate a complete break with the historical roots of the tradition that modern practitioners nonetheless refer back to when the occasion suits? The chapters in this book seek to contribute to answering that question.

Bibliography for chapters 1–7

Select bibliography chapter 1

SECONDARY SOURCES

Dean-Jones, L. A. *Women's Bodies in Classical Greek Science*, Oxford, Clarendon Press, 1994.

Edelstein, E. J. and L. *Asclepius*, Baltimore, Johns Hopkins University Press, 1945.

Edelstein, L. *Ancient Medicine*, Baltimore, Johns Hopkins University Press, 1967.

Fraser, P. M. *Ptolemaic Alexandria*, Oxford, Clarendon Press, 1972.

Gotthelf, A. *Aristotle on Nature and Living Things*, Bristol University Press, 1992.

Grmek, M. D. *Diseases in the Ancient Greek World*, Johns Hopkins University Press, Baltimore, 1989.

Hanson, A. E. 'The medical writers' woman', in D. Halperin (ed.), *Before Sexuality*, Princeton University Press, 1990, pp. 309–37.

Harris, C. R. S. *The Heart and the Vascular System in Ancient Greek Medicine*, Oxford, Clarendon Press, 1973.

Langholf, V. *Medical theories in Hippocrates*, Berlin, De Gruyter, 1990.

Lloyd, G. E. R. *Early Greek Science*, London, Chatto, 1982.

Lloyd, G. E. R. *Greek Science after Aristotle*, London, Chatto, 1982.

Lloyd, G. E. R. *The Revolutions of Wisdom*, Berkeley, University of California Press, 1987.

Longrigg, J. N. ' The great plague of Athens', *History of Science*, 18 (1980), 209–25.

Longrigg, J. N. *Greek Rational Medicine*, London, Routledge, 1993.

Majno, G. *The Healing Hand*, Cambridge, Mass., Harvard University Press, 1976.

Nutton, V. *From Democedes to Harvey*, London, Variorum, 1988.

Nutton, V. 'Healers in the medical market place', in A. Wear (ed.), *Medicine in Society*, Cambridge University Press, 1992, pp. 15–59.

Parker, R. *Miasma*, Oxford, Clarendon Press, 1983.

Potter, P. *A Short Handbook of Hippocratic Medicine*, Quebec, Les Editions du Sphinx, 1988.

Sallares, R. *The Ecology of the Ancient Greek World*, London, Duckworth, 1991.

Simon, B. *Mind and Madness in Ancient Greece*, Ithaca, Cornell University Press, 1978.

Smith, W. D. *The Hippocratic Tradition*, Ithaca, Cornell University Press, 1979.

Temkin, O. *The Double Face of Janus*, Baltimore, Johns Hopkins University Press, 1977.

Von Staden, H. *Herophilus. The Art of Medicine in Early Alexandria*, Cambridge University Press, 1989.

TRANSLATIONS

There is no complete English translation of the Hippocratic Corpus. There are partial translations by Francis Adams (London, The Sydenham Society, 1849, and often reprinted); by W. H. S. Jones, E. T. Withington, and P. Potter in the Loeb series (London, Heinemann, 1927); and by J. Chadwick, W. N. Mann, and I. M. Lonie in G. E. R. Lloyd (ed.), *The Hippocratic Writings* (Harmondsworth, Penguin, 1978, and reprinted). The works of Plato and Aristotle are printed with an English version in the Loeb Classical Library series; and there are translations of the fragments of Herophilus, by H. von Staden (Cambridge University Press, 1989); and the *Anonymus Londinensis* papyrus, by W. H. S. Jones (Cambridge University Press, 1948).

Many of the works referred to in the bibliography to Chapter 2 are also relevant.

Select bibliography chapter 2

SECONDARY SOURCES

Amundsen, D. W. 'Images of the physician in classical times', *Journal of Popular Culture* 11 (1977), 643–655.

Benz, H. G. *The Greek Magical Papyri*, Chicago University Press, 1985.

Boon, G. C. 'Potters, oculists, and eye-troubles', *Britannia*, 14 (1983), 1–12.

Bowersock, G. W. *Greek Sophists in the Roman Empire*, Oxford, Clarendon Press, 1969.

Davies, R. W. *Service in the Roman Army*, Edinburgh University Press, 1989.

Duff, J. W. *A Literary History of Rome*, London, Benn, 1964.

French, R. and Greenaway, F. *Science in the Early Roman Empire*, London, Croom Helm, 1986.

Jackson, R. *Doctors and Diseases in the Roman Empire*, London, British Museum, 1988.

Lloyd, G. E. R. *Science, Folklore, and Ideology*, Cambridge University Press, 1983.

Lane-Fox, R. *Pagans and Christians*, Harmondsworth, Penguin, 1988.

Nutton, V. 'The patient's choice', *Classical Quarterly*, 40 (1990), 236–57.

Parkin, T. G. *Demography and Roman Society*, Baltimore, Johns Hopkins University Press, 1992.

Riddle, J. M. *Dioscorides on Pharmacy and Medicine*, Austin, University of Texas Press, 1985.

Rousselle, A. *Porneia*, Oxford, Blackwell, 1988.

Saxl, F. *Saturn and Melancholy*, London, Constable, 1964.

Temkin, O. *Galenism: Rise and Decline of a Medical Philosophy*, Ithaca, Cornell University Press, 1973.

Temkin, O. *The Falling Sickness*, Baltimore, Johns Hopkins University Press, 1971.

Toledo-Pereyra, L. 'Galen's contribution to surgery', *Journal of the History of Medicine and Allied Sciences*, 28 (1973), 357–75.

Vallance, J. R. *The Lost Theory of Asclepiades of Bithynia*, Oxford, Clarendon Press, 1990.

TRANSLATIONS

Two thirds of the Galenic Corpus has still to be translated into English.

English versions of the rest include: *Anatomical Procedures*, Books 1–9, by C. Singer (Oxford University Press, 1956); Books 9–15, by W. H. L. Duckworth *et al.* (Cambridge University Press, 1962); *On the Usefulness of the Parts of the Body*, by M. T. May (Ithaca, Cornell University Press, 1968); *On the Opinions of Hippocrates and Plato*, by P. DeLacy (Berlin, Akademie Verlag, 1978–84); *On Prognosis*, by V. Nutton (Berlin, Akademie Verlag, 1979); *Three Treatises on the Nature of Science*, by R. Walzer and M. Frede (Indianapolis, Hackett, 1985); *On Venesection*, by P. Brain (Cambridge University Press, 1986); *On Examinations by which the Best Physicians are Recognised*, by A. Z. Iskandar (Berlin, Akademie Verlag, 1988); and *On the Therapeutic Method*, Books 1–2, by R. J. Hankinson (Oxford, Clarendon Press, 1991). The best selection of Galenic passages in translation is provided by A. J. Brock in his *Greek Medicine* (London, Dent, 1929; repr. New York, AMS Press, 1977), which also includes the *Medical Questions* of Rufus of Ephesus. The relevant treatises of Cato, Celsus, and the Elder Pliny are included with an English translation in the Loeb Classical Library series. In the last century Francis Adams translated for the Sydenham Society Aretaeus (London, 1856), and there is a more recent English version of Soranus, by O. Temkin (Baltimore, Johns Hopkins University Press, 1956, and reprinted).

Many of the works and translations listed in the bibliography to Chapter 1 are also relevant.

Select bibliography chapter 3

SECONDARY SOURCES

Allen, N. 'Hospice to hospital in the Near East', *Bulletin of the History of Medicine*, 64 (1990), 446–62.

Brown, P. *The Body and Society*, New York, Knopf, 1988.

Brown, P. *Society and the Holy in Late Antiquity*, Berkeley, University of California Press, 1982.

Cameron, M. L. *Anglo-Saxon Medicine*, Cambridge University Press, 1993.

Ferngren, G. B. 'Early Christianity and healing', *Bulletin of the History of Medicine*, 66 (1992), 1–15.

Horden, P. 'The Byzantine welfare state: image and reality', *Society of the Social History of Medicine Bulletin*, 37 (1985), 7–10.

Jacquart, D. and Thomasset, C. *Sexuality and Medicine in the Middle Ages*, Cambridge, Polity Press, 1988.

MacKinney, L. C. *Early Medieval Medicine*, Baltimore, Johns Hopkins University Press, 1937.

Miller, T. S. *The Birth of the Hospital in the Byzantine Empire*, Baltimore, Johns Hopkins University Press, 1985.

Nutton, V. *Galen, Problems and Prospects*, London, The Wellcome Institute, 1981.

Nutton, V. *From Democedes to Harvey*, London, Variorum, 1988.

Park, K. 'Medicine and society in medieval Europe, 500–1500', in A. Wear (ed.), *Medicine in Society*, Cambridge University Press, 1992, pp. 59–90.

Preuss, J. *Biblical and Talmudic Medicine*, New York, Sanhedrin Press, 1978.

Riché, P. *Education and Culture in the Barbarian West*, New York, Columbia University Press, 1976.

Scarborough, J. *Symposium on Byzantine Medicine, Dumbarton Oaks Papers* 38 (1984).

Sears, E. *The Ages of Man*, Princeton University Press, 1986.

Sheils, W. J. *The Church and Healing*, Oxford, Blackwell, 1982.

Siraisi, N. G. *Medieval and Early Renaissance Medicine*, Chicago University Press, 1990.

Stancliffe, C. *St. Martin and his Hagiographer: History and Miracle in Sulpicius Severus*, Oxford, Clarendon Press, 1983.

Sternberg, T. *Orientalium More Secutus*, Munster, Aschendorff, 1991.

Temkin, O. *The Double Face of Janus*, Baltimore, Johns Hopkins University Press, 1977.

Temkin, O. *Hippocrates in a World of Pagans and Christians*, Baltimore, Johns Hopkins University Press, 1992.

TRANSLATIONS

Few texts from this period are available in English. As well as the versions of Caelius Aurelianus, by I. E. Drabkin (Chicago University Press, 1950) and Paul of Aegina, by Francis Adams (London, Sydenham Society, 1844–47), the latter with a magnificent commentary, note Agnellus of Ravenna, *Lectures on Galen's De Sectis* (Buffalo, University of New York at Buffalo Press, 1982); W. D. Sharpe, *Isidore, The Medical Writings* (Philadelphia, American Philosophical Society, 1964).

Many secondary works listed in the bibliographies to Chapters 1 and 2 are also relevant.

Select bibliography chapter 4

SECONDARY SOURCES

Browne, Edward G. *Arabian Medicine*, Cambridge University Press, 1921.

Conrad, Lawrence I. 'Arab-Islamic Medicine', in W. F. Bynum and Roy Porter (eds.), *Companion Encyclopaedia in the History of Medicine*, London, Routledge, 1993, 676–727.

Conrad, Lawrence I. *Before the Black Death: Epidemic Disease and Society in the Early Medieval Near East*. Aldershot, Variorum, 1994. (In Press.)

Conrad, Lawrence I. *The Plague in the Early Medieval Near East*. Handbuch der Orientalistik. Leiden, E. J. Brill, 1995. (In Press.)

Dols, Michael W. *The Black Death in the Middle East*, Princeton University Press, 1977.

Dols, Michael W. *Majnun: the Madman in Medieval Islamic Society*, Oxford, Clarendon Press, 1992.

Dunlop, D. M. 'Science and medicine', in D. M. Dunlop (ed.), *Arab Civilization to AD 1500*, London, Longman's, 1971, pp. 204–50.

Elgood, Cyril. *A Medical History of Persia and the Eastern Caliphate*, Cambridge University Press, 1951.

Goitein, S. D. F. 'The medical profession' and 'Druggists and Pharmacists', in S. D. F. Goitein (ed.), *A Mediterranean Society: the Jewish Communities of the Arab World as Portrayed in the Documents of the Cairo Geniza*, II, Berkeley and Los Angeles, University of California Press, 1971, pp. 240–72.

Hamarneh, Sami K. *Health Sciences in Early Islam*, ed. Munawar A. Anees, 2 vols, Blanco, Texas, Noor Health Foundation and Zahra Publications, 1984.

Jacquart, Danielle and Micheau, Françoise. *La médecine arabe et l'occident médiéval*, Paris, Maisonneuve et Larose, 1990.

Klein-Franke, Felix. *Vorlesungen über die Medizin im Islam*, Wiesbaden, Franz Steiner Verlag, 1982.

Leclerc, Lucien. *Histoire de la médecine arabe*, Paris, Ernest Leroux, 1876.

Leiser, Gary. 'Medical education in Islamic lands from the seventh to the fourteenth century', *Journal of the History of Medicine*, 38 (1983), 48–75.

Levey, Martin. *Early Arabic Pharmacology*, Leiden, E. J. Brill, 1973.

Meyerhof, Max. *Studies in Medieval Arabic Medicine*, ed. Penelope Johnstone, London, Variorum, 1984.

Rahman, Fazlur. *Health and Medicine in the Islamic Tradition: Change and Identity*, New York, Crossroad, 1989.

Rosenthal, Franz. *Science and Medicine in Islam*, Aldershot, Variorum, 1990.

Sezgin, Fuat (ed.). *Beiträge zur Geschichte der arabisch-islamischen Medizin. Aufsätze aus den Jahren 1819–1920*, 4 vols, Frankfurt, Institut für Geschichte der arabisch-islamischen Wissenschaften, 1980.

Sezgin, Fuat. *Geschichte des arabischen Schrifttums*, 3. *Medizin – Zoologie – Tierheilkunde bis ca. 430 H*, Leiden, E. J. Brill, 1970.

Ullmann, Manfred. *Islamic Medicine*, Edinburgh University Press, 1978.

Ullmann, Manfred. *Die Medizin im Islam*, Leiden, E. J. Brill, 1970.

Walzer, Richard. *Greek into Arabic*, Oxford, Bruno Cassirer, 1962.

Young, M. J. L., Latham, J. D. and Sergeant, R. B. (eds.), *Religion, Learning and Science in the 'Abbasid Period* (Cambridge History of Arabic Literature, 3), Cambridge University Press, 1990.

TRANSLATIONS

Bar-Sela, Ariel. *Moses Maimonides' Two Treatises on the Regimen of Health*, Philadelphia, American Philosophical Society, 1964.

Bos, Gerrit. *Qusta Ibn Luqa's Medical Regime for the Pilgrims to Mecca*, Leiden, E. J. Brill, 1992.

Gohlman, William E. *The Life of Ibn Sina*, Albany, State University of New York Press, 1974.

Dols, Michael W. *Medieval Islamic Medicine: Ibn Ridwan's Essay 'On the Prevention of Bodily Ills in Egypt'*, Los Angeles and Berkeley, University of California Press, 1984.

Elgood, Cyril. 'Tibb-ul-Nabbi or medicine of the prophet, being a translation of two works of the same name', *Osiris*, 14 (1962), 33–192.

Graziani, Joseph Salvatore. *Arabic Medicine in the Eleventh Century as Represented in the Works of Ibn Jazlah*, Karachi, Hamdard Academy, 1980.

Greenhill, William Alexander. *A Treatise on the Small-Pox and Measles, by Abú Becr Mohammed ibn Zacaríyá ar-Rází*, London, Sydenham Society, 1848.

Gruner, O. Cameron. *A Treatise on the Canon of Medicine of Avicenna, Incorporating a Translation of the First Book*, London, Luzac, 1930.

Meyerhof, Max. *The Book of the Ten Treatises on the Eye Ascribed to Hunain ibn Ishaq*, Cairo, Government Press, 1928.

Meyerhof, Max. 'Thirty-Three clinical observations by Rhazes (circa AD 900)', *Isis*, 23 (1935), 321–56.

Rosenthal, Franz. *The Classical Heritage in Islam*, trans. Emile and Jenny Marmorstein, London, Routledge and Kegan Paul, 1975.

Salem, Sema'an and Kumar, Alok. *Science in the Medieval World, 'Book of the Categories of Nations' by Sa'id al-Andalusi*, Austin, University of Texas Press, 1991.

Schacht, Joseph and Meyerhof, Max. *The Medico-Philosophical Controversy between Ibn Butlan of Baghdad and Ibn Ridwan of Cairo: a Contribution to the History of Greek Learning among the Arabs*, Cairo, Egyptian University, 1937.

Spink, M. S. and Lewis, G. L. *Albucasis: On Surgery and Instruments*, London, Wellcome Institute for the History of Medicine, 1973.

Zand, Kamal Hafuth, Videan, John A. and Videan, Ivy E. *The Eastern Key: Kitab al-Ifadah wa'l-I'tibar of 'Abd al-Latif al-Baghdadi*, London, George Allen and Unwin, 1965.

Select bibliography chapter 5

SECONDARY SOURCES

Amundsen, D. W. 'Medieval Canon law on medical and surgical practice by the clergy', *Bulletin of the History of Medicine*, 52 (1978), 22–44.

Bloch, H. W. *Monte Cassino in the Middle Ages*, Cambridge, Mass., Harvard University Press, 1986.

Bynum, C. W. *Fragmentation and Redemption. Essays on Gender and the Human Body in Medieval Religion*, New York, Zone Books, 1991.

Campbell, S., Hall, B. and Klausner, D. *Health, Disease and Healing in Medieval Culture*, New York, St. Martin's Press, 1992.

Carmichael, A. G. *Plague and the Poor in Renaissance Florence*, Cambridge University Press, 1986.

Clarke, B. *Mental Disorder in Earlier Britain*, Cardiff, University of Wales Press, 1975.

Finucane, R. C. *Miracles and Pilgrims*, London, Dent, 1977.

French, R. K. 'An origin for the bone text of the "Five-figure series",' *Sudhoffs Archiv*, 68 (1984), 143–56.

Garcia Ballester, L., French, R. K., Arrizabalaga, J., and Cunningham, A. *Practical Medicine from Salerno to the Black Death*, Cambridge University Press, 1993.

Grant, E. M. *A Sourcebook in Medieval Science*, Cambridge, Mass., Harvard University Press, 1974.

Green, M. 'Women's medical practice and medical care in medieval Europe', *Signs*, 14 (1989), 434–73.

Greilsammer, M. 'The midwife, the priest, and the physician', *Journal of Medieval and Renaissance Studies*, 21 (1991), 285–329.

Horden, P. 'A discipline of relevance: the historiography of the later medieval hospital', *Social History of Medicine*, 1 (1988), 359–74.

Jacquart, D. and Thomasset, C. *Sexuality and Medicine in the Middle Ages*, Cambridge, Polity Press, 1988.

Jones, P. M. *Medieval Medical Miniatures*, London, The British Library, 1984.

Laharie, M. *La folie au Moyen Age*, Paris, Le léopard d'or, 1991.

Lang, S. J. 'John Bradmore and his book Philomena', *Social History of Medicine*, 5 (1992), 121–30.

McVaugh, M. R. *Medicine in the Crown of Aragon*, Cambridge University Press, 1993.

McVaugh, M. R. and Siraisi, N. G. 'Renaissance medical learning: evolution of a tradition', *Osiris*, 6 (1990).

MacKinney, L. C. *Medical illustrations in medieval manuscripts*, London, The Wellcome Historical Medical Library, 1965.

Nutton, V. 'Medicine at the German universities, 1348–1500', *Sudhoffs Archiv* 80 1996.

Origo, I. *The Merchant of Prato*, Harmondsworth, Penguin, 1963.

Orme, N. and Webster, M., *The English Hospital, 1070–1570*, New Haven, Yale University Press, 1995.

Ottosson, P. G. *Scholastic Medicine and Philosophy*, Naples, Bibliopolis, 1984.

Palmer, R. J. *The Control of Plague in Venice and Northern Italy, 1348–1600*, Ph.D. Diss., Univ. of Kent, Canterbury, 1978.

Park, K. 'Medicine and society in medieval Europe, 500–1500', in A. Wear, *Medicine in Society*, Cambridge University Press, 1992, 59–90.

Park, K. *Doctors and Medicine in Early Renaissance Florence*, Princeton University Press, 1985.

Park, K. and Henderson, J. 'The first hospital among Christians', *Medical History*, 35 (1991), 164–88.

Rawcliffe, C. *Medicine and Society in Late Medieval England*, Stroud, A. Sutton, 1995.

Richards, P. *The Medieval Leper and his Northern Heirs*, Cambridge University Press, 1977.

de Ridder-Symoens, H. *A History of the University in Europe*, Cambridge University Press, 1992.

Riddle, J. M. *Quid Pro Quo: Studies in the History of Drugs*, Aldershot, Variorum, 1992.

Russell, A. W. *The Town and State Physician in Europe*, Wolfenbüttel, Herzog-August-Bibliothek, 1981.

Siraisi, N. G. *Medieval and Early Renaissance Medicine*, Chicago University Press, 1990.

Siraisi, N. G. *Taddeo Alderotti and his Pupils*, Princeton University Press, 1981.

Talbot, C. H. *Medicine in Medieval England*, London, Oldbourne, 1967.

Tester, S. J. *A History of Western Astrology*, Woodbridge, Boydell and Brewer, 1987.

Thorndike, L. *Science and Thought in the Fifteenth Century*, New York, Columbia University Press, 1929.

Weiss, R. *Medieval and Humanist Greek*, Padua, Antenore, 1977.

Ziegler, P. *The Black Death*, Harmondsworth, Penguin, 1969.

TRANSLATIONS

Access to mediaeval medical writings is far from easy. A few texts, incuding Johannitius, are translated in E. M. Grant, *A Source Book in Medieval Science* (Cambridge, Mass., Harvard University Press, 1974). Some idea of scholastic theory and practice can be gained from Maurus of Salerno, tr. M. H. Saffron (Philadelphia, American Philosophical Society, 1972), and the selection in D. P. Lockwood, *Ugo Benzi, 1376–1439* (Chicago University Press, 1951). Anatomy is served by G. W. Corner, *Anatomical Texts of the Earlier Middle Ages* (Washington, American Philosophical Society, 1927), and by C. Singer,. *The Fascicolo di medicina, 1493* (Florence, R. Lier, 1925), which includes Mondino. For medieval surgery, see Theodoric, *Surgery*, tr. E. Campbell (New York, Hafner, 1955); and John of Mirfield, *Surgery*, tr. J. B. Colton (New York, Hafner, 1969). The brave may explore the Middle English versions of Guy de Chauliac, ed. M. Ogden (Oxford, Early English Text Society, 1961); of Gilbertus Anglicus, ed. F. M. Getz (Madison, University of Wisconsin Press, 1991); and some anonymous texts, Beryl Rowland, *Medieval Woman's Guide to Health* (Kent, University of

Ohio Press, 1981); L. E. Voigts and M. R. McVaugh, *A Latin Technical Phlebotomy and its Middle English Translation*, (Philadelphia, American Philosophical Society, 1984); Tony Hunt, *Popular Medicine in Thirteenth-Century England* (Woodbridge, D. S. Brewer, 1990). Interesting documents from the world of learned medicine may be found in Lynn Thorndike, *University records and life in the Middle Ages* (New York, Norton, 1975).

Select bibliography for chapter 6

MEDICINE AND SOCIETY

Demography

Flinn, Michael *The European Demographic System 1500–1800*, Brighton, Harvester Press, 1981.

Wrigley, E. A. and Schofield, R. S. *The Population History of England 1541–1871*, London, Arnold, 1981.

Wrigley, E. A. 'No death without birth: the implications of English mortality in the early modern period', in R. Porter and A. Wear (eds.) *Problems and Methods in the History of Medicine*, London, Croom Helm, 1987, pp. 133–50. (Discusses the case of Hartland.)

Diseases

Camporesi, Piero *Bread of Dreams*, Oxford, Polity Press, 1989.

Cipolla, Carlo *Public Health and the Medical Profession in the Renaissance*, Cambridge, Cambridge University Press, 1976.

Massimo Livi-Bacci gives population figures for Europe: *Population and Nutrition. An Essay on European Demographic History*, Cambridge University Press, 1991.

Slack, Paul *The Impact of Plague in Tudor and Stuart England*, London, Routledge and Kegan Paul, 1985.

Walter, John, and Schofield, Roger, (eds.) *Famine, Disease and the Social Order in Early Modern Society*, Cambridge University Press, 1989.

Europeans abroad

Brooks, Francis 'Revising the conquest of Mexico: smallpox, sources, and populations', *Journal of Interdisciplinary History*, 24, 1993, 1–29.

Carpenter, Kenneth *The History of Scurvy and Vitamin C*, Cambridge University Press, 1986.

Crosby, Alfred W. *Ecological Imperialism: The Biological Expansions of Europe, 900–1900*. Cambridge University Press, 1986.

Dobson, Mary 'Mortality gradients and disease exchanges: comparisons from Old England and Colonial America', *Social History of Medicine*, 2 (1989), 259–97.

Kupperman, Karen 'Fear of hot climates in the Anglo-American experience', *William and Mary Quarterly*, 41 (1984), 213–40.

Numbers, Ronald L. (ed.) *Medicine in the New World*, Knoxville, University of Tennessee, 1987.

The world of the sick

Ariès, Philippe *The Hour of Our Death*, Harmondsworth, Penguin Books, 1983.

Black, Christopher *Italian Confraternities in the Sixteenth Century*, Cambridge University Press, 1989.

Crawford, Catherine 'Medicine and the law' in W. F. Bynum and Roy Porter (eds.) *Companion Encyclopaedia of the History of Medicine*, London, Routledge, 1993, vol. 2, pp. 1619–40.

Fildes, Valerie (ed.) *Women as Mothers in Pre-Industrial England*, London, Routledge, 1990.

Gélis, Jacques *History of Childbirth*, Oxford, Polity Press, 1991.

Grell, Ole and Cunningham, Andrew (eds.), *Medicine and the Reformation*, London, Routledge, 1993.

Jones, Colin *The Charitable Imperative. Hospitals and Nursing in Ancien Régime and Revolutionary France*, London, Routledge, 1989.

MacDonald, Michael *Mystical Bedlam, Madness, Anxiety, and Healing in Seventeenth-Century England*, Cambridge University Press, 1981.

McCray Beier, Lucinda *Sufferers and Healers, The Experience of Illness in Seventeeth-Century England*, London, Routledge and Kegan Paul, 1987.

Marland, Hilary (ed.), *The Art of Midwifery. Early Modern Midwives in Europe*, London, Routledge, 1993.

Martz, Linda *Poverty and Welfare in Habsburg Spain*, Cambridge University Press, 1983.

Nagy, Doreen G. *Popular Medicine in Seventeenth-Century England*, Bowling Green, 1988.

Pelling, Margaret 'Healing the sick poor: social policy and disability in Norwich 1550–1640', *Medical History*, 29 (1985), 115–37.

Pelling, Margaret and Webster, Charles, 'Medical Practitioners' in Charles Webster (ed.), *Health, Medicine and Mortality in the Sixteenth Century*, Cambridge University Press, 1979 pp. 165–235. (Give the figures for London practitioners.)

Porter, Roy (ed.) *Patients and Practitioners. Lay Perceptions of Medicine in Pre-Industrial Society*, Cambridge Univesity Press, 1985.

Porter, Roy (ed.), *The Popularisation of Medicine 1650–1850*, London, Routledge, 1992. (See chapters by Andrew Wear 'The popularisation of medicine in early modern England', pp. 17–41; and Philip Wilson 'Acquiring surgical know-how. Occupational and lay instruction in early eighteenth-century London', pp. 42–71

Pullan, Brian *Rich and Poor in Renaissance Venice*, Oxford, Basil Blackwell, 1971.

Russell, Andrew (ed.) *The Town and State Physician in Europe from the Middle Ages to the Enlightenment*, Wolfenbütteler Forschungen, vol. 17, Wolfenbüttel, Herzog August Bibliothek, 1981. (The essays by Richard Palmer and by Jose Maria López Piñero give the figures of physicians to population for Italy and Spain respectively.)

Sheils, W. J. (ed.), *The Church and Healing*, Studies in Church History, 19, Oxford, Basil Blackwell, 1982.

Slack, Paul *Poverty and Policy in Stuart England*, London, Longmans, 1988.

Solomon, Howard *Public Welfare, Science and Propaganda in Seventeenth Century France: The Innovations of Théophraste Renaudot*, Princeton University Press, 1972.

Stannard, David *The Puritan Way of Death*, New York, Oxford University Press, 1977.

Thomas, Keith *Religion and the Decline of Magic*, Harmondsworth, Penguin Books, 1978.

Vovelle, Michel *La Morte en l'Occident de 1300 à Nos Jours*, Paris, Gallimard, 1983.

Wear, Andrew, Geyer-Kordesch, Johanna and French, Roger, (eds.) *Doctors and Ethics: the Earlier Historical Setting of Professional Ethics*, Amsterdam, Rodopi, 1993.

Wear, Andrew 'Caring for the sick poor in St Bartholomew's exchange: 1580–1676', in W. F. Bynum and Roy Porter (eds.), *Living and Dying in London, Medical History* Supplement No. 11, 1991, pp. 41–60.

Sixteenth-century learned medicine in general

Bylebyl, Jerome 'Teaching Methodus Medendi, in the Renaissance' in F. Kudlien and R. J. Durling (eds.), *Galen's Method of Healing*, Leiden, E. J. Brill, 1991, pp. 157–89.

Durling, R. J. 'A chronological census of Renaissance editions and translations of Galen', *J. Warburg and Courtauld Institutes*, 24 (1961), 230–305.

Siraisi, Nancy *Avicenna in Renaissance Italy*, Princeton University Press, 1987.

Siraisi, Nancy *Medieval and Early Renaissance Medicine*, Chicago, University of Chicago Press, 1990.

Wear, A. 'Galen in the Renaissance', in V. Nutton (ed.), *Galen: Problems and Prospects*, London, 1981, pp. 229–62.

Wear, A., French, R. and Lonie, I. (eds.) *The Medical Renaissance of the Sixteenth Century*, Cambridge University Press, 1985.

Webster, C. (ed), *Health, Medicine and Mortality in the Sixteenth Century*, Cambridge University Press, 1979.

Sixteenth-century anatomy

Choulant, Ludwig *History and Bibliography of Anatomic Illustration*, N. York, Schuman's 1945.

Herrlinger, Robert *History of Medical Illustration from Antiquity to AD 1600*, London, Pitman Medical, 1970.

Lind, L. R. *Studies in Pre-Vesalian Anatomy*, Philadelphia, American Philosophical Society, 1975.

Kemp, Martin *Leonardo da Vinci, The Marvellous Works of Nature and Man*, London, J. M. Dent, 1981.

O'Malley, C. D. *Andreas Vesalius of Brussels 1514–1564*, University of California Press, 1964.

Schulz, B. *Art and Anatomy in Renaissance Italy*, Ann Arbor, University of Michigan Press, 1985.

See also the essay by J. Bylebyl 'The school of Padua: humanistic medicine in the sixteenth century' in C. Webster (ed.), *Health, Medicine and Mortality in the Sixteenth Century*, pp. 335–370.

Surgery

Lawrence, Christopher, (ed.) *Medical Theory, Surgical Practice*, London, Routledge, 1992. (See the essay by Lucinda McCray Beier on Joseph Binn's casebook, pp. 48–84.)

Jütte, Robert 'A Seventeenth-Century German Barber-Surgeon and His Patients', *Medical History*, 33 (1989), 184–98.

See also the essay by V. Nutton, 'Humanistic surgery' in A. Wear, R. French and I. Lonie (eds.), *The Medical Renaissance of the Sixteenth Century*, pp.75–99.

Medicine and botany

Arber, Agnes *Herbals*, Cambridge University Press, 3rd edition, 1986.

Faust, Clifford *Rhubarb. The Wonder Drug*, Princeton University Press, 1992.

Griggs, Barbara *Green Pharmacy. A History of Herbal Medicine*, London, Robert Hale, 1981.

Palmer, Richard 'Medical botany in Northern Italy in the Renaissance', *Journal of the Royal Society of Medicine*, 78 (1985), 149–57.

Prest, John *The Garden of Eden. The Botanic Garden and the Re-Creation of Paradise*, New Haven, Yale University Press, 1981.

Reeds, Karen M. *Botany in Medieval and Renaissance Universities*, New York, Garland, 1991. (This also includes her important article, 'Renaissance humanism and botany' which was published in *Annals of Science*, 33 (1979), 519–42.

See also Richard Palmer, 'Pharmacy in the Republic of Venice in the sixteenth-century', in Wear, A., French, R. and Lonie, I (eds.), *The Medical Renaissance of the Sixteenth Century*, Cambridge University Press, pp. 100–117.

Paracelsianism

Debus, Allen *The English Paracelsians*, London, Oldbourne Press, 1965.

Debus, Allen *The French Paracelsians*, Cambridge University Press, 1991.

Nutton, Vivian (ed.) *Medicine at the Courts of Europe 1500–1837*, London, Routledge, 1990. (See especially the essays by Hugh Trevor Roper, 'The court physician and Paracelsianism' and by Bruce Moran, 'Prince-practitioning and the direction of medical roles at the German court: Maurice of Hesse-Kassel and his physicians'.)

Pagel, Walter *Paracelsus*, Basel, Karger, 1958.

Vickers, Brian (ed.), *Occult and Scientific Mentalities in the Renaissance*, Cambridge University Press, 1984.

Webster, Charles *From Paracelsus to Newton. Magic and the Making of Modern Science*, Cambridge University Press, 1982.

Webster, Charles *The Great Instauration, Science, Medicine and Reform 1626–1660*, London, Duckworth, 1975.

Discovery of circulation

Keynes, Geoffrey *The Life of William Harvey*, Oxford, Clarendon Press, 1978.

Pagel, Walter *William Harvey's Biological Ideas*, Basel, Karger, 1967.

Wear, Andrew 'William Harvey and the 'Way of the Anatomists'', *History of Science*, 21 (1983), 223–49.

Whitteridge, Gweneth *William Harvey and the Circulation of the Blood*, London, Macdonald, and New York, American Elsevier, 1971.

Seventeenth-century medicine and the new science

Brockliss, L. W. B. *French Higher Education in the Seventeenth and Eighteenth Centuries*, Oxford, Clarendon Press, 1987.

Cook, Harold J. *The Decline of the Old Medical Regime in Stuart London*, Ithaca and London, Cornell University Press 1986; and idem, 'The new philosophy and medicine in seventeenth-century England' in David Lindberg and Robert Westman (eds.) *Reappraisals of the Scientific Revolution*, Cambridge University Press, 1990, pp. 397–436.

Frank, Robert *Harvey and the Oxford Physiologists*, Berkeley, University of California Press, 1980.

French, Roger and Wear, Andrew (eds.) *The Medical Revolution of the Seventeenth-Century*, Cambridge University Press, 1989. (See also the essays by H. Cook, R. Porter and A. Wear on medicine and the new science, and that by Andrew Cunningham on 'Thomas Sydenham: Epidemics, Experiment and the "Good Old Cause"'.)

Guerrini, Anita 'Archibald Pitcairne and Newtonian Medicine', *Medical History*, 31 (1987), 70–83. (See also her essay in Roger French and Andrew Wear (eds.), *The Medical Revolution of the Seventeenth Century* on 'Isaac Newton, George Cheyne and the 'Principia Medicinae',' Cambridge University Press, pp. 222–45.

Hall, A. R. *The Revolution in Science, 1500–1750*, London, Longman, 1983.

King, Lester *The Road to Medical Enlightenment 1650–1695*, London, Macdonald; New York, American Elsevier, 1970.

Porter, Roy and Teich, Mikulas (eds.) *The Scientific Revolution in National Context*, Cambridge University Press, 1992.

TRANSLATIONS

Translations and Texts: L. R. Lind, *Studies in Pre-Vesalian Anatomy* (Philadelphia, American Philosophical Society, 1975), has translations of late fifteenth and early sixteenth century anatomical texts; Berengario da Carpi, *A Short Introduction to Anatomy*, translated by L. R. Lind, (Chicago, University of Chicago Press, 1959 and New York, Kraus Reprint, 1969); Berengario da Carpi, *On Fracture of the Skull or Cranium*, translated by L. R. Lind (Philadelphia, American Philosophical Society, 1990); Andreas Vesalius, *The Epitome of Andreas Vesalius*, translated by L. R. Lind, (New York, Macmillan, 1949); Charles Singer (ed. and trans.), *Vesalius on the Human Brain* (Oxford, Oxford University Press, 1952); Geoffrey Keynes (ed.), *The Apologie and Treatise of Ambroise Paré* (New York, Dover Publications, 1968); Ambroise Paré, *The Collected Works of Ambroise Paré*, facsimile of 1634 translation by Thomas Johnson (New York, Milford House, 1968); Henry Sigerist (ed. and trans.), *Four Treatises of Theophrastus von Hohenheim, called Paracelsus* (New York, Arno Press reprint, 1979); Nicholas Goodrick-Clarke (ed.), *Paracelsus Essential Readings* (Wellingborough, U.K., Crucible, 1990); William Harvey, *The Circulation of the Blood and Other Writings*, translated by Kenneth J. Franklin (London, Everyman, J. M. Dent, 1993); John Frampton, *Joyfull Newes out of the Newe Founde Worlde. Written in Spanish by Nicholas Monardes and Englished by John Frampton* (London, Constable; New York, A. Knopf, 1925); Thomas Willis, *The Anatomy of the Brain and Nerves*, translated by Samuel Pordage and edited by William Feindel (Montreal, McGill University Press, 1965); Giovanni Borelli, *On the Movement of Animals*, translated by Paul Maquet (Berlin, Springer Verlag, 1989) Friedrich Hoffman, *Fundamenta Medicinae*, Introduction and translated by Lester King (London, Macdonald and New York, American Elsevier, 1971).

Select bibliography chapter 7

GENERAL

Background reading and works of reference

The following reference books provide backgrounds to many aspects of eighteenth-century history.

Black, Jeremy *Eighteenth Century Europe*, London, Macmillan, 1990.

Foucault, M. *The Order of Things: An Archaeology of the Human Sciences*, London: Routledge, 1989.

Fox, Christopher, Porter, Roy and Wokler, Robbey (eds.) *Inventing Human Science: Eighteenth Century Domains*, Berkeley, University of California Press, 1995. (In Press.)

Gay, Peter *The Enlightenment: An Interpretation*, 2 vols., New York, Vintage, 1966–69.

Landes, David S. *The Unbound Prometheus: Technological Change and Industrial Development in Western Europe from 1750 to the Present*, London, Cambridge University Press, 1960.

Stone, Lawrence *The Family, Sex and Marriage in England, 1500–1800*, London, Weidenfeld and Nicolson, 1977.

Williams, E. N. *The Penguin Dictionary of English and European History 1485–1789*, Harmondsworth, Penguin, 1980.

Yolton, John, Porter, Roy, Rogers, Pat and Stafford, Barbara (eds), *Blackwell Companion to the Enlightenment*, Oxford, Basil Blackwell, 1991.

General accounts of medical history

Bynum, W. F. 'Health, disease and medical care', in G. S. Rousseau and R. Porter (eds.), *The Ferment of Knowledge*, Cambridge University Press, 1980, pp. 211–54.

Cunningham, Andrew and French, Roger (eds), *The Medical Enlightenment of the Eighteenth Century*, Cambridge University Press, 1990.

Gay, Peter 'The Enlightenment as medicine and as cure', in W. H. Barber (ed.), *The Age of the Enlightenment: Studies Presented to Theodore Besterman*, Edinburgh, St Andrews University Publications, 1967, pp. 375–86.

King, Lester S. *The Medical World of the Eighteenth Century*, University of Chicago Press, 1958.

King, Lester S. *The Growth of Medical Thought*, University of Chicago Press, 1963.

King, Lester S. *The Road to Medical Enlightenment, 1650–1695*, London, Macdonald; New York, American Elsevier, 1970.

King, Lester S. *The Philosophy of Medicine: the Early Eighteenth Century*, Cambridge, Mass., Harvard University Press, 1978.

King, Lester S. *Transformations in American Medicine: From Benjamin Rush to William Osler*, Baltimore, Johns Hopkins University Press, 1990.

LeFanu, W. R. 'The lost half-century in English medicine, 1700–1750', *Bulletin of the History of Medicine*, 46 (1972), 319–48.

Risse, Guenter B. 'Medicine in the age of Enlightenment', in A. Wear (ed.), *Medicine in Society: Historical Essays*, Cambridge University Press, 1992, pp. 149–95.

SPECIFIC ISSUES

The legacy of the scientific revolution and the Enlightenment

Frängsmyr, Tore, Heilbron, J. L. and Rider, Robin E. (eds.), *The Quantifying Spirit in the Eighteenth Century*, Berkeley, Los Angeles and Oxford, University of California Press, 1990.

French, Roger and Wear, Andrew (eds), *The Medical Revolution of the Seventeenth Century*, Cambridge University Press, 1989.

Hacking, Ian *The Taming of Chance*, Cambridge University Press, 1990.

Holmes, F. L. *Lavoisier and the Chemistry of Life: An Exploration in Scientific Creativity*, Madison, University of Wisconsin Press, 1985.

Hankins, Thomas *Science and the Enlightenment*, Cambridge University Press, 1985.

Gasking, E. B. *Investigations into Generation 1651–1828*, London, Hutchinson, 1964.

Roe, Shirley A. *Matter, Life and Generation: Eighteenth-Century Embryology and the Haller-Wolff Debate*, Cambridge University Press, 1981.

Roger, J. *Les Sciences de la Vie dans la Pensée Française du XVIIIè siècle*, Paris, A. Colin, 1971.

Anatomy and physiology

Choulant, Ludwig *History and Bibliography of Anatomic Illustration*, translated by M. Frank, revised edition, New York, Henry Schuman, 1945.

Lindeboom, G. A. *Hermann Boerhaave: The Man and His Work*, London, Methuen, 1968.

Spillane, J. *The Doctrine of the Nerves*, London, Oxford University Press, 1981.

Clinical medicine and disease theory

Bynum, W. F. and Nutton, V. (eds.) *Theories of Fever from Antiquity to the Enlightenment*, *Medical History*, Supplement No. 1, London, Wellcome Institute for the History of Medicine, 1981.

Bynum, W. F. and Porter, Roy (eds), *Brunonianism in Britain and Europe*, *Medical History*, Supplement 8, London, Wellcome Institute for the History of Medicine, 1989.

Heberden, Ernest *William Heberden 1710–1801: Physician of the Age of Reason*, London and New York, Royal Society of Medicine Services, 1990.

Loudon, Irvine *Medical Care and the General Practitioner 1750–1850*, Oxford, Clarendon Press, 1986.

Risse, Guenter B. 'A shift in medical epistemology: clinical diagnosis, 1770–1828' in Y. Kawakita (ed.), *History of Diagnosis*, Japan, Taniguchi Foundation, 1987.

Therapeutics

Bynum, W. F. 'Treating the wages of sin: venereal disease and specialism in eighteenth-century Britain', in W. F. Bynum and R. Porter (eds.), *Medical Fringe and Medical Orthodoxy, 1750–1850*, London, Croom Helm, 1987, pp. 5–28.

Bynum, W. F. and Nutton, Vivian (eds.), *Essays on the History of Therapeutics*, *Clio Medica*, 22 (1991).

Bynum, W. F. and Porter, R. (eds.) *William Hunter and The Eighteenth-Century Medical World*, Cambridge University Press, 1985.

Worth Estes, J. *Dictionary of Protopharmacology: Therapeutic Practices, 1700–1850*, Canton, MA, Science History Publications, USA, 1990.

Fisher, R. B. *Edward Jenner 1749–1823*, London, Andre Deutsch, 1991.

Foucault, M. *Folie et Déraison: Histoire de la Folie à l'age Classique*, Paris, Plon, Abridged edition, 1964, translated as *Madness and Civilization*, New York, Pantheon Books 2nd edition, 1971; English edition, London, Tavistock, 1967.

Hembry, Phyllis *The English Spa 1560–1815: A Social History*, London, Althone Press, 1990.

Marland, Hilary (ed.), *The Art of Midwifery*, London, Routledge, 1993.

Miller, G. *The Adoption of Inoculation for Smallpox in England and France*, London, Oxford University Press, 1957.

Porter, Roy *Mind Forg'd Manacles: Madness and Psychiatry in England from Restoration to Regency*, London, Athlone Press, 1987; paperback edition, Penguin, 1990.

Wilson, Adrian *The Making of Man Midwifery*, London, University College Press, 1995.

Surgery

Gelfand, Toby *Professionalizing Modern Medicine: Paris Surgeons and Medical Science and Institutions in the Eighteenth Century*, Westport, Conn., Greenwood Press, 1982.

Laget, Mireille and Luu, Claudine (eds.) *Médecine et Chirurgie des Pauvres au 18e Siècle d'Après le Livret de Dom Alexandre*, Toulouse: Privat, 1984.

Wilson, Philip K. 'Acquiring surgical know-how: occupational and lay instruction in early eighteenth-century London', in Roy Porter (ed.), *The Popularization of Medicine, 1650–1850*, London, Routledge, 1992, pp. 42–71.

Popular medicine: elite and plebeian culture

Bloch, M. *The Royal Touch: Sacred Monarchy and Scrofula in England and France*, London, Routledge & Kegan Paul, 1973.

Duden, Barbara *Geschichte unter der Haut*, Stuttgart, Klett, Cotta, 1987, translated as *The Woman Beneath the Skin. A Doctor's Patients in Eighteenth-Century Germany*, translated by Thomas Dunlap, Cambridge, Mass., Harvard University Press, 1991.

Loux, F. *Sagesse du Corps: Santé et Maladie dans les Proverbs Réginaux Françaises*, Paris, Masionneuve et Larose, 1978.

McManners, J. *Death and the Enlightenment: Changing Attitudes Towards Death Among Christians and Unbelievers in Eighteenth-Century France*, Oxford, Clarendon Press, 1981.

Porter, Dorothy and Porter, Roy *Patient's Progress: Doctors and Doctoring in Eighteenth-Century England*, Cambridge, Polity Press, 1989.

Porter, Roy (ed.) *Patients and Practitioners: Lay Perceptions of Medicine in Pre-Industrial Society*, Cambridge University Press, 1985.

Porter, Roy (ed.) *The Popularization of Medicine, 1650–1850*, London, Routledge, 1992.

Porter, Roy and Porter, Dorothy *In Sickness and in Health: The British experience 1650–1850*, London, Fourth Estate, 1988.

The profession and medical education

Burnby, Juanita G. L. *A Study of the English Apothecary from 1660 to 1760, Medical History*, Supplement No. 3, London, Wellcome Institute for the History of Medicine, 1983.

Hannaway, Caroline C. 'The Société Royale de Médecine and Epidemics in the Ancien Régime', in *Bulletin of the History of Medicine*, 44 (1972), 257–73.

Lesky, Erna *The Vienna Medical School of the 19th Century*, translated from the German by L. Williams and I. S. Levij, Baltimore, Johns Hopkins University Press, 1965.

Lawrence, S. 'Entrepreneurs and private enterprise: the development of medical lecturing in London, 1775–1820', *Bulletin of the History of Medicine*, 57 (1988), 171–92.

Numbers, Ronald L. (ed.), *Medicine in the New World: New Spain, New France, and New England*, Knoxville, University of Tennessee Press, 1987.

Poynter, F. N. L. (ed.) *The Evolution of Medical Education in Britain*, London: Pitman, 1966.

Ramsey, Matthew *Professional and Popular Medicine in France, 1770–1830*, New York, Cambridge University Press, 1988.

Rosner, Lisa *Medical Education in the Age of Improvement: Edinburgh Students and Apprentices 1760–1826*, Edinburgh, Edinburgh University Press, 1991.

Waddington, Ivan *The Medical Profession in the Industrial Revolution*, Dublin, Gill & Macmillan, 1984.

Quackery

Bynum, W. F. and Porter, R. (eds.) *Medical Fringe and Medical Orthodoxy 1750–1850*, London, Croom Helm, 1987.

Cooter, R. (ed.) *Studies in the History of Alternative Medicine*, London, Macmillan, 1988.

Huisman, Frank 'Itinerant medical practitioners in the Dutch Republic: the case of Groningen', *Tractrix*, 1 (1980), 63–84.

Porter, Roy *Health for Sale: Quackery in England 1650–1850*, Manchester, Manchester University Press, 1989.

Medicine and the State: hospitals

Lloyd, C. and Coulter, J. L. S. *Medicine and the Navy 1200–1900*, vol.3, *1714–1815*, Edinburgh: Livingstone, 1961.

Jones, Colin *The Charitable Imperative: Hospitals and Nursing in Ancien Régime and Revolutionary France*, Wellcome Institute Series in the History of Medicine, London and New York, Routledge, 1990.

Riley, James C. *The Eighteenth Century Campaign to Avoid Disease*, Basingstoke, Macmillan, 1987.

Risse, Guenter *Hospital Life in Enlightenment Scotland: Care and Teaching at the Royal Infirmary of Edinburgh*, Cambridge University Press, 1986.

Rosen, George *From Medical Police to Social Medicine*, New York, Science History Publications, 1974.

Weiner, Dora *The Citizen-Patient in Revolutionary and Imperial Paris*, Baltimore, Johns Hopkins University Press, 1993.

Woodward, J. *To Do The Sick No Harm. A Study of the British Voluntary Hospital System to 1875*, London, Routledge & Kegan Paul, 1974.

Conclusion: disease, medicine, and society

Anderson, Michael *Population Change in North-Western Europe, 1750–1850*, London, Macmillan Education Ltd., 1988.

Clarkson, L. *Death, Disease and Famine in Pre-Industrial England*, Dublin, Gill & Macmillan, 1975.

Floud, Roderick, Wachter, Kenneth and Gregory, Annabel *Height, Health and History: Nutritional Status in the United Kingdom, 1750–1980*, Cambridge University Press, 1990.

Goubert, J.-P. (ed.) *La Médicalisation de la Société Française 1770–1830*, Waterloo, Ont., Historical Reflections Press, 1982.

Komlos, John *Nutrition and Economic Development in the Eighteenth-Century Habsburg Monarchy: An Anthropometric History*, Princeton University Press, 1989.

McKeown, T. *The Modern Rise of Population*, London, Edward Arnold; New York, Academic Press, 1976.

McKeown, T. *The Role of Medicine: Dream, Mirage or Nemesis?*, London, Nuffield Provincial Hospitals Trust, 1976.

Walter, John and Schofield, Roger (eds.) *Famine, Disease and the Social Order in Early Modern Society*, Cambridge University Press, 1989.

Wrigley, E. A. and Schofield, R. S. *The Population History of England 1541–1971: A Reconstruction*, London, Edward Arnold, 1981.

Translations

Recent translations of non-English language texts for this period include the following:

Frank, Johann P. *A System of Complete Medical Police*, Erna Lesky (ed.), translated by E. Vilim, Baltimore, Johns Hopkins University Press, 1976.

Hoffmann, Friedrich *Fundamenta Medicinae*, translated and edited by Lester S. King, London, Macdonald, 1971.

Jarcho, Saul (trans. and ed.) *The Clinical Consultations of Giambattista Morgagni*, Boston, Countway Library of Medicine, 1984.

General bibliography

GENERAL HISTORIES OF MEDICINE

Ackerknecht, Erwin H. *A Short History of Medicine*, Baltimore, Johns Hopkins University Press, 1968.

Ackerknecht, Erwin H. *Medicine and Ethnology*, H.H. Walser and H.M. Koelbing (eds.), Baltimore, Johns Hopkins University Press, 1971.

Ackerknecht, Erwin H. *Therapeutics From the Primitives to the 20th Century*, New York, Hafner, 1973.

Ackerknecht, Erwin H. *History and Geography of the Most Important Diseases*, New York, Hafner, 1972.

Bariety, M. and Courcy, C. *Histoire de la Médecine*, Paris, Fayard, 1967.

Bouissou, P. *Histoire de la Médecine*, Paris, Larousse, 1967.

Bynum, W.F. and Porter, Roy (eds.) *Companion Encyclopedia of the History of Medicine*, 2 vols., London, Routledge, 1993.

Carmichael, A.G. and Ratzan, R.M. (eds.) *Medicine: A Treasury of Art and Literature*, New York, Levin/Macmillan, 1991.

Cartwright, F.F. *A Social History of Medicine*, London, Longman, 1972.

Castiglioni, Arturo *A History of Medicine*. 2nd edition. Translated by E.B. Krumbhaar, New York, Alfred A. Knopf, 1947.

Cid, F. *Reflexiones sobre histoira de la medicina*, Barcelona, Anagrama, 1974.

Clarke, Edwin. (ed.) *Modern Methods in the History of Medicine*, London, Athlone Press University of London, 1971.

Cohen, Mark Nathan *Health and the Rise of Civilization*, New Haven, Yale University Press, 1989.

Currer, C. and Stacey, M. (eds.) *Concepts in Health, Illness and Disease: A Comparative Perspective*. Leamington Spa, Berg, 1986.

Diepgen, Paul *Geschichte der Medizin: Die historische Entwicklung der Heikunde und des ärztlichen Lebens*. 2 vols., Berlin, W. de Gruyter, 1949–55.

Duden, B. 'A repertory of body history' in Feher, M. (ed.), *Fragments for a History of the Human Body*, vol. 3., New York, Zone, 1989, pp. 470–554.

Duin, N., Sutcliffe, J. *et al. A History of Medicine: From Pre-history to the Year 2020*, New York, Simon and Schuster, 1992.

Fischer-Homberger, E. *Geschichte der Medizin*, New York, Springer-Verlag, 1977.

Garrison, Fielding H. *An Introduction to the History of Medicine*, 4th edition, Philadelphia and London: W.B. Saunders, 1917; Philadelphia: W.B. Saunders, 1929; reprinted Philadelphia: W.B. Saunders, 1960.

Helman, C. *Body Myths*, London, Chatto and Windus, 1991.

Kiple, Kenneth F. (ed.) *The Cambridge World History of Human Disease*, Cambridge, University Press, 1992.

Kleinman, A. *The Illness Narratives: Suffering, Healing and the Human condition*, New York, Basic Books, 1988.

Lain Entralgo, P. *Historia de la medicina moderna y contemporanea.* 2nd edition, Barcelona, Editorial Cientifico Medica, 1963.

Landy, David (ed.) *Culture, Disease and Healing. Studies in Medical Anthropology,* New York, Macmillan, 1977.

Lilienfeld, Abraham, M. (ed.) *Times, Places and Persons. Aspects of the History of Epidemiology.* Baltimore, Johns Hopkins University Press, 1980.

Lyons, A.S. and Petrucelli, R.J. *Medicine: An Illustrated History,* New York, Abrams, 1978; reprinted 1987.

McGrew, R. *Encyclopedia of Medical History,* London, Macmillan, 1985.

McKeown, Thomas *The Origins of Human Disease,* Oxford, Blackwell, 1988.

McKeown, Thomas *The Role of Medicine. Dreams, Mirage or Nemesis?* Princeton University Press, 1979.

McNeill, William H. *Plagues and Peoples,* Garden City, N.Y., Doubleday Anchor, 1976.

Magner, L.A. *A History of Medicine,* New York/Basel, Marcel Dekker, 1992.

Neuburger, Max *History of Medicine,* 2 vols., translated by Ernest Playfair, London, H. Frowde, 1910–25.

Neuburger, Max *The Doctrine of the Healing Power of Nature Throughout the Course of Time,* translated by L.J. Boyd, New York, 1932. (Privately printed.)

Porter, R. (ed.) *The Cambridge Illustrated History of Medicine,* Cambridge University Press.

Puschmann, Theodor, Neuburger, Max and Pagel, Julius *Handbuch der Geschichte der Medizin.* 3 vols. Jena, Gustav Fischer, 1902–5.

Riley, James *Sickness, Recovery and Death: A History and Forecast of Ill Health.* Iowa, University of Iowa Press, 1989.

Rosenberg, C. and Golden, J. (eds.) *Framing Disease: Studies in Cultural History,* New Brunswick, Rutgers University Press, 1992.

Shryock, Richard H. *The Development of Modern Medicine,* 2nd edition, New York, Alfred A. Knopf, 1947.

Shryock, Richard H. *Medicine in America: Historical Essays,* Baltimore, Johns Hopkins University Press, 1966.

Sigerist, Henry E. *Great Doctors: A Biographical History of Medicine,* translated by E. & C. Paul, London, Allen and Unwin, 1933.

Sigerist, Henry E. *A History of Medicine,* 2 vols., New York, Oxford University Press, 1951–61.

Sigerist, Henry E. *Sigerist On the Sociology of Medicine,* edited by Milton I. Roemer, New York, M.D. Publications, 1960.

Sigerist, Henry E. *Civilisation and Disease,* Ithaca, Cornell University Press, 1943; reprinted, University of Chicago Press, Phoenix, 1962.

Singer, Charles and Underwood, E. Ashworth. A Short History of Medicine, 2nd edition. New York, Oxford University Press, 1962.

Sournia, J.-C. *The Illustrated History of Medicine,* London, Harold Starke, 1992.

Sprengel, K. *Versuch einer pragmatischen Geschichte der Arzneykunde,* 5 vols., Halle, Gebauer, 1792–1803.

Stevenson, L.G. and Multhauf, R. (eds.) *Medicine, Science and Culture: Historical Essays in Honour of Owsei Temkin,* Baltimore, Johns Hopkins University Press, 1977.

Walton, J, Beeson, P.B. and Scott, R.B. (eds.) *The Oxford Companion to Medicine,* 2 vols., Oxford, Oxford University Press, 1986.

GENERAL HISTORICAL BACKGROUND

Achterberg, J. *Woman as Healer: A Panoramic Survey of the Healing Activities of Women from Prehistoric Times to the Present*, Boston, Shambhala, 1991.

Ackerknecht, Erwin H. *Medicine at the Paris Hospital 1794–1848*, Baltimore: Johns Hopkins University Press, 1967.

Attali, J. *L'ordre Cannibale: vie et mort de la médecine*, Paris, Grasset, 1979.

Boyden, Stephen *Western Civilization in Biological Perspective, Patterns in Biohistory*. Oxford, Clarendon Press, 1987.

Cipolla, Carlo M. *The Economic History of World Population*, 6th edn. Baltimore, Penguin Books, 1974.

Cipolla, Carlo M. *Before the Industrial Revolution: European Society and Economy, 1000–1700*, 2nd edition. New York, Norton, 1980.

Crosby, Alfred W., Jr. *The Columbian Exchange: Biological and Cultural Consequences of 1492*, Westport, Conn., Greenwood Press, 1972.

Crosby, Alfred W., Jr. *Ecological Imperialism: The Biological Expansion of Europe, 900–1900*. Cambridge University Press, 1986.

Floud, Roderick, Wachter, Kenneth and Gregory, Annabel *Height, Health and History. Nutritional Status in the United Kingdom, 1750–1980*. Cambridge University Press, 1990.

Forster, Robert and Ranum, Orest (eds.) *Biology of Man in History: Selections from the Annales - Economies, Societies, Civilisations*, Baltimore, Johns Hopkins University Press, 1975.

Geertz, C. *The Interpretation of Cultures*, New York, Basic Books, 1973.

Glacken, Clarence J. *Traces on the Rhodian Shore: Nature and Culture in Western Thought from Ancient Times to the End of the Eighteenth Century*. Berkeley, University of California Press, 1967.

Herzlich, C. and Pierret, J. *Illness and Self in Society*, translated by E. Foster, Baltimore, Johns Hopkins University Press, 1987.

Kearney, Hugh. *Science and Change 1500–1700*, New York, McGraw-Hill, 1971.

Kleinman, A. *Patients and Healers in the Context of Culture*, Berkeley, University of California Press, 1980.

Laslett, P. *The World We Have Lost*, London, Methuen, 1965.

Livi-Bacci, Massimo. *Population and nutrition. An essay on European demographic history*, translated by Tania Croft-Murray, Cambridge University Press, 1991.

Ranger, T. and Slack, P. *Epidemics and Ideas*, Cambridge University Press, 1992.

Rotberg, Robert I. and Rabb, Theodore K. (eds.) *Hunger and History. The Impact of Changing Food Production and Consumption Patterns of society*. Cambridge University Press, 1983.

Zinsser, Hans *Rats, Lice and History*. Boston, Atlantic Monthly Press, 1934.

HISTORIES OF SCIENCE AND IDEAS

Abt, A.F. and Garrison, F.H. *History of Paediatrics*, Philadelphia, Saunders, 1965.

Boas, Marie *The Scientific Renaissance 1450–1630*, New York, Harper & Row, 1962.

Bowler, Peter *The Fontana History of the Environmental Sciences*, London, Harper Collins, 1992.

Brock, W. *The Fontana History of Chemistry*, London, Harper Collins, 1992.

Lovejoy, A.O. *The Great Chain of Being: A Study of the History of an Idea*, New York, Harper, 1960.

513

Sarton, George *A History of Science*. 2 vols., Cambridge, Mass., Harvard University Press, 1952–59.

Thorndike, Lynn *A History of Magic and Experimental Science*, 8 vols., New York, Columbia University Press, 1923–58.

HISTORIES OF SPECIALISED MEDICAL FIELDS

Biraben, Jean Noel *Les Hommes et la peste en France et dans les pays européens et méditerranéens*, Paris, Mouton, 1975.

Bloch, Marc *The Royal Touch: Sacred Monarchy and Scrofula in England and France*, translated by J.E. Anderson, London, Routledge and Kegan Paul, 1973.

Bremner, Robert H. (ed.) *Children and Youth in America: A Documentary History*, 5 vols., Cambridge, Mass, Harvard University Press, 1970–74.

Bynum, W.F. and Porter Roy, eds. *Living and Dying in London, Medical History*, Supplement 11, London, Wellcome Institute for the History of Medicine, 1991.

Bynum, W.F. and Nutton, V. *Theories of Fever from Antiquity to the Enlightenment. Medical History*, Supplement 1, London, Wellcome Institute for the History of Medicine, 1981.

Carpenter, Kenneth J. *The History of Scurvy and Vitamin C*, Cambridge University Press, 1986.

Creighton, Charles *A History of Epidemics in Britain*, 2 vols., Cambridge University Press, 1891–94; reprinted with additional material, New York, Barnes and Noble, 1965.

Crellin, John K. and Philpott, Jane *Herbal Medicine Past and Present*, 2 vols., Durham, NC, Duke University Press, 1991.

Ellenberger, Henri F. *The Discovery of the Unconscious: The History and Evolution of Dynamic Psychiatry*, New York, Basic Books, 1970.

Faber, K. *Nosography*, New York, P.B. Hoeber, 1923.

Granshaw, L. and Porter, R. (eds.) *The Hospital in History*, London, Routledge, 1989.

Grmek, M. *Diseases in the Ancient Greek World*, translated by M. Muellner and L. Muellner, Baltimore, Johns Hopkins University Press, 1989.

Hall, Thomas *Ideas of Life and Matter: Studies in the History of General Physiology 600 BC to AD 1900* 2 vols., Chicago, University of Chicago Press, 1969.

Hirsch, August *Handbook of Geographical and Historical Pathology*, 3 vols., translated by Charles Creighton, London, The New Sydenham Society, 1883–86.

Hopkins, D. *Princes and Peasants: Smallpox in History*, Chicago, University of Chicago Press, 1983.

Jetter, Dieter *Geschichte des Hospitals*, Wiesbaden, Franz Steiner Verlag, 1966–72.

Lawrence, C. (ed.) *Medical Theory, Surgical Practice: Studies in the History of Surgery*, London, Routledge, 1992.

May, Jacques M. *Studies in Disease Ecology*, New York, Hafner, 1961.

O'Malley, Charles D. (ed.) *The History of Medical Education*, Berkeley, University of California Press, 1970.

Puschmann, Theodor *A History of Medical Education from the Most Remote to the Most Recent Times*, translated by E.H. Hare, London, H.K. Lewis, 1896; reprinted, New York, Hafner, 1966.

Quétel, C.F. *A History of Syphilis*, translated by J. Braddock and B. Pike, Oxford, Blackwell, 1990.

Rather, L.J. *The Genesis of Cancer: A Study of the History of Ideas*, Baltimore, Johns Hopkins University Press, 1978.

Rosen, George *A History of Public Health*, New York, M.D. Publications, 1958.

Rosen, George *Preventive Medicine in the United States 1900–1975: Trends and Interpretations*, New York, Science History Publications, 1975.

Ruffie, J. and Sournia, J.C. *Les Epidémies dans l'Histoire de l'Homme*, Paris, Flammarion, 1984.

Sallares, R. *The Ecology of the Ancient Greek World*, London, Duckworth, 1991.

Schouten, J. *The Rod and Serpent of Asklepios: Symbol of Medicine*, New York, Elsevier, 1967.

Shrewsbury, J.F.D. *A History of Bubonic Plague in the British Isles*, Cambridge University Press, 1970.

Sournia, Jean Charles *A History of Alcoholism*, translated by N. Hindley and G. Stanton, Oxford, Blackwell, 1990.

Still, George F. *The History of Paediatrics; the Progress of the Study of Diseases of Children up to the End of the Eighteenth Century*, London, Oxford University Press, 1931; London, Dawsons, 1965.

Walter, J. and Schofield, R. (eds.) *Famine, Disease, and the Social Order in Early Modern Society*, Cambridge University Press, 1989.

Wangensteen, O.H. and Wangensteen, S.D. *The Rise of Surgery: From Empiric Craft to Scientific Discipline*, University of Minnesota/Dawson, Folkestone, 1978.

Zilboorg, Gregory *A History of Medical Psychology*, New York, W.W. Norton, 1941.

Zimmerman, Leo M. and Veith, Ilza *Great Ideas in the History of Surgery*, 2nd edition New York, Dover, 1967.

METHODS AND PHILOSOPHY

Porter, R. and Wear, A. (eds.) *Problems and Methods in the History of Medicine*, London, Croom Helm, 1987.

GENERAL MEDICAL REFERENCES AND BIBLIOGRAPHICAL WORKS

Austin, Robert B. *Early American Medical Imprints: A Guide to Works Printed in the United States 1668–1820*, Washington, Department of H.E.W., 1961.

Besson, Alain (ed.) *Thornton's Medical Books, Libraries and Collectors*, 3rd edition Aldershot; Brookfield, Vermont, Gower, 1990.

Besterman, Theodore *Medicine, a Bibliography of Bibliographies*. Totowa, New Jersey, Rowman and Littlefield, 1971.

Bibliography of the History of Medicine. No. 1– Bethesda, Maryland, National Library of Medicine, 1965–.

Blake, John B. and Roos, C. *Medical Reference Works, 1676–1966: A Selected Bibliography*, Chicago, Medical Library Association, 1967; with supplements in 1970, 1973, 1975.

Brodman, Estelle *The Development of Medical Bibliography*, Washington, Medical Library Association, 1954.

Choulant, Ludwig *History and Bibliography of Anatomic Illustration*, translated by M. Frank, revised edition, New York, Henry Schuman, 1945.

Corsi, P. and Weindling, P. (eds.) *Information Sources in the History of Science and Medicine*. London, Butterworth Scientific, 1983.

Current Work in the History of Medicine: An International Bibliography, London, The Wellcome Institute for the History of Medicine, 1954–.

Durbin, P.T. (ed.) *A Guide to the Culture of Science, Technology and Medicine*, New York, Free Press, 1980.

Erlen, J. *The History of the Health Care Sciences and Health Care, 1700–1980; A Selective Bibliography*, New York, Garland, 1984.

Gilbert, Judson B. *Diseases and Destiny: A Bibliography of Medical References to the Famous*, London, Dawson, 1962.

Guerra, Francisco (comp.) *American Bibliography 1639–1783*, New York, Lathrop C. Harper, 1962.

Index Catalog of the Library of the Surgeon General's Office, 61 vols., 5 series, Washington, US Government Printing Office, 1880–1961.

Index Medicus. 21 vols. New York, 1879–1899; 1903–1920; 1921–1927; Washington, National Library of Medicine, 1960–.

Isis. Cumulative Bibliography, London, Mansell, 1971–.

Jordanova, L.J. 'The Social Sciences and History of Science and Medicine', in P. Corsi and P. Weindling (eds.), *Information Sources in the History of Science and Medicine*, London, Butterworth Scientific, 1983, pp. 81–98.

Kelly, Emerson C. *Encyclopedia of Medical Sources*, Baltimore, Williams and Wilkins, 1948.

Le Fanu, W.R. *British Medical Periodicals: a Chronological List 1640–1899*, Oxford, Wellcome Unit for History of Medicine, Research Publications 6, 1984.

Miller, G. (ed.) *Bibliography of the History of Medicine of the United States and Canada, 1939–1960*, Baltimore, Johns Hopkins University Press, 1964.

Morton, L.T. (comp). *Garrison and Morton's Medical bibliography: an annotated check-list of texts illustrating the history of medicine*, 4th edn. Aldershot, Gower 1983.

Morton, L.T. and Godbolt, S. (eds.) *Information sources in the Medical Sciences*, 4th edition, London, Bowker-Saur, 1992.

Morton, L.T. and Moore, Robert J. *A Bibliography of Medical and Biomedical Biography*, 2nd edn., Aldershot, Scolar Press; Brookfield, Vermont, Gower; 1994.

National Library of Medicine. *Bibliography of the History of Medicine*, Washington, 1964–.

Olby, R.C., Cantor, G.N., Christie,, J.R.R. and Hodge, M.J.S. (eds.) *Companion to the History of Modern Science*, London, Routledge, 1989.

Pelling, Margaret 'Medicine Since 1500', in P. Corsi and Paul Weindling (eds.) *Information Sources in the History of Science and Medicine*, London, Butterworth Scientific, 1983, pp. 379–407.

Quarterly Cumulative Index Medicus. 60 vols., AMA and Army Medical Library, 1927–56.

Trautmann, Joanne and Pollard, Carol (comp.) *Literature and Medicine: An Annotated Bibliography*. 2nd edition, Pittsburg, Contemporary Community Health Series, 1982.

Webster, Charles. 'The Historiography of Medicine', in P. Corsi and P. Weindling (eds.) *Information Sources in the History of Science and Medicine*. London, Butterworth Scientific, 1983, pp. 29–43.

MEDICAL BIOGRAPHICAL COLLECTIONS AND DICTIONARIES

Bayle, A.L.J. and Thillaye, A.J. *Biographie Médicale*, 2 vols., Paris, A. Delahaye, 1855.

Fischer, Isidor. *Biographisches Lexikon der hervorragenden Ärzte der letzten fünfzig Jahre*, 2 vols., Berlin, Urban and Schwarzenberg, 1932–33.

Hirsch, August *Biographisches Lexikon der hervorragenden Ärzte aller Zeiten and Völker*, 2nd edition, 5 vols., Vienna, Urban and Schwarzenberg, 1884–88.

Hutchinson, Benjamin *Biographica Medica*; or, *Historical and Critical Characters that Have*

Existed from the Earliest Account of Time to the Present Period; with a Catalog of their Literary Productions, 2 vols., London, J. Johnson, 1799.

MacMichael, William *The Gold Headed Cane*. London, J. Murray, 1827; new edition, Springfield, Ill., Charles C. Thomas, 1953.

Munk, William *Roll of the Royal College of Physicians of London*, 8 vols. London, The College, 1878–1989.

Pagel, Julius *Biographisches Lexikon hervorragenden Ärzte des neunzehnten Jahrhunderts* 5 vols., Berlin, Urban and Schwarzenberg, 1901.

Plarr, Victor G. *Plarr's Lives of the Fellows of the Royal College of Surgeons of England*, revised by Sir D'Arcy Power, 2 vols., Bristol, John Wright and Sons, 1930.

Power, Sir D'A. *Lives of the Fellows of the Royal College of Surgeons of England 1930 to 1951*, London, Royal College of Surgeons of England, 1953.

Talbott, John H. *A Biographical History of Medicine*, New York, Grune and Stratton, 1970.

Thatcher, James *American Medical Biography*, 2 vols., Boston, Richardson, 1828.

Wickersheimer, Ernest *Dictionnaire biographique des médecins en France au moyen age*, 2 vols., Paris, E. Droz, 1936; supplement by D. Jacquart, Geneva, Droz; Paris, Champion, 1979; and D. Jacquart, *Le milieu médical en France du XIIe au XVe siècle*, Geneva, Droz; Paris, Champion, 1981.

Index